Pancreatic Diseases: Diagnosis and Treatment

Pancreatic Diseases: Diagnosis and Treatment

Edited by Rosie Mason

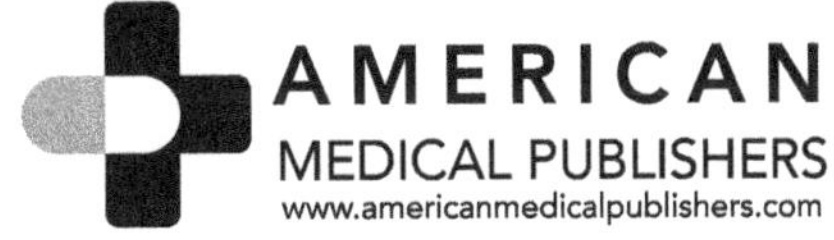

American Medical Publishers,
41 Flatbush Avenue,
1st Floor, New York,
NY 11217, USA

Visit us on the World Wide Web at:
www.americanmedicalpublishers.com

ISBN: 978-1-63927-198-6

Cataloging-in-Publication Data

Pancreatic diseases : diagnosis and treatment / edited by Rosie Mason.
p. cm.
Includes bibliographical references and index.
ISBN 978-1-63927-198-6
1. Pancreas--Diseases. 2. Pancreas--Diseases--Diagnosis.
3. Pancreas--Diseases--Treatment. I. Mason, Rosie.
RC857 .P36 2022
616.37--dc23

Table of Contents

Preface

It is often said that books are a boon to mankind. They document every progress and pass on the knowledge from one generation to the other. They play a crucial role in our lives. Thus I was both excited and nervous while editing this book. I was pleased by the thought of being able to make a mark but I was also nervous to do it right because the future of students depends upon it. Hence, I took a few months to research further into the discipline, revise my knowledge and also explore some more aspects. Post this process, I begun with the editing of this book.

The pancreas is an endocrine and exocrine gland that is responsible for the secretion of insulin, glucagon, pancreatic juice, somatostatin and pancreatic polypeptide. It regulates blood sugar levels and breaks down proteins, carbohydrates and fats entering the duodenum from the stomach. The pancreas is susceptible to several kinds of diseases-pancreatitis, diabetes mellitus, cystic fibrosis, congenital malformations, neoplasms and cysts, etc. Pancreatitis is the chronic or acute inflammation of the pancreas. When food is not properly digested owing to a lack of digestive enzymes secreted by the pancreas, a condition known as exocrine pancreatic insufficiency occurs. Certain congenital malformations of the pancreas include annular pancreas and pancreas divisum. The diagnosis of pancreatic diseases is based on a physical examination, blood tests, computed tomography scan, magnetic resonance imaging and endoscopic ultrasound. Endoscopic retrograde cholangiopancreatography and magnetic resonance cholangiopancreatography, allow the evaluation of the pancreatic ducts. Oral pancreatic enzyme supplements and insulin therapy are often prescribed to manage pancreatitis and diabetes, respectively. This book aims to shed light on some of the unexplored aspects of pancreatic diseases and the recent researches in their pathophysiology. The objective of this book is to give a general view of the different kinds of pancreatic disorders, and their diagnosis and management. It aims to serve as a resource guide for students and experts alike.

I thank my publisher with all my heart for considering me worthy of this unparalleled opportunity and for showing unwavering faith in my skills. I would also like to thank the editorial team who worked closely with me at every step and contributed immensely towards the successful completion of this book. Last but not the least, I wish to thank my friends and colleagues for their support.

Editor

1

Clinical significance of serum triglyceride elevation at early stage of acute biliary pancreatitis

Long Cheng[1†], Zhulin Luo[1†], Ke Xiang[1†], Jiandong Ren[2], Zhu Huang[1], Lijun Tang[1*] and Fuzhou Tian[1*]

Abstract

Background: Pancreatitis induced by hypertriglyceridemia (HTG) has gained much attention. However, very limited numbers of studies have focused on the clinical significance of TG elevation in non-HTG induced pancreatitis, such as acute biliary pancreatitis (ABP). This study aimed to study the clinical significances of triglyceride (TG) elevation in patients with ABP.

Methods: We retrospectively analyzed a total of 426 ABP cases in our research center. According to the highest TG level within 72 h of disease onset, the patients were divided into a normal TG group and an elevated TG group. We analyzed the differences between the two groups of patients in aspects such as general information, disease severity, APACHE II (acute physiology and chronic health evaluation II) and Ranson scores, inflammatory cytokines, complications and prognosis.

Results: Compared with the normal TG group, patients in the elevated TG group showed a significantly higher body mass index and were significantly younger. TG elevation at the early stage of ABP was associated with higher risk of severe pancreatitis and organ failures, especially respiratory failure. For patients with severe pancreatitis, those with elevated TG levels were more likely to have a larger area of necrosis, and higher incidence of pancreatic abscess as well as higher mortality (17.78% versus 9.80%, $P < 0.05$).

Conclusions: In ABP patients, TG elevation might participate in the aggravation of pancreatitis and the occurrence of systemic or local complications. Thus, the TG level may serve as an important indicator to determine the prognosis of patients with ABP.

Keywords: Acute pancreatitis, Biliary pancreatitis, Hypertriglyceridemia, Triglyceride

Background

Acute pancreatitis (AP) is a life-threatening inflammatory disease involving the pancreas as well as peripancreatic and even distant organs [1]. The main causes of AP include biliary tract disease, alcohol abuse, congenital anomaly, drugs, etc. [2]. In recent years, the relationship between hypertriglyceridemia (HTG) and AP has received widespread attention from scholars, and it is generally believed that blood triglyceride (TG) levels greater than 11.3 mmol/L can directly induce AP [3,4]. However, HTG-induced AP is uncommon, accounting for only 1-4% of AP cases. On the other hand, HTG is commonly present at the early stage of non-HTG-induced AP, such as acute biliary pancreatitis (ABP), and its clinical significance remains unclear.

It has been reported that more than 50% of non-HTG-induced AP patients demonstrate mild-to-moderate TG elevation [5]. However, the relationship between the elevated TG level and severity of non-HTG-induced AP is not well documented. Some studies reported that when non-HTG-induced AP was accompanied by TG elevation, the disease course of AP shows a trend for aggravation; in particular, if the serum TG level is reduced under 5.65 mmol/L, the disease condition will be gradually stabilized and improved [6-8]. However, some other studies showed that an increased TG level might just represent a symptom associated with AP, and there is no significant relationship between an elevated TG level and the severity and prognosis of AP patients [9]. This discrepancy may be due to the fact that the AP cases included in these studies

* Correspondence: whjtlj1251@163.com; tfz3006101@163.com
†Equal contributors
[1]Department of General Surgery, Chengdu Military General Hospital, Jinniu District, Chengdu, Sichuan Province, PR China, 610083
Full list of author information is available at the end of the article

were induced by different causes, and HTG might play different roles in AP cases induced by different causes.

Therefore, investigating the clinical significance of an elevated TG level in AP induced by a single homogeneous cause could more accurately illustrate the effects of mild-to-moderate HTG on the severity and prognosis of AP patients. As acute biliary pancreatitis (ABP) remains the main type of AP in China and many other countries, the current study focused on the clinical significance of HTG in ABP patients.

Methods

Patients

Patient selection

This study retrospectively analyzed 426 ABP cases that were treated in our hospital. The diagnosis and classification of the severity of AP were performed according to the 2012 revision of the Atlanta Classification [10]. The diagnosis of ABP was based on the standards proposed in the literature with the following minor amendments [11]: 1) confirmed diagnosis of AP; 2) no history of hyperlipidemia or alcohol abuse; 3) abdominal ultrasonography (AUS), computed tomography (CT), magnetic resonance cholangiopancreatography (MRCP), and endoscopic ultrasound (EUS) detection of gallstones or biliary sludge, or laboratory tests showing two of the following items: ALT >75U/L, ALP >125 U/L, and TBIL >2.3 mg/dl. This study was performed according to the principles of the Declaration of Helsinki (modified 2000) and was approved by the ethics committee of Chengdu Military General Hospital (No. 2013037).

Treatment protocols

At the outset, all patients were treated in a conservative manner, with fluid resuscitation and antibiotics, as described in the literature [12,13]. Endoscopic retrograde cholangiopancreatography (ERCP) and endoscopic sphincterotomy (EST) were performed in patients with jaundice and cholangitis. Percutaneous catheter drainage (PCD) were carried out to eliminate the debris and collections in the (peri)pancreas, similar to other reports [14]. The number and size of the catheters were determined by the size, viscosity, and location of the debris and collections. In accordance with widely accepted consensus [15], if there was no clinical improvement or if ongoing necrosis with bowel complications was present, open necrosectomy with closed lesser-sac drainage and postoperative lavage was performed.

Methods

Group division

According to the highest TG level within 72 h of disease onset, the patients were divided into a normal TG group (<1.88 mmol/L) and an elevated TG group (≥1.88 mmol/L).

Data collection

In addition to the collection of general information including sex, age, body mass index (index), etc., we specially analyzed differences between the normal TG group and the elevated TG group in aspects such as pancreatitis severity score, incidence of systemic complications, incidence of local complications, mortality, days in hospital and intensive care unit and care cost. Differences in levels of inflammatory cytokines within 72 h of disease onset—C-reaction protein (CRP), interleukin 6 (IL-6), IL-10, tumor necrosis factor-alpha (TNF-α) —between the two groups were also analyzed. Initial contrast-enhanced computed tomography was performed within the first week of the onset of disease and repeated depending on the indication. The images obtained were double-checked by two experienced radiologists. Meanwhile, extent of necrosis were measured and classified into three grades, <30%, 30-50% and >50%, according to Balthazar classification. Acute physiology and chronic health evaluation II (APACHE II) score and CTSI were calculated for each patient at the time of admission and serially calculated before and after each type of intervention.

Definition and criteria

The classification of AP severity was based on the 2012 revision of the Atlanta Classification, and the Ranson score and APACHE II (acute physiology and chronic health evaluation II) score were calculated within 24 ~ 48 h after patient admission.

The diagnostic criteria for systemic complications of AP were as follows: shock, with systolic blood pressure ≤80 mmHg and a duration of 15 min; respiratory failure, with PaO2 ≤ 60 mmHg; renal failure, with serum creatinine >176.8 μmol/L; coagulation disorders, with prothrombin time (PT) less than 70% that of normal people and/or partial thromboplastin time (PTT) > 45 s; sepsis, with a body temperature (T) > 38.5°C, white blood cell (WBC) count >6.0 × 10^9/L, base excess ≤ 4 μmol/L, a duration of 48 h, and positive blood/ aspirate bacterial culture; systemic response syndrome, with T >38.5°C or <36°C, WBC count >12.0 × 10^9/L or <4.0 × 10^9/L, pulse >90 beats/min, and respiratory rate >20 breaths/min or PCO2 < 32 mmHg; upper gastrointestinal bleeding; and pancreatic encephalopathy. Local complications of AP included pancreatic necrosis, inanimate pancreatic tissue, or peripancreatic fat as revealed by enhanced CT and pancreatic pseudocyst, with liquid accumulation wrapped in a complete and non-epithelial envelope and enclosed pancreatic secretions, granulation tissue, and fibrous tissue.

Statistical methods

The statistical analysis was carried out using SPSS version 16.0 for Windows (SPSS Inc., Chicago, IL). Normality of data was determined by Kolmogorov–Smirnov tests of normality. Data were expressed as mean ± standard deviation for normally distributed data and median and interquartile range for non-normally distributed data. For normally distributed data, variables were compared using Student's t test for two groups. For skewed data, the Mann–Whitney test was used. Qualitative or categorical variables were described as frequencies and proportions. Proportional variables were compared using the $\chi2$ test or Fisher's exact test. All statistical tests were two-tailed and performed at a significance level of $P < 0.05$.

Results

Comparison of general information of patients

There were 426 ABP cases included, of which 289 (67.84%) were assigned to the normal TG group and 137 (32.16%) to the elevated TG group. The mean levels of TG in the two groups were 1.21 mmol/L and 6.52 mmol/L, respectively. This cohort included 188 male and 238 female patients, and the male/female ratio of the elevated TG group was significantly higher than that of the normal TG group (72/65 versus 116/173, $p < 0.05$). In addition, the age of the patients in the elevated TG group was significantly lower than that in the normal TG group (46.35 ± 7.26 versus 54.89 ± 7.84, $p < 0.05$), while the body mass index (BMI) of the elevated TG group was significantly higher than that of the normal TG group (28.35 ± 5.13 versus 22.57 ± 4.42, $p < 0.01$), Table 1. Meanwhile, the frequencies of manifestation of cholangitis between the two groups were not significantly different, 22.15% (64/289) versus 23.36% (32/137). These results showed that younger male ABP patients with a higher BMI were more likely to be complicated with TG elevation.

Relationship between TG level and ABP severity

The total incidence rate of moderately severe acute pancreatitis (MSAP) and severe acute pancreatitis (SAP) in this study group was 22.54% (96/426); in particular, SAP and MSAP patients accounted for 32.85% (45/137) of the cases in elevated TG group, and this rate was significantly higher than that in the normal TG group ($p < 0.05$). Laboratory detection showed that the CRP level in elevated TG group was remarkably higher than that in normal TG group ($p < 0.05$). Meanwhile, patients in the elevated TG group had APACHE II scores and Ranson scores that were significantly higher than those of patients in the normal TG group (p values were <0.01 and <0.05, respectively), Table 2. Correlation analysis showed that TG levels and APACHE II scores were significantly correlated ($p < 0.05$, $R = 0.665$) in patients in the elevated TG group, whereas TG levels were not significantly correlated with the Ranson score. These results suggest that elevated TG levels in the early phase of ABP may be involved in the progress of the disease.

Involvement of TG elevation in the occurrence of systemic complications in severe ABP patients

With regard to the severe cases (including MSAP and SAP), the incidence of systemic organ failure in elevated TG group (33.33%, 17/51) was significantly higher than that in the normal TG group (46.67%, 21/45), $p < 0.05$), Table 3. Statistical analysis showed that severe ABP patients with elevated TG levels had a significantly increased risk of organ failures involving single organ failure. Among patients with moderate-severe degrees of severe pancreatitis, the incidence of respiratory failure was significantly higher in the elevated TG group than the normal TG group (28.89% (13/45) versus 13.73% (7/51), $p < 0.05$). However, these two groups did not show significant differences in the incidence rates of renal failure, circulatory

Table 1 The characteristics of ABP patients enrolled in this study

characteristic	Normal TG group	Elevated TG group	P value
Number of patients	289	137	
Demographic data			
Age (mean ± SD)	54.89 ± 7.84	46.35 ± 7.26	0.011*
Male/female	116/173	72/65	0.027*
BMI	22.57 ± 4.42	28.35 ± 5.13	0.001*
Referral after onset of symptoms (hours) (mean ± SD)	26.8 ± 16.8	24.5 ± 15.2	0.402
TG level (mmol/L)	1.21 ± 0.56	6.52 ± 1.52	0.001*
Manifestation of cholangitis (%)	22.15% (64/289)	23.36% (32/137)	0.435
Medical economics (median ± interquartile range)			
Days in hospital	34.7 ± 16.42	39.5 ± 18.54	0.375
Days in intensive care unit (ICU)	5.2 ± 2.36	6.4 ± 3.46	0.562
Total cost during hospitalization (Dollars)	5646.1 ± 1432.32	6103.2 ± 2140.29	0.781

TG, triglyceride; BMI, body mass index. *Significant difference.

Table 2 The Laboratory and clinical parameters between two groups

Items	Normal TG group	Elevated TG group	P value
Number of patients	289	137	
Severity classification			
MAP	238 (82.35%)	94 (68.61%)	0.157
MSAP	32 (11.07%)	28 (20.44%)	0.021*
SAP	19 (6.57%)	17 (12.41%)	0.015*
Laboratory parameters			
C.reaction protein (CRP) (mg/L)	36.2 ± 15.33	61.2 ± 18.41	0.038*
IL-6 (pg/L)	54.5 ± 20.41	62.6 ± 22.42	0.241
IL-10 (pg/L)	30.6 ± 17.48	35.1 ± 18.59	0.672
TNF-α (pg/L)	8.2 ± 3.53	9.8 ± 3.77	0.521
Severity scores			
APACHIIscore (mean ± SD)	6.26 ± 3.48	10.11 ± 3.62	0.007*
Ranson score (mean ± SD)	1.68 ± 0.79	2.34 ± 0.93	0.042*
Marshall score (mean ± SD)	2.1 ± 0.57	2.6 ± 0.68	0.142

TG, triglyceride; MAP, mild acute pancreatitis; MSAP, moderately severe acute pancreatitis; SAP, severe acute pancreatitis; APACHE II, acute physiology and chronic health evaluation II. *Significant difference.

failure, coagulation disorders, and other types of organ failure ($p > 0.05$). These results suggest that ABP patients with elevated TG levels are more likely to develop organ failure, particularly respiratory failure.

Effect of TG elevation on the development of local complications in patients with ABP

Among patients with moderate-severe degrees of severe ABP, 55.56% of patients with elevated TG levels had pancreatic necrosis, and 50.98% of patients with normal TG had pancreatic necrosis, with no significant difference between these two groups. However, patients with elevated TG levels showed significantly higher probabilities of developing necrosis over a relatively large area (with a necrotic area greater than 30%) and a higher incidence of pancreatic abscess compared to patients with normal TG levels, Table 4. For patients with moderate-severe degrees of severe ABP, there was no significant difference in the incidence rates of pseudocysts between patients with elevated TG and patients with normal TG levels. These results suggest that although TG elevation did not increase the total incidence of pancreatic necrosis in ABP patients, TG elevation may increase the scope and extent of pancreatic necrosis once necrosis occurs.

Table 3 Incidence of organ failure in MSAP or SAP patients

Items	Normal TG group	Elevated TG group	P value
Number of patients	51	45	
Total organ failure	17 (33.33%)	21 (46.67%)	0.036*
Single	11 (21.57%)	15 (33.33%)	0.047*
Multiple	6 (11.76%)	6 (13.33%)	0.761
Respiration	7 (13.73%)	13 (28.89%)	0.022*
Circulation	5 (9.80%)	3 (6.67%)	0.535
Kidney	6 (11.76%)	5 (11.11%)	0.882
Coagulation	4 (7.84%)	3 (6.67%)	0.682
Other organ or system	4 (7.84%)	3 (6.67%)	0.682

TG, triglyceride; MSAP, moderately severe acute pancreatitis; SAP, severe acute pancreatitis. *Significant difference.

Association of TG level with treatments and prognosis of ABP patients

All mild ABP patients were treated in a conservative manner and were discharged after rehabilitation. There were 41.87 % of mild ABP patients (139/332) underwent ERCP/EST, and no significant difference was observed between normal TG group and elevated TG group. Besides ERCP/EST,PCD and open necrosectomy were also performed in some of patients with moderate or severe ABP. For patients with MSAP/SAP, although the frequencies of ERCP/EST were not significantly different between normal TG group and elevated TG group (47.06% (24/51) versus 46.67% (21/45)), more patients in elevated TG group underwent PCD and open necrosectomy, Table 5. The mortality rate of severe ABP patients with elevated TG was 17.78% (8/45), whereas that of severe ABP patients with normal serum TG was 9.80% (5/51); the difference between the two groups was significant ($p < 0.05$). The patients were followed for 1 year, and we found no significant differences in the recurrence rate and life quality of patients after discharge. These results showed that TG elevation may be a manifestation indicating poor prognosis in patients with ABP.

Discussion

In recent years, the relationship between HTG and AP has received widespread attention from scholars, and it

Table 4 Occurrence of local complications in MSAP or SAP patients

Items	Normal TG group	Elevated TG group	P value
Number of patients	51	45	
Incidence of necrosis	34 (66.67%)	36 (80.00%)	0.253
Maximum extent of necrosis			
Less than 30%	18 (35.29%)	12 (26.67 %)	0.137
30% ~ 50%	10 (19.61 %)	15 (33.33%)	0.027*
More than 50%	6 (11.76 %)	9 (20.00%)	0.002*
Pancreatic abscess	4 (7.84 %)	8 (17.78%)	0.001*
Pseudocyst	6 (11.76 %)	5 (11.11%)	0.683

*Significant difference.

Table 5 Treatment and prognosis for MSAP or SAP patients

Items	Normal TG group	Elevated TG group	P value
Number of patients	51	45	
ERCP or EST	24 (47.06%)	21 (46.67%)	0.566
PCD	20 (39.12%)	27 (60.00%)	0.033*
Open necrosectomy	3 (5.88%)	9 (13.33%)	0.037*
mortality	5 (9.80%)	8 (17.78%)	0.011*
recurrence rate within 1 year	10 (19.61%)	11 (24.44 %)	0.372

ERCP, Endoscopic retrograde cholangiopancreatography; and EST, endoscopic sphincterotomy; PCD, Percutaneous catheter drainage. *Significant difference.

is generally believed that a serum TG level >11.3 mmol/L can directly induce AP. However, despite the increasing incidence of AP induced by HTG, this type of AP is not the major type observed in clinical practice. The more common clinical situation is that non-HTG-induced AP patients were complicated with TG elevation, and it has been reported in the literature that approximately 50% of non-HTG-induced AP patients demonstrate mild-moderate TG elevation. However, there have been only limited numbers of studies on the significance of TG elevation in non-HTG induced pancreatitis, such as acute biliary pancreatitis (ABP), and the results were inconsistent.

It also remains controversial whether TG elevation is an associated etiological factor or a concomitant symptom in non-HTG induced AP patients. In alcoholic pancreatitis, alcohol can directly affect the metabolism of TG, causing elevated TG levels, and is therefore directly involved in the occurrence of pancreatitis. Thus, an elevated TG level can be seen as an associated etiological factor of alcoholic pancreatitis [16], whereas it may be considered as concurrent symptom of biliary pancreatitis [17]. In addition, the relationships between TG elevation and the severity and prognosis of AP, as reported in the literature, are also inconsistent. For example, studies have reported that when AP induced by non-HTG causes is complicated with TG elevation, the disease course of AP shows a trend for aggravation [7,8]. However, other studies show that an increased TG level may only represent a symptom associated with AP, as there is no significant relationship between TG level and the severity and prognosis of AP patients [9]. The presence of these controversies is likely due to the analysis of different compositions of AP patient, including patients with biliary AP, alcoholic AP, cryptogenic AP, and AP due to other factors, as HTG is known to play different roles in AP caused by different factors.

Therefore, the study of the clinical significance of an elevated TG level in AP due to a single etiological factor could accurately illustrate the effects of mild-moderate HTG on AP disease condition and prognosis. Because biliary tract disease is a major cause of AP in China and other Eastern countries, we chose to study the effects of TG elevation on the disease condition and prognosis of patients with ABP. When selecting cases, we excluded patients with a history of hyperlipidemia and alcoholism, aiming to exclude cases with elevated TG levels before the onset of pancreatitis. During the occurrence of AP, due to the body's stress response, serum catecholamine and glucagon levels, as well as lipase activity, are increased, leading to accelerated break down of fat tissue and the subsequent release of TG and increase in serum lipid concentrations [18,19]. In this study group, the incidence of SAP in ABP patients associated with elevated TG was significantly higher compared to that in patients without elevated TG; in addition, ABP patients with elevated TG levels also showed more severe pancreatic necrosis. These results may be due to the fact that elevated TG might lead to increased blood viscosity, which further promotes blood circulation disorders of the pancreas. In addition, large quantities of free fatty acids released from TG breakdown damage the pancreatic acinar cells and capillaries, leading to a higher likelihood of SAP [20,21]. Furthermore, this result might also be related to the participation of cholecystokinin, as some studies have shown that in the presence of TG elevation, free fatty acids produced in the body can strengthen the stimulation of cholecystokinin on the excretion function of pancreatic acinar cells, which subsequently activates the endoplasmic reticulum stress phenomenon and thereby damages pancreatic acinar cells [22].

This study also found that ABP patients with elevated TG levels were more prone to organ failure, particularly respiratory failure. In the AP disease course, respiratory complications primarily include hypoxemia, acute respiratory distress syndrome, atelectasis, and pleural effusion. Respiratory failure is largely due to the large number of toxic cytokines produced during the AP disease course, mainly including platelet-activating factor, TNF-α, IL-1, IL-6, IL-8, NO, P substance, and macrophage-secreted cytokines, which can cause systemic inflammatory response syndrome and respiratory dysfunction. The reason why ABP patients with elevated TG levels were more likely to experience respiratory failure is related to the functions of free fatty acids. In the presence of elevated TG, serum TG is broken down under the action of lipoprotein lipase in the lung, leading to the production of large quantities of free fatty acids. Subsequently, free fatty acids dissociate from albumin in the blood, enter the alveolar capillary membrane, and destruct the pulmonary blood microcirculation, leading to respiratory failure [23,24].

It remains unclear why some ABP patients show elevated TG levels while others have normal TG levels, and why the degree of elevated TG varies among patients. We believe that this difference may be related to a number of factors. First, the local or whole body fat distribution of patients may be associated with elevated TG levels and the degree of such elevation. When the body has high levels of fat, under the same level of stress and level of lipase activity, the amount of involved fat tissue is increased, and the amount of TG release is increased. In the present study, the BMI of ABP patients with elevated TG levels was significantly higher than that in patients with normal TG levels. Indeed, previous studies have shown that obesity is closely associated with AP aggravation, and some scholars have suggested that obesity should be considered an independent risk factor of AP aggravation, which is consistent with the results of this study. In addition, in recent years, some scholars have found that genetic polymorphisms are associated with the pathogenesis of AP with HTG [25]. For example, Chang and his colleagues [26] first reported that in HTG-induced AP patients, lipoprotein lipase gene mutation was significantly increased, and the probability of AP was 77.8% in patients with hyperlipidemia caused by the mutation in this gene. In short, there may be a mutually reinforcing cycle between elevated TG levels and pancreatitis, such that the occurrence of pancreatitis leads to elevated TG levels, which further increase the severity of pancreatitis. This cycle may represent another important vicious cycles in AP pathogenesis, and timely blockade of this cycle may hold important significance for reducing the degree of AP aggravation and improving the efficacy and prognosis for patients with SAP.

The general treatment protocol of ABP was similar to AP induced by other causes. At the outset, all patients were treated in a conservative manner, and subsequently so-called step-up approach was carried out [27,28]. Meanwhile, ERCP and EST were selectively performed in some ABP patients, especially for patients with jaundice and cholangitis. However, there were still controversies on the indications and outcomes of ERCP and EST in ABP treatment [29,30]. In the current study, no significant difference of the frequencies of ERCP/EST was observed between normal TG group and elevated TG group. For patients with MSAP/SAP, the frequencies of ERCP/EST were also not significantly different between normal TG group and elevated TG group, but more patients in elevated TG group underwent PCD and open necrosectomy. These results indicated that the ABP patients with TG elevation might be liable to undergo PCD and open necrosectomy. However, as the patients were divided into two groups according to the highest TG level within 72 h of disease onset, we presumed that the raised TG level might be responsible for the liability of PCD and open necrosectomy.

Conclusions

In summary, when ABP is accompanied with TG elevation, the risks of SAP and organ failure (especially respiratory failure) are significantly higher compared to patients with normal TG levels. In particular, elevated TG levels and pancreatitis may form a mutually reinforcing cycle, and timely implementations of measures to block this vicious cycle may hold important significance for reducing the rate of AP aggravation and improving the treatment effects and prognosis of SAP patients. Nevertheless, further research is needed to reveal the pathophysiological mechanisms for why elevated TG levels are present in ABP patients, as well as the mechanism by which elevated TG cause injury to specific tissues and organs.

Abbreviations

AP: Acute pancreatitis; TG: Triglyceride; ABP: Acute biliary pancreatitis; HTG: Hypertriglyceridemia; APACHE II: Acute physiology and chronic health evaluation II; AUS: Abdominal ultrasonography; CT: Computed tomography; MRCP: Magnetic resonance cholangiopancreatography; EUS: Endoscopic ultrasound.

Competing interests

The authors declare that they have no competing interests.

Authors' contributions

LC contributed to the design of the study and direction of its implementation. FZT and LJT conceived and designed the experiments and supervision of the field activities. LC and ZLL carried out the prepared the Materials of patient and prepared the literature review as well as the Discussion sections of the text. JDR, KX and ZH conducted the data analysis. All authors read and approved the final version of the manuscript.

Acknowledgements

This work was supported by the National Scientific Foundation Committee of China (No. 81300280).

Author details

[1]Department of General Surgery, Chengdu Military General Hospital, Jinniu District, Chengdu, Sichuan Province, PR China, 610083. [2]Department of Pharmacy, Chengdu Military General Hospital, Chengdu, Sichuan Province, People's Republic of China.

References

1. Wu BU, Conwell DL. Update in acute pancreatitis. Curr Gastroenterol Rep. 2010;12:83–90.
2. Waldthaler A, Schutte K, Malfertheiner P. Causes and mechanisms in acute pancreatitis. Dig Dis. 2010;28:364–72.
3. Murphy MJ, Sheng X, MacDonald TM, Wei L. Hypertriglyceridemia and acute pancreatitis. JAMA Internal Med. 2013;173:162–4.
4. Scherer J, Singh VP, Pitchumoni CS, Yadav D. Issues in hypertriglyceridemic pancreatitis: an update. J Clin Gastroenterol. 2014;48:195–203.
5. Ewald N, Hardt PD, Kloer HU. Severe hypertriglyceridemia and pancreatitis: presentation and management. Curr Opin Lipidol. 2009;20:497–504.
6. Lindberg DA. Acute pancreatitis and hypertriglyceridemia. Gastroenterol Nurs. 2009;32:75–82.
7. Deng LH, Xue P, Xia Q, Yang XN, Wan MH. Effect of admission hypertriglyceridemia on the episodes of severe acute pancreatitis. World J Gastroenterol. 2008;14:4558–61.
8. Anderson F, Thomson SR, Clarke DL, Buccimazza I. Dyslipidaemic pancreatitis clinical assessment and analysis of disease severity and outcomes. Pancreatology. 2009;9:252–7.
9. Preiss D. Triglyceride levels, pancreatitis and choice of lipid-modifying therapy. Expert Rev Gastroenterol Hepatol. 2013;7:193–5.
10. Banks PA, Bollen TL, Dervenis C, Gooszen HG, Johnson CD, Sarr MG, et al. Classification of acute pancreatitis–2012: revision of the Atlanta classification and definitions by international consensus. Gut. 2013;62:102–11.

11. van Geenen EJ, van der Peet DL, Bhagirath P, Mulder CJ, Bruno MJ. Etiology and diagnosis of acute biliary pancreatitis. Nat Rev Gastroenterol Hepatol. 2010;7:495–502.
12. Babu RY, Gupta R, Kang M, Bhasin DK, Rana SS, Singh R. Predictors of surgery in patients with severe acute pancreatitis managed by the step-up approach. Ann Surg. 2013;257:737–50.
13. van Santvoort HC, Besselink MG, Bakker OJ, Hofker HS, Boermeester MA, Dejong CH, et al. A step-up approach or open necrosectomy for necrotizing pancreatitis. N Engl J Med. 2010;362:1491–502.
14. Baudin G, Chassang M, Gelsi E, Novellas S, Bernardin G, Hebuterne X, et al. CT-guided percutaneous catheter drainage of acute infectious necrotizing pancreatitis: assessment of effectiveness and safety. AJR Am J Roentgenol. 2012;199:192–9.
15. Bausch D, Wellner U, Kahl S, Kuesters S, Richter-Schrag HJ, et al. Minimally invasive operations for acute necrotizing pancreatitis: comparison of minimally invasive retroperitoneal necrosectomy with endoscopic transgastric necrosectomy. Surgery. 2012;152:S128–34.
16. Klop B, Rego AT, Cabezas MC. Alcohol and plasma triglycerides. Curr Opin Lipidol. 2013;24:321–6.
17. Stefanutti C, Labbadia G, Morozzi C. Severe hypertriglyceridemia-related acute pancreatitis. Ther Apher Dial. 2013;17:130–7.
18. Murad MH, Hazem A, Coto-Yglesias F. The association of hypertriglyceridemia with cardiovascular events and pancreatitis: a systematic review and meta-analysis. BMC Endocr Disord. 2012;12:2.
19. Brunzell JD, Schrott HG. The interaction of familial and secondary causes of hypertriglyceridemia: role in pancreatitis. J Clin Lipido. 2012;6:409–12.
20. Kota SK, Krishna SV, Lakhtakia S, Modi KD. Metabolic pancreatitis: Etiopathogenesis and management. Indian J Endocrinol Metab. 2013;17:799–805.
21. Yang F, Wang Y, Sternfeld L, Rodriguez JA, Ross C, Hayden MR, et al. The role of free fatty acids, pancreatic lipase and Ca + signalling in injury of isolated acinar cells and pancreatitis model in lipoprotein lipase-deficient mice. Acta Physiol (Oxf). 2009;195:13–28.
22. Zeng Y, Wang X, Zhang W, Wu K, Ma J. Hypertriglyceridemia aggravates ER stress and pathogenesis of acute pancreatitis. Hepatogastroenterology. 2012;59:2318–26.
23. Zhou MT, Chen CS, Chen BC, Zhang QY, Andersson R. Acute lung injury and ARDS in acute pancreatitis: mechanisms and potential intervention. World J Gastroenterol. 2010;16:2094–9.
24. Patel AD. Hypertriglyceridemia-induced acute pancreatitis treatment with insutin and heparin. Indian J Endocrinol Metab. 2012;16:671–2.
25. Lloret Linares C, Pelletier AL, Czernichow S, Vergnaud AC, Bonnefont-Rousselot D, Levy P, et al. Acute pancreatitis in a cohort of 129 patients referred for severe hypertriglyceridemia. Pancreas. 2008;37:13–22.
26. Chang YT, Chang MC, Su TC, Liang PC, Su YN, Kuo CY, et al. Lipoprotein lipase mutation S447X associated with pancreatic calcification and steatorrhea in hyperlipidemic pancreatitis. J Clin Gastroenterol. 2009;43:591–6.
27. Zerem E, Imamovic G, Susic A, Haracic B. Step-up approach to infected necrotizing pancreatitis: a 20-year experience of percutaneous drainage in a single centre. Dig Liver Dis. 2011;43:478–83.
28. van Baal MC, van Santvoort HC, Bollen TL, Bakker OJ, Besselink MG, Gooszen HG, et al. Systematic review of percutaneous catheter drainage as primary treatment for necrotizing pancreatitis. Br J Surg. 2011;98:18–27.
29. Kuo VC, Tarnasky PR. Endoscopic management of acute biliary pancreatitis. Gastrointest Endosc Clin N Am. 2013;23:749–68.
30. van Geenen EJ, van Santvoort HC, Besselink MG, van der Peet DL, van Erpecum KJ, Fockens P, et al. Lack of consensus on the role of endoscopic retrograde cholangiography in acute biliary pancreatitis in published meta-analyses and guidelines: a systematic review. Pancreas. 2013;42:774–80.

2

Continuous suturing with two anterior layers reduces post-operative complications and hospitalization time in pancreaticoenterostomy

Guoliang Yao, Yonggang Fan and Jingming Zhai*

Abstract

Background: Most complications after pancreaticoduodenectomy (PD) were relation to pancreaticoenterostomy. We improved a new method of pancreaticoenterostomy that included the continuous suturing of the jejunum and the stump of the pancreas end-to-side with one layer posteriorly and two layers anteriorly. To evaluate the safety and efficiency of this new method, we introduced this retrospectively compared trial.

Methods: We compared 45 patients who had undergone pancreaticoduodenectomy with either the regular interrupted suturing method or the new continuous mattress suturing method in our hospital from September 2011 to March 2014.

Results: Although the total operation times were not reduced, the suturing time for the pancreaticoenterostomies in the continuous suture group (11.3 ± 1.8 min) was greatly reduced compared with that for the interrupted suture group (14.1 ± 2.9 min, $p = 0.045$). Importantly, the continuous mattress suturing method significantly decreased short-term post-operative complications, including pancreatic leakage ($p = 0.042$). Furthermore, shorter hospitalization times were observed in the continuous mattress suture group (12.3 ± 5.0 d) than in the interrupted suture group (24.2 ± 11.6 d, $p = 0.000$).

Conclusions: Continuous mattress suturing is a safe and effective pancreaticoenterostomy method that leads to reduced complications and hospitalization times.

Keywords: Pancreaticoenterostomy, Pancreaticoduodenectomy, Pancreatic leakage, Continuous mattress suturing

Background

Pancreaticoduodenectomy (PD) has been rapidly developed since it was first introduced. PD is used not only for peri-ampullary malignant tumors but also for certain benign pancreatic disorders. PD is a relatively safe surgery because its recent mortality rate has been reported to be only approximately 3–5 % [1–3]. However, the post-operative complications of PD have not been greatly reduced [4, 5]. Several modifications have been used to produce better outcomes, but they are complicated and time consuming [6]. Thus far, there is still no worldwide-accepted procedure to reduce complications. Here, we introduce a safe and effective procedure to reduce the complications and provided better outcomes.

Methods

Patient characteristics

We retrospectively analyzed all PDs performed because of peri-ampullary tumors in our hospital between September 2011 and March 2014. Patients with diffused metastases in the abdomen were excluded. Patients with severe diseases in other systems were also excluded because of their poor tolerances. From September 2011 to

* Correspondence: 15237917026@163.com
Yao Guoliang is the first author.
Department of General Surgery, The First Affiliated Hospital of Henan University of Science and Technology, 24 Jinghua Road, Luoyang 471003, People's Republic of China

August 2013, 29 patients underwent PD with interrupted suturing. Because two patients died after their second laparotomies in August 2013 because of hemorrhaging secondary to pancreatic leakage, we modified the pancreaticoenterostomy procedure to include a new method of continuous suturing. By March 2014, 16 patients had undergone PD with continuous suturing by the same surgeon, who had more than 10 years' experience with PD. The patient information, including basic characteristics, such as age and gender, and operation-related characteristics, such as the operation time, pancreaticoenterostomy time, hospitalization time, blood lost during the operation, and complications including pancreatic leakage and mortality were analyzed. According to the International Study Group for Pancreatic Fistula, pancreatic leakage was defined as drainage of any volume on or after postoperation d 3 with an amylase content greater than 3-fold the upper normal serum value.

Operation procedure

The patients were sufficiently physiologically and psychologically prepared before the operations. During the operations, the transfixations of the upper and lower edges of the stump of the pancreas were emphasized to decrease blood loss before the transection of the pancreas. A pancreatic duct stent was used to the fix the stump of pancreas for at least 15 cm to drain the pancreatic jaundice to the distal end of the jejunum and was placed at least 10 cm away from the anastomosis of the cholangioenterostomy. The stump of the jejunum was pulled to the stump of the pancreas behind the transverse mesocolon without tension. The stump of the pancreas was invaginated into the jejunum by at least 2–3 cm and fixed with 3-0 polypropylene suture (Prolene, Ethicon). The difference between the continuous suturing and interrupted suturing was limited to the procedure of suturing the pancreaticoenterostomy. The interrupted suturing involved one layer of discontinuous sutures with distances of 2–3 mm between each pair of stitches. The continuous suturing involved one layer posteriorly and two layers anteriorly. A 3-0 polypropylene suture was used to complete the suturing from the very upper edge of the pancreas to the lower edge through the posterior edge of the pancreas, and the anterior suture was then completed with the suture. Finally, a knot was tied at the upper edge of the pancreas with the very end of the suture (Figs. 1, 2, 3 and 4). After the first-layer suture, a second-layer suture was applied from at the end edge of the lateral opening of the jejunum anteriorly from the very lower edge of the pancreas to the very upper edge (Fig. 5).

Statistical analysis

SPSS 16.0 was used to analyze the data. The measurement data, including age, operation time, pancreaticoenterostomy time, blood loss, and hospitalization time, were compared with t tests. The numerical data, such as tumor location, pancreas texture, American Society of Anesthesiologists (ASA) classification, and complications, were compared with chi square tests. $P < 0.05$ was considered to be significant.

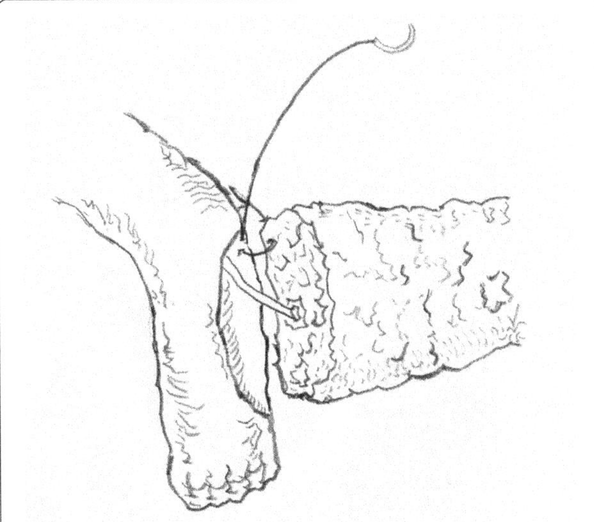

Fig. 1 The first stitch was located at the upper edge of the pancreas. It's beginning from the outside to the inside of the pancreas, and then from the inside to the outside of the jejunum and then a knot was tied outside

Results

The basic characteristics of the two groups, including gender, age, carcinoma location, pancreas texture and

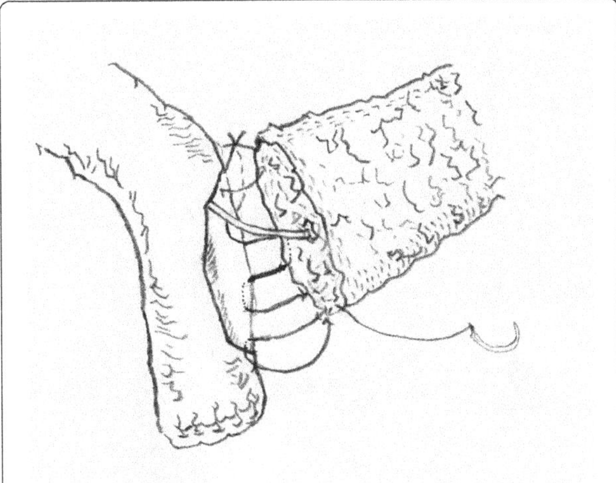

Fig. 2 The posterior of the anastomosis was from upper edge to the lower edge. All the stitches were from the outside to the inside of the jejunum and then transfix the pancreas, and then the stump of pancreas was sutured with jejunum from the inside to the outside. The procedure was repeated until the very lower edge of the pancreas

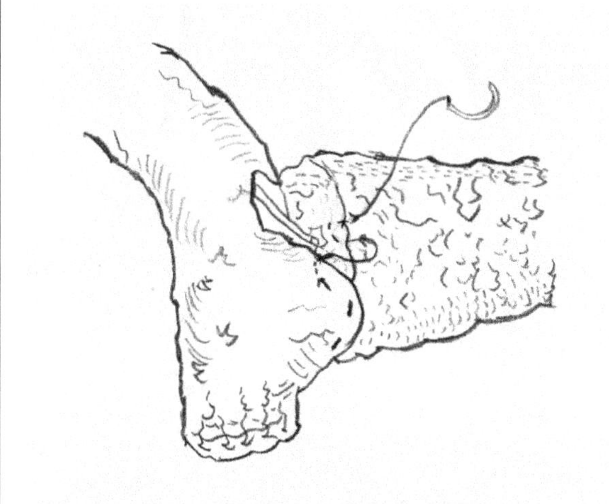

Fig. 3 The anterior side of the anastomosis was continuously sutured just like the posterior side. All the stitches were from the outside to the inside of the jejunum and then transfix the pancreas. Then the stump of pancreas was sutured with jejunum from the inside to the outside. The procedure was repeated until the very upper edge of the pancreas. A knot was tied at the very end of the suture shown in Fig. 4 blow

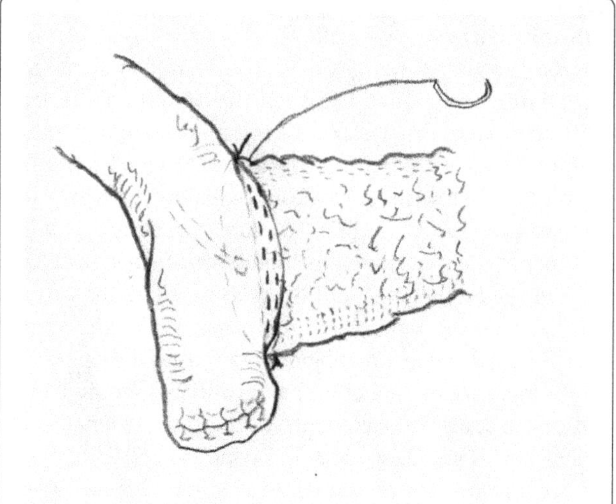

Fig. 5 The second layer suture of the anterior side was location at the very edge of the jejunum just like the first layer. After this suture, the whole anastomosis was finished

ASA classification, are presented in Table 1. Two duodenal interstitialomas were found in the interrupted suture group, and one duodenal carcinoid was found in the continuous suture group. Advanced stage patients with portal vein or inferior vena cava invasion were excluded. There were no significant differences between the two groups in terms of age, gender, tumor location, degree of anemia, pancreatic texture, ASA score, blood loss or total operation time (Table 2). However, the pancreaticoenterostomy time in the continuous suture group was 11.3 ± 1.8 min, which was significantly shorter than the 14.1 ± 2.9 min observed in the interrupted suture group ($p = 0.045$). The hospitalization time was also significantly shorter for the continuous suture group (12.3 ± 5.0 d) than the interrupted suture group (24.2 ± 11.6 d, $p = 0.000$). Furthermore, the total

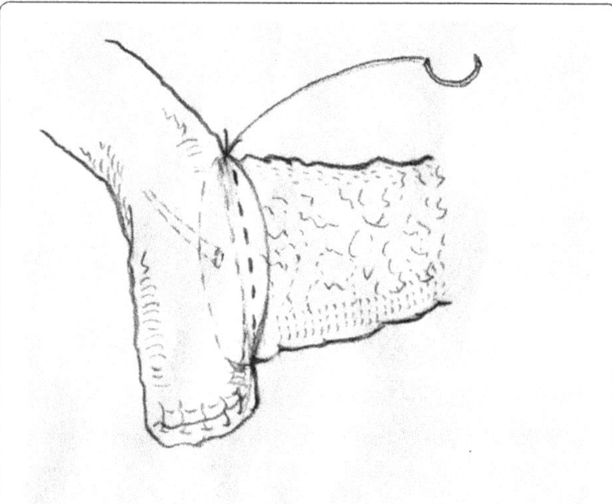

Fig. 4 A knot was tied at the very upper edge of the pancreas and the first layer suture was finished

Table 1 Basic clinic characteristics of the patients

Characteristics	Interrupt suturing ($N = 29$)	Continuous suturing ($N = 16$)	P
Gender (M/F)	18/11	11/5	0.752
Age (y)	67.3 ± 7.4	61.2 ± 6.2	0.482
Location			0.676
Jejunum	14[a]	5[b]	
Lower bile duct	4	4	
Ampulla	8	5	
Head of pancreas	3	2	
Anemia	86.3 ± 17.5	83.9 ± 18.3	0.793
ASA stage			0.901
I	5	2	
II	13	8	
III	11	6	
Pancreas texture			0.868
Hard	7	5	
Firm	17	7	
Soft	5	4	

[a]Including two cases of duodenal interstitialomas. One presented with melena, and the other was discovered via an upper digestive tract endoscopy examination for a non-specific abdominal distension syndrome
[b]Including a duodenal carcinoid that was discovered via an upper digestive tract endoscopy examination for abdominal distension and interrupted melena

Table 2 The operative characteristics of the patients

Characteristics	Interrupt suturing (*N* = 29)	Continuous suturing (*N* = 16)	P
Operation time (min)	260.8 ± 35.6	249.5 ± 31.7	0.731
Pancreaticoenterostomy time (min)	14.1 ± 2.9	11.3 ± 1.8	0.045
Blood lost (ml)	465.4 ± 72.3	426.1 ± 57.6	0.672
Hospitalization time (d)	24.2 ± 11.6	12.3 ± 5.0	0.000
Complications[a]			0.042
Death	3	1[b]	
Pancreatic leakage	8	2	
Bleeding	7	2	
Pneumonia	2	1	

[a] The complications were varied. In the interrupted suture group, two of the three deaths were due to pancreatic leakage followed by severe hemorrhaging, as revealed by secondary laparotomy, and active bleeding occurred at the stomas of the pancreaticojejunostomies. The other death was due to hemorrhaging without pancreatic leakage. Two cases of bleeding that presented with post-operative blood drainage were cured conservatively and were secondary to pancreatic leakage. The remaining two cases of bleeding were also cured conservatively, and these cases presented with hematemesis and melena without pancreatic leakage. The remaining cases of pancreatic leakage were cured conservatively, and secondary injuries were not found
[b] The death in the continuous group was also due to a large hemorrhage secondary to pancreatic leakage. The other case of pancreatic leakage was cured conservatively. The other case of bleeding in continuous group presented with melena and was cured conservatively. The case with pneumonia was cured by the time of discharge

complications were significantly decreased in the continuous suture group compared with the interrupted suture group ($p = 0.042$). There were three cases of death in the interrupted suture group and one case of death in the continuous suture group. Two out of these three deaths occurred after the second laparotomies, owing to hemorrhaging secondary to pancreatic leakage. The other death in the interrupted suture group was due to hemorrhaging without pancreatic leakage. The death in the continuous suture group occurred because of hemorrhaging secondary to pancreatic leakage without a second laparotomy. Regarding pancreatic leakage, according to the criteria of the International Study Group on Pancreatic Fistula (ISGPF), we defined leakage as a drain output of any measurable volume of fluid on or after postoperation day 3 with an amylase activity three times greater than that in the serum [4]. There were eight cases of pancreatic leakage in the interrupted suture group and two cases in the continuous suture group (Table 3). According to the ISGPF, one case was grade A, three cases were grade B and four cases were grade C in the interrupted suture group, whereas one case was grade B and one case was grade C in the continuous suture group (Table 3). However, neither the incidence ($p = 0.585$) nor the severity ($p = 0.292$) of pancreatic leakage was significantly different between groups. In the eight cases of

Table 3 Pancreatic leakage classification according to the ISGPF

	Interrupt suturing (*N* = 29)	Continuous suturing (*N* = 16)	P
Pancreatic leakage	8(27.6 %)	2(12.5 %)	0.585
Severity classification			0.292
Grade A	1	0	
Grade B	4	1	
Grade C	3	1	

pancreatic leakage in the interrupted suture group, two died after the second laparotomies, two exhibited bleeding secondary to leakage and were cured conservatively, and the other four were cured without other secondary injuries. In the continuous suture group, one case of pancreatic leakage died because of a secondary injury of a large hemorrhage, and the other case was cured conservatively.

Discussions

PD is the optimal choice for the peri-ampullary tumors [7]. Although the mortality after PD is low, the post-operative morbidity remains as high as 30–65 % [3, 8–13]. Pancreatic fistulae are the most serious postoperative complication and may cause a series of secondary injuries, and even death [14]. Many efforts have been made to reduce the occurrence of pancreatic fistulae. Baki Topal et al [7] have reported that pancreaticogastrostomy can reduce the clinical and biochemical pancreatic fistulae compared with pancreaticojejunostomy. However, pancreaticogastrostomy has no advantage in reducing the overall postoperative complications. Moreover, Bassi C et al [15] have reported contradictory results and have found no significant differences in pancreatic leakage between pancreaticogastrostomy and pancreaticojejunostomy. Pancreatic duct stent placement is a widely adopted improvement that may reduce pancreatic leakage, morbidity and mortality after PD [16–18]. However, stenting increases the operation cost. Additionally, Seung Eun Lee et al [19] have found that continuous stitching is more feasible and safe than interrupted stitching during the performance of duct-to-mucosa pancreaticojejunostomy. However, this modification is a complicated procedure with an extended operation time.

Here, we introduced a small modification that led to a substantial improvement in postoperative morbidity. We performed continuous stitching of the pancreaticojejunal anastomosis involving one layer posteriorly and two layers anteriorly rather than interrupt sutures. We used two layers anteriorly because two of the patients who died in the interrupt suture group had ulcers located at the anterior of the pancreaticojejunal anastomotic stoma with active bleeding. This enhanced anterior suturing with two layers is a very simple procedure that requires only a 3-0 polypropylene suture. We sutured the jejunum and the stump of pancreas from the very upper edge of the pancreas to the lower edge through the posterior edge of the pancreas and then continuously completed the anterior suture with the same suture. Finally, a knot was tied at the upper edge of pancreas with the very end of the suture. In the first layer, only two knots were needed. Moreover, the second anterior layer was also continuously completed. Continuous suturing has at least four advantages: First, a more even distribution of tension can be achieved between the pancreatic parenchyma and the jejunum [20]. Second, owing to the coiled spring effect, the continuous suturing method also provides a reduction in the likelihood of focal tissue ischemia, an increase in tensile strength, and a reduction of the risk of pancreaticojejunal rupture [20]. Third, continuous suturing reduces the anastomosis time. Finally, continuous suturing is technically easier and costs less [21].

Our results revealed a shortened pancreaticojejunostomy time due to the simple procedure involving the end-to-side invagination technique. This technique required only 11.3 ± 1.8 min to complete the anastomosis. Because of the advantages of the continuous suturing, fewer cases with severe complications and shorter hospitalization times were achieved. Although neither the incidence nor severity of pancreatic leakage were different between the two groups, our results revealed a trend toward a decline (27.6 % vs 12.5 %). This trend may explain the decline in the total complications, which led to shorter hospitalizations. As a preliminary investigation, our study included a relatively small number of patients, and this may have influenced the results.

Conclusions

Continuous mattress suturing is a safe and effective pancreaticoenterostomy method that leads to reduced complications and hospitalization times.

Abbreviations

ASA, American Society of Anesthesiologists; ISGPF, the International Study Group on Pancreatic Fistula; PD, pancreaticoduodenectomy

Acknowledgements

Not applicable.

Funding

Not applicable.

Authors' contributions

YGL and FYG extracted the data. YGL and FYG were responsible for the analysis. ZJM explained the results and completed this manuscript. All authors read and approved the final manuscript.

Competing interests

The authors declare that they have no competing interests.

Consent for publication

All the authors, including Yao Guoliang, Fan Yonggang and Zhai Jingming approve to publish this paper on BMC gastroenterology.

References

1. Gouma DJ, van Geenen RC, van Gulik TM, et al. Rates of complications and death after pancreaticoduodenectomy: risk factors and the impact of hospital volume. Ann Surg. 2000;232(6):786–95.
2. Michalski CW, Kleeff J, Wente MN, et al. Systematic review and meta-analysis of standard and extended lymphadenectomy in pancreaticoduodenectomy for pancreatic cancer. Br J Surg. 2007;94(3):265–73.
3. Cameron JL, Riall TS, Coleman J, et al. One thousand consecutive pancreaticoduodenectomies. Ann Surg. 2006;244(1):10–5.
4. Grobmyer SR, Rivadeneira DE, Goodman CA, et al. Pancreatic anastomotic failure after pancreaticoduodenectomy. Am J Surg. 2000;180(2):117–20.
5. Grobmyer SR, Pieracci FM, Allen PJ, et al. Defining morbidity after pancreaticoduodenectomy: use of a prospective complication grading system. J Am Coll Surg. 2007;204(3):356–64.
6. Katsaragakis S, Larentzakis A, Panousopoulos SG, et al. A new pancreaticojejunostomy technique: a battle against postoperative pancreatic fistula. World J Gastroenterol. 2013;19(27):4351–5.
7. Topal B, Fieuws S, Aerts R, et al. Pancreaticojejunostomy versus pancreaticogastrostomy reconstruction after pancreaticoduodenectomy for pancreatic or periampullary tumours: a multicentre randomised trial. Lancet Oncol. 2013;14(7):655–62.
8. Bassi C, Dervenis C, Butturini G, et al. Postoperative pancreatic fistula: an international study group (ISGPF) definition. Surgery. 2005;138(1):8–13.
9. Callery MP, Pratt WB, Vollmer CM, et al. Prevention and management of pancreatic fistula. J Gastrointest Surg. 2009;13(1):163–73.
10. Yang YM, Tian XD, Zhuang Y, et al. Risk factors of pancreatic leakage after pancreaticoduodenectomy. World J Gastroenterol. 2005;11(16):2456–61.
11. Shrikhande SV, D'Souza MA. Pancreatic fistula after pancreatectomy: evolving definitions, preventive strategies and modern management. World J Gastroenterol. 2008;14(38):5789–96.
12. Lai EC, Lau SH, Lau WY. Measures to prevent pancreatic fistula after pancreatoduodenectomy: a comprehensive review. Arch Surg. 2009;144(11):1074–80.
13. Schmidt CM, Powell ES, Yiannoutsos CT, et al. Pancreaticoduodenectomy: a 20-year experience in 516 patients. Arch Surg. 2004;139(7):718–27.
14. Zhou YM, Zhang XF, Wu LP, et al. Pancreatic fistula after central pancreatectomy: case series and review of the literature. Hepatobiliary Pancreat Dis Int. 2014;13(2):203–8.
15. Bassi C, Falconi M, Molinari E, et al. Reconstruction by pancreaticojejunostomy versus pancreaticogastrostomy following pancreatectomy: results of a comparative study. Ann Surg. 2005;242(6):767–73.
16. Poon RT, Fan ST, Lo CM, et al. External drainage of pancreatic duct with a stent to reduce leakage rate of pancreaticojejunostomy after pancreaticoduodenectomy : a prospective randomized trial. Ann Surg. 2007; 246(3):425–35.
17. Mok KT, Wong BW, Liu SI. Management of pancreatic remnant with strategies according to the size of pancreatic duct after pancreaticoduodenectomy. Br J Surg. 1999;86(8):1018–9.
18. Hong S, Wang H, Yang S, et al. External stent versus no stent for pancreaticojejunostomy: A Meta-analysis of randomized controlled trail. J Gastrointest Surg. 2013;17(8):1516–25.
19. Lee SE, Yang SH, Jang JY, et al. Pancreatic fistula after pancreaticoduodenectomy: A comparison between the two pancreaticojejunostomy methods for approximating the pancreatic parenchyma to the jejunal seromuscular layer: Interrupted vs continuous stitches. World J Gastroenterol. 2007;13(40):5351–6.

3

Associations between polymorphisms in folate-metabolizing genes and pancreatic cancer risk in Japanese subjects

Haruhisa Nakao[1], Kenji Wakai[2], Norimitsu Ishii[1], Yuji Kobayashi[1], Kiyoaki Ito[1], Masashi Yoneda[1], Mitsuru Mori[3], Masanori Nojima[3], Yasutoshi Kimura[4], Takao Endo[5], Masato Matsuyama[6], Hiroshi Ishii[7], Makoto Ueno[8], Sawako Kuruma[9], Naoto Egawa[10], Keitaro Matsuo[11,12], Satoyo Hosono[13], Shinichi Ohkawa[8], Kozue Nakamura[14], Akiko Tamakoshi[15], Mami Takahashi[16], Kazuaki Shimada[17], Takeshi Nishiyama[18], Shogo Kikuchi[18] and Yingsong Lin[18*]

Abstract

Background: Evidence supporting the associations between folate metabolizing gene polymorphisms and pancreatic cancer has been inconclusive. We examined their associations in a case-control study of Japanese subjects.

Methods: Our case-control study involved 360 newly diagnosed pancreatic cancer cases and 400 frequency-matched, non-cancer control subjects. We genotyped four folate metabolizing gene polymorphisms, including two polymorphisms (rs1801133 and rs1801131) in the methylenetetrahydrofolate (*MTHFR*) gene, one polymorphism (rs1801394) in the 5-methyltetrahydrofolate-homocysteine methyltransferase reductase (*MTRR)* gene and one polymorphism (rs1805087) in the 5-methyltetrahydrofolate-homocysteine methyltransferase (*MTR*) gene. Genotyping was performed using Fluidigm SNPtype assays. Unconditional logistic regression methods were used to estimate odds ratios (ORs) and 95 % confidence intervals (CIs) for the associations between folate metabolizing gene variants and pancreatic cancer risk.

Results: Overall we did not observe a significant association between these four genotypes and pancreatic cancer risk. For rs1801133, compared with individuals with the CC genotype of *MTHFR* C677T, the OR for those with the CT genotype and TT genotype was 0.87 (0.62-1.22) and 0.99 (0.65-1.51), respectively. For rs1801131, individuals with the CC genotype had approximately 1.2-fold increased risk compared with those with the AA genotype, but the association was not statistically significant. In analyses stratified by smoking and drinking status, no significant associations were noted for C677T genotypes. No significant interactions were observed with smoking and drinking with respect to pancreatic cancer risk.

Conclusions: Our data did not support the hypothesis that *MTHFR* polymorphisms or other polymorphisms in the folate metabolizing pathway are associated with pancreatic cancer risk.

Keywords: Folate, Polymorphism, Pancreatic cancer, Risk, Case-control study

* Correspondence: linys@aichi-med-u.ac.jp
[18]Department of Public Health, Aichi Medical University School of Medicine, Nagakute 480-1195, Japan
Full list of author information is available at the end of the article

Background

Pancreatic cancer is often diagnosed at an advanced stage and has the poorest 5-year survival rate of any cancer. There is no effective screening method to identify apparently healthy individuals who are at risk for pancreatic cancer. The etiology of pancreatic cancer remains largely unknown, with only cigarette smoking and long standing diabetes being established as risk factors [1]. The role of diet in carcinogenesis has been recognized for a long time. Evidence on the diet-pancreatic cancer associations from epidemiologic studies remains elusive, in part because of wide variation in dietary habits and the difficulty of accurate diet measurement. In nutrient-based studies, there has been much research interest in folate, a water soluble vitamin B that is abundant in green leafy vegetables, citrus fruit, legumes and cereals [2]. Folate plays a vital role in maintaining health because it is closely involved in two vital cellular processes, DNA methylation and DNA synthesis [2]. Epidemiologic studies have linked folate deficiency to a variety of conditions, including cardiovascular diseases and cancer [3–5]. For pancreatic cancer, previous studies have shown mixed findings on the association between dietary folate intake and pancreatic cancer risk [6–9], although a 2014 meta-analysis reported an inverse association [10]. One possible reason for the inconsistent findings is that folate status is determined by both dietary folate intake and folate metabolism, making it difficult to accurately quantify folate intake. Of numerous genes involved in the folate metabolizing pathway, *MTHFR* has been the most extensively studied [11, 12]. *MTHFR* irreversibly converts 5,10-methylenetetrahydrofolate to 5-methyltetrahydrofolate, the predominant form of folate in the circulation. Two variants in the *MTHFR*, namely C677T (rs1801133) and A1298C (rs1801131), have been the focus of most studies [11] because the variations are associated with a small change in protein structure. Compared with the CC genotype (wild-type), the TT genotype (minor homozygotes) of C677T has approximately 35 % lower enzyme activity and 10 % lower levels of methylhydrolate folate [11]. The 677 T variant has been associated with numerous conditions, including elevated homocysteine, spinal bifida, colon cancer, and Down syndrome [3] As for *MTHFR* A1298C, the homozygous CC genotype has approximately 60 % of normal *MTHFR* activity [12].

Evidence supporting the associations between folate metabolizing gene polymorphisms and pancreatic cancer has been inconclusive. To date, five case-control studies have examined the association between the polymorphisms in *MTHFR*, *MTR*, or *MTRR* genes and pancreatic cancer risk, with conflicting results [13–17]. Of them, two case-control studies conducted in Japan found no main effects for polymorphisms in *MTHFR* (rs1801133, rs1801131), *MTR* (rs1805087) or MTRR (rs1801394) genes [15, 17]. However, rs162049 in the *MTRR* gene, which encodes enzymes responsible for DNA methylation, has been shown to be associated with the susceptibility to pancreatic cancer in one previous Japanese case-control study [17]. The significance of these polymorphisms in the folate metabolizing pathway on pancreatic cancer remains to be determined.

Given that substantial evidence from epidemiologic and laboratory research supports an important role of folate in carcinogenesis [18], we genotyped several genetic polymorphisms in the folate metabolizing pathway and examined their associations with pancreatic cancer risk in Japanese subjects. We hypothesized that the variant *MTHFR* C667T and A1298C genotypes resulting in decreased enzyme activity are associated with an increased risk for pancreatic cancer. Additionally, we performed analyses stratified by cigarette smoking and alcohol drinking to address the possibility that these two lifestyle factors may modify the associations between genetic polymorphisms and pancreatic cancer risk.

Methods

Study subjects

This case-control study was designed to address the role of genetic variations in determining pancreatic cancer risk in Japanese subjects. A detailed description of the study method has been published elsewhere [19]. In brief, eligible cases were defined as newly diagnosed pancreatic cancer patients at five participating hospitals from April 1, 2010, through May 15, 2012. Those who had received chemotherapy for pancreatic cancer prior to the study entry were excluded. The diagnosis was based on imaging modalities and pathology reports (if available) were further reviewed for final diagnosis. Control subjects, who had no history of cancer, were recruited from inpatients and outpatients at each participating hospital, as well as from individuals who underwent medical checkups at one of the participating hospitals. The response rate was 85 % for cases and 98 % for control subjects. The control subjects were frequency matched to the case patients according to sex and age (within 10-year categories). Finally, 360 case patients and 400 control subjects were included in the present analysis. Approximately 90 % of tumors were histologically confirmed, with all tumors being adenocarcinomas.

For the main effect of genotypes, the sample size was estimated using the following assumptions: multiplicative genetic model, 10 % minor allele frequency, 0.1 % disease prevalence, 1:1 case-control ratio, and OR = 2.0. Then the number of cases required to achieve 90 % power at a significance threshold of $\alpha = 0.05$ was 190 cases [20]. This study was conducted in accordance with the Helsinki Declaration. All the study subjects provided written informed consent. The Ethics Board of Aichi Medical University and the Institutional Review Board of all the participating hospitals approved this study.

Data collection

A self-administered questionnaire was used to solicit detailed information on demographic characteristics, medical history, and lifestyle factors such as smoking, drinking and dietary habits. Dietary habits were surveyed using a validated food frequency questionnaire (FFQ), in which the study subjects were asked to describe the usual intake frequency of 36 foods during the previous year prior to the study entry [21]. After written informed consent was obtained from the study subjects, a 7 mL venous blood sample was collected. Genomic DNA was extracted using the same protocol for cases and controls, and subsequently stored at -30 °C until analysis.

Genotyping assays

The genotyping of folate-metabolizing gene polymorphisms was performed using Fluidigm 192.24 Dynamic Array with BioMark HD Systems and EP1 (Fluidigm Corp., CA). SNPtype assay (Fluidigm Corp., CA), which employs allele-specifically designed fluorescences (FAM or VIC) primers and a common reverse primer, was used in this study. Genotype calls were obtained using the BioMark SNP Genotyping Analysis software. This software defined the genotype of each sample based on the relative intensities of fluorescences. The laboratory staff members were blinded to case or control status. Four quality control samples (negative control and positive controls for major homozygote, heterozygote and minor homozygote) were included in each assay, and the successful genotyping rate was 100 %.

Statistical analysis

The differences in the characteristics of case patients and control subjects were tested using t-test, Mann-Whitney test, or chi-square test. The amount of daily ethanol intake was calculated based on the frequency and amount of alcohol beverages reported by the study subjects. The amount of daily dietary folate intake was estimated based on the responses to FFQ. A chi-square test was used to assess the Hardy-Weinberg equilibrium (HWE) in control subjects. Because the biological function of most SNPs has not been clearly defined, a co-dominant genomic model was assumed for SNP effects. Unconditional logistic regression models were used to estimate odds ratios (ORs) and 95 % confidence intervals (CIs) for the associations between folate metabolism-associated genetic polymorphisms and pancreatic cancer risk. All analyses were adjusted for age (continuous), sex (male or female), BMI (<20, 20-22.4, 22.5-24.9, or ≥25.0), and cigarette smoking (current, former, or never smokers). All tests were two-tailed; a P value less than 0.05 was used to define statistical significance. The interaction of genotype and smoking and drinking with regard to pancreatic cancer risk was assessed using a likelihood ratio test. All statistical analyses were performed using SAS 9.12 (SAS Institute, Inc., Cary, North Carolina, USA).

Results

The distribution of genotypes for all SNPs among control subjects did not deviate from HWE. The selected characteristics of cases and controls are presented in Table 1. Compared with control subjects, the cases were more likely to have a history of diabetes and to be current smokers. The proportion of current drinkers is higher in control subjects than in case patients. The daily ethanol intake was 24.1 g/d among case patients and 17.5 g/d among control subjects. The median of daily folate intake was 338.9 μg for case patients and 359.5 μg for control subjects. High intake of dietary folate was inversely associated with pancreatic cancer risk, with OR of 0.52 (95 % CI: 0.33-0.82) among individuals falling into the highest quartile when compare with those falling into the lowest quartile.

Table 2 shows the ORs of pancreatic cancer in relation to individual polymorphisms in the following genes: *MTHFR* (rs1801133, rs1801131), *MTRR* (rs1801394), and *MTR* (rs1805087). Overall no significant associations were noted between any single genotype and risk of pancreatic cancer. For rs1801133, compared with individuals with the CC genotype of *MTHFR* C677T, the OR for those with the CT genotype and TT genotype was 0.87 (0.62–1.22) and 0.99 (0.65–1.51), respectively. For rs1801131, individuals with the CC genotype had approximately 1.2-fold increased risk compared with those with the AA genotype, but the association was not statistically significant.

Table 3 shows the associations of pancreatic cancer with folate metabolizing gene polymorphisms by smoking and drinking status. There were no significant associations in either never smokers or current smokers. Similarly, there were no significant associations in either never drinkers or current drinkers.

Table 4 shows the joint effects of smoking, drinking and *MTHFR* genotypes on pancreatic cancer risk. No significant interactions were observed for C667T genotypes and cigarette smoking; the OR of pancreatic cancer was 1.94 (1.05–3.57) for individuals who had the TT genotype and were ever smokers. Similarly, no significant interactions were noted for C677T genotypes and alcohol drinking; the OR of pancreatic cancer was 1.05 (95 % CI: 0.62-1.78) for individuals who had the TT genotype and were ever smokers.

Discussion

In this genetic case-control association study, we found no statistically significant associations between polymorphisms in folate metabolizing gene pathways, including *MTHFR* C677T and A1298C, and the risk of pancreatic

Table 1 Characteristics of case patients and control subjects

Characteristics	Case patients (*N* = 360)	Control subjects (*N* = 400)	P
Age (mean ± SD)	67.8 ± 8.8	64.8 ± 9.5	<0.0001
Male, *N* (%)	215 (59.7)	226 (56.5)	0.58
Body mass index (kg/m2) (mean ± SD)	22.9 ± 3.3	22.8 ± 3.2	0.62
History of diabetes, *N* (%)			<0.0001
No	269 (74.7)	362 (90.5)	
Yes	87 (24.2)	35 (8.7)	
Unknown	4 (1.1)	3 (0.8)	
Smoking status, *N* (%)			<0.0001
Non-smokers	145 (40.2)	202 (50.5)	
Former smokers	119 (33.1)	140 (35.0)	
Current Smokers	96 (26.7)	58 (14.5)	
Alcohol drinking, *N* (%)			0.23
Non-drinkers	134 (37.2)	147 (36.8)	
Former drinkers	24(6.7)	16 (4.0)	
Current Drinkers	202(56.1)	237(59.2)	
Ethanol intake (g/d), median (25th, 75th percentile)	24.1 (7.8, 48.9)	17.5 (5.7, 43.4)	0.02
Dietary folate intake (μg), median (25th, 75th percentile)	338.9 (280.9, 407.6)	359.2 (293.0, 438.8)	0.0007

SD, standard deviation

cancer. Previous studies on the associations of *MTHFR* (C677T) with pancreatic cancer risk have shown inconsistent results [13–16]. A hospital-based case-control study, conducted at the MD Anderson Cancer Center in the United States, found that individuals with the TT variant genotype had a 2-fold increased risk for pancreatic cancer when compared with individuals with the CC genotype [13]. A stronger association was reported in a case-control study of Chinese population, in which the OR was 5.12 for individuals with the TT genotype

Table 2 Associations of pancreatic cancer with folate metabolizing gene polymorphisms

	Case patients (*n* = 360)	Control subjects (*n* = 400)	Crude OR	95 % CI	Multivariable-adjusted OR*	95 % CI	P for trend**
*MTHFR*_C677T rs1801133							
CC	127	124	1.00		1.00		
CT	161	194	0.81	0.59-1.12	0.87	0.62-1.22	
TT	72	82	0.86	0.57-1.28	0.99	0.65-1.51	0.86
*MTHFR*_A1298C rs1801131							
AA	240	285	1.00		1.00		
AC	107	102	1.25	0.90-1.72	1.28	0.91-1.80	
CC	13	13	1.19	0.54-2.61	1.22	0.53-2.80	0.17
*MTRR*_A66G rs1801394							
AA	167	206	1.00		1.00		
AG	157	158	1.23	0.91-1.66	1.29	0.94-1.77	
GG	36	36	1.23	0.74-2.04	1.12	0.66-1.91	0.27
*MTR*_A2756G rs1805087							
AA	224	241	1.00		1.00		
AG	117	142	0.89	0.65-1.20	0.87	0.63-1.21	
GG	19	17	1.20	0.61-2.37	1.53	0.75-3.12	0.89

OR odds ratio, *CI* confidence interval
*OR was adjusted for age, sex, cigarette smoking, BMI, and history of diabetes
**P for trend is shown for multivariable-adjusted OR

Table 3 Associations of pancreatic cancer with polymorphisms in genes involved in folate metabolism by smoking and drinking status

	Case patients ($n = 360$)	Control subjects ($n = 400$)	Multivariable-adjusted OR	95 % CI	Casepatients ($n = 360$)	Control subjects ($n = 400$)	Multivariable-adjusted OR	95 % CI	P for interaction
*MTHFR*_C677T rs1801133	Never smokers			Ever smokers					
CC	48	63	1.00		79	61	1.00		
CT	61	89	0.83	0.49-1.40	100	105	0.80	0.51-1.26	
TT	36	50	0.91	0.50-1.66	36	32	1.02	0.55-1.87	0.94
*MTHFR*_A1298C rs1801131									
AA	95	143	1.00		145	142	1.00		
AC	45	53	1.39	0.84-2.29	62	49	1.24	0.78-1.96	
CC	5	6	1.71	0.49-6.00	8	7	1.12	0.38-3.28	0.83
*MTRR*_A66G rs1801394									
AA	61	101	1.00		106	105	1.00		
AG	69	82	1.37	0.86-2.18	88	76	1.16	0.75-1.79	
GG	15	19	1.21	0.56-2.62	21	17	1.09	0.52-2.26	0.46
*MTR*_A2756G rs1805087									
AA	98	127	1.00		126	114	1.00		
AG	41	69	0.73	0.44-1.19	76	73	1.08	0.70-1.66	
GG	6	6	1.61	0.48-5.40	13	11	1.35	0.56-3.24	0.93
*MTHFR*_C677T rs1801133	Never drinkers			Ever drinkers					
CC	47	54	1.00		80	70	1.00		
CT	58	66	1.05	0.60-1.82	103	128	0.74	0.48-1.16	
TT	29	27	1.33	0.67-2.64	43	55	0.81	0.47-1.40	0.41
*MTHFR*_A1298C rs1801131									
AA	88	101	1.00		152	184	1.00		
AC	39	40	1.16	0.67-2.01	68	62	1.40	0.90-2.16	
CC	7	6	1.43	0.44-4.61	6	7	1.06	0.32-3.55	0.78
*MTRR*_A66G rs1801394									
AA	58	67	1.00		109	139	1.00		
AG	56	66	1.03	0.61-1.73	101	92	1.45	0.96-2.19	
GG	20	14	1.61	0.73-3.56	16	22	0.78	0.37-1.65	0.15
*MTR*_A2756G rs1805087									
AA	87	86	1.00		137	155	1.00		
AG	43	57	0.78	0.47-1.32	74	85	0.98	0.64-1.50	
GG	4	4	1.49	0.35-6.38	15	13	1.59	0.69-3.65	0.57

OR was adjusted for age, sex, BMI and history of diabetes

Table 4 Joint effects of smoking, drinking and MTHFR C677T on pancreatic cancer risk

C677T Genotype	Smoking	Case patients	Control subjects	OR (95 % CI)
CC + CT	Never	109	152	1.00
TT	Never	36	50	1.04 (0.62-1.73)
CC + CT	Ever	179	166	1.69 (1.13-2.54)
TT	Ever	36	32	1.94 (1.05-3.57)
				P for interaction = 0.79
	Drinking	Case patients	Control subjects	OR* (95 % CI)
CC + CT	Never	105	120	1.00
TT	Never	29	27	1.33 (0.72-2.45)
CC + CT	Ever	183	198	1.10 (0.75-1.61)
TT	Ever	43	55	1.05 (0.62-1.78)
				P for interaction = 0.38

OR odds ratio, *CI* confidence interval
*OR was adjusted for age, sex, body mass index, cigarette smoking and history of diabetes

compared with individuals with the CC genotype [14]. By contrast, two previous case-control studies in Japan did not find significant main effects for *MTHFR* C677T and A1298C genotypes [15, 17]. Our null findings were in agreement with results of these two previous studies. Our null findings were also consistent with the conclusion of a recent meta-analysis, which included all previous studies and showed no significant main effects for both *MTHFR* C677T and A1298C genotypes [22]. Furthermore, a recent study has sought to examine 37 genes and 834 SNPs related to one-carbon metabolism. There were no significant associations for any of the SNPs after correction for multiple comparisons [23]. However, in the case-control study by Ohnami et al, rs162049 (intronic SNP) in the *MTRR* gene showed significant associations after multiple testing [17]. One strength of their study is that functional tests were performed to collaborate the SNP-phenotype association. Unfortunately, we did not genotype rs162049 in the *MTRR* gene, but further studies needs to replicate their positive finding.

Given the lower enzymatic activity in individuals with the variant TT genotype of *MTHFR* C677T, a key enzyme in the folate metabolizing pathway, we hypothesized that the TT genotype carriers have an increased risk of pancreatic cancer. Our results, however, showed that case patients had a similar distribution of the TT genotypes with that of control subjects, and neither CT nor TT genotypes were significantly associated with the risk when compared with CC genotypes. The reason for our null findings on the associations between *MTHFR* genotypes and pancreatic cancer risk is not clear, but the differences observed in minor allele frequencies among ethnic groups may in part account for the conflicting results. The genotype frequencies of *MTHFR* C677T differed between our case-control study and the previous case-control study that involved a US population [13]. Even though there may be no main effects for the genotypes themselves, previous studies have shown that the *MTHFR* 677C→T polymorphism is only associated with increased coronary heart disease risk in a setting of low folate intake [4]. This finding suggested that the effect modification by dietary folate intake is important when interpreting the genotype-disease associations. If nutritional folate status is poor, the 677 T variant might promote the misincorporation of uracil into DNA, leading to genomic instability, a hallmark of cancer [3]. This mechanism may, in part, account for the increased cancer risk among individuals with the 677 T variant of *MTHFR*. On the other hand, if folate intake is adequate, the 677 T variant of *MTHFR* preferentially routes one-carbon units to DNA synthesis at the expense of methionine, which is involved in DNA methylation [3]. To address the possible effect modification by dietary folate intake, we evaluated their associations in low- versus high- dietary intake group, and found no significant effect modifications (data not shown). One possible reason is that most subjects in our study had adequate dietary folate intake because the estimated amount was comparable to 240 μg per day for Japanese adults recommended by the government.

In addition to dietary folate intake, other lifestyle factors that may modify the associations between *MTHFR* C677T and pancreatic cancer risk are smoking and drinking. Because alcohol is known as a folate antagonist and because smoking may impair folate status, several studies have evaluated the joint effects of the *MTHFR* polymorphisms with cigarette smoking or alcohol consumption in relation to pancreatic cancer risk [13–15]. In one hospital-based case-control study conducted in Japan, the risk of pancreatic cancer increased by 4.5-fold among heavy drinkers with the *MTHFR* 677 CC genotype [15]. Similarly, another two case-control studies found that individuals with the 677 T variant combined with heavy smoking or drinking had significantly increased risk for pancreatic cancer [13, 14]. In contrast to their findings, we failed to observe the synergistic effect of the genotypes with either cigarette smoking or heavy alcohol consumption. It is worth noting that the analysis of gene-environment interaction was limited by a small sample size in our study, as well as in those previous studies. So the probability that the positive interaction was due to chance cannot be ruled out.

Our study has several limitations. First, we had sufficient number of cases required to detect significant associations for the main effect of genotypes based on sample size estimation; however, we did not have sufficient power to detect significant associations in the analyses examining the synergistic effect of genotypes and exposure of interest. Assuming a dominant genetic model, a dichotomous exposure prevalence of 10 %, a relative risk for a genotype of 1.5, a relative risk for exposure of 1.5, and 1:1 case-control ratio, we need thousands of cases and controls to detect multiplicative interactions with relative risk of 2.0 [24]. Second, environmental exposure (folate) assessment or environmental exposure (folate)-pancreatic cancer association could have been affected by selection or recall bias inherent in case-control studies; however, the genotype-pancreatic cancer association was generally not affected by bias due to differential environmental exposure assessment between cases and control subjects. Third, the lack of the data on plasma folate levels did not allow us to address the relationship among *MTHFR* genotypes, plasma levels and pancreatic cancer risk. It has been shown that DNA methylation was affected by genotype among only those with lower plasma folate levels [25]. Moreover, it is expected that multifactorial interactions may exist among *MTHFR* genotypes, dietary folate, circulating folate level, alcohol, and/or other relevant nutrients including vitamin B2 and B12. Further studies need to develop a novel analytical method addressing the complex gene-environment interaction pathways involved in folate-derived carcinogenesis.

Conclusions

In conclusion, our case-control study suggests that there is no association between genetic polymorphisms in folate-metabolizing genes and the risk of pancreatic cancer in Japanese subjects. The results may not be generalizable in view of limited sample size. Our study is also limited to address effect modification by alcohol, smoking or folate intake (gene-environment interaction) because of inadequate statistical power.

Abbreviations

BMI, body mass index; CI, confidence interval; FFQ, food frequency questionnaire; HWE, Hardy-Weinberg equilibrium; *MTHFR*, methylenetetrahydrofolate; MTR, 5-methyltetrahydrofolate-homocysteine methyltransferase; *MTRR*, 5-methyltetrahydrofolate-homocysteine methyltransferase reductase; ORs, odds ratios.

Acknowledgements

We thank Kiyoko Yagyu for the contribution to the study design and data collection. We thank Mayuko Masuda, Kikuko Kaji, Kazue Ando, Etsuko Ohara, and Sumiyo Asakura for assisting us with data collection. We also thank Miki Watanabe, Tomoko Ito, Sanae Inui, and Sachiko Mano for technical assistance with genotyping.

Funding

This work was supported by Grants-in-Aid for Cancer Research from the Ministry of Health, Labour and Welfare, Japan. The funding body had no role in the design of the study and collection, analysis, and interpretation of data and in writing the manuscript.

Authors' contributions

KS supervised the study; KS, HN, KW, MM, MN, KN, AT, MT and KS designed the study; YL, TN and HN conducted the statistical analysis and drafted the manuscript; KM and SH performed genotyping and SNP data analysis; NI, YK, KI, MY, YK, TE, MM, HI, MU, SK, NE and SO collected the data. All authors read and approved the final version of the manuscript.

Competing interest

The authors declare that they have no competing interests.

Consent for publication

Not applicable.

Author details

[1]Division of Gastroenterology, Department of Internal Medicine, Aichi Medical University School of Medicine, Nagakute 480-1195, Japan. [2]Department of Preventive Medicine, Nagoya University Graduate School of Medicine, Nagoya 466-8550, Japan. [3]Department of Public Health, Sapporo Medical University School of Medicine, Sapporo 060-0061, Japan. [4]Department of Surgery, Surgical Oncology and Science, Sapporo Medical University, Sapporo 060-8543, Japan. [5]Sapporo Shirakaba-dai Hospital, Sapporo 062-0052, Japan. [6]Hepatobiliary and Pancreatic Section, Gastroenterological Division, Cancer Institute Hospital, Tokyo 135-8550, Japan. [7]Clinical Research Center, National Hospital Organization Shikoku Cancer Center, Matsuyama 791-0280, Japan. [8]Hepatobiliary and Pancreatic Medical Oncology Division, Kanagawa Cancer Center Hospital, Kanagawa 241-8515, Japan. [9]Department of Internal Medicine, Tokyo Metropolitan Komagome Hospital, Tokyo 113-8677, Japan. [10]Tokyo Metropolitan Otsuka Hospital, Tokyo 170-8476, Japan. [11]Division of Molecular Medicine, Aichi Cancer Center Research Institute, Nagoya 762-6111, Japan. [12]Department of Epidemiology, Nagoya University Graduate School of Medicine, Nagoya 466-8550, Japan. [13]Division of Epidemiology and Prevention, Aichi Cancer Center Research Institute, Nagoya 762-6111, Japan. [14]Department of Food and Nutrition, Gifu City Women's College, Gifu 501-2592, Japan. [15]Department of Public Health, Hokkaido University Graduate School of Medicine, Sapporo 060-8638, Japan. [16]Central Animal Division, National Cancer Center Research Institute, Tokyo 104-0045, Japan. [17]Department of Hepatobiliary and Pancreatic Surgery, National Cancer Center Hospital, Tokyo 104-0045, Japan. [18]Department of Public Health, Aichi Medical University School of Medicine, Nagakute 480-1195, Japan.

Reference

1. Michaud DS. Epidemiology of pancreatic cancer. Minerva Chir. 2004;59:99–111.
2. Choi SW, Mason JB. Folate and carcinogenesis: an integrated scheme. J Nutr. 2000;130:129–32.

3. Lucock M, Yates Z. Folate acid-vitamin and panacea or genetic time bomb? Nat Rev Genetics. 2005;6:235–40.
4. Klerk M, Verhoef P, Clarke R, Blom HJ, Kok FJ, Schouten EG, MTHFR Studies Collaboration Group. MTHFR 677C–>T polymorphism and risk of coronary heart disease: a meta-analysis. JAMA. 2002;288:2023–31.
5. Larsson SC, Giovannucci E, Wolk A. Folate intake, MTHFR polymorphisms, and risk of esophageal, gastric, and pancreatic cancer: a meta-analysis. Gastroenterology. 2006;131:1271–83.
6. Schernhammer E, Wolpin B, Rifai N, Cochrane B, Manson JA, Ma J, et al. Plasma folate, vitamin B6, vitamin B12, and homocysteine and pancreatic cancer risk in four large cohorts. Cancer Res. 2007;67:5553–60.
7. Gong Z, Holly EA, Bracci PM. Intake of folate, vitamins B6, B12 and methionine and risk of pancreatic cancer in a large population-based case-control study. Cancer Causes Control. 2009;20:1317–25.
8. Bao Y, Michaud DS, Spiegelman D, Albanes D, Anderson KE, Bernstein L, et al. J Natl Cancer Inst. 2011;103:1840–50.
9. Keszei AP, Verhage BA, Heinen MM, Goldbohm RA, van den Brandt PA. Dietary folate and folate vitamers and the risk of pancreatic cancer in the Netherlands cohort study. Cancer Epidemiol Biomarkers Prev. 2009;18:1785–91.
10. Tio M, Andrici J, Cox MR, Eslick GD. Folate intake and the risk of upper gastrointestinal cancers: a systematic review and meta-analysis. J Gastroenterol Hepatol. 2014;29:250–8.
11. Frosst P, Blom HJ, Milos R, Goyette P, Sheppard CA, Matthews RG, et al. A candidate genetic risk factor for vascular disease: a common mutation in methylenetetrahydrofolate reductase. Nat Genet. 1995;10:111–3.
12. Weisberg I, Tran P, Christensen B, Sibani S, Rozen R. A second genetic polymorphism in methylenetetrahydrofolate reductase (MTHFR) associated with decreased enzyme activity. Mol Genet Metab. 1998;64:169–72.
13. Li D, Ahmed M, Li Y, Jiao L, Chou TH, Wolff RA, et al. 5,10-Methylenetetrahydrofolate reductase polymorphisms and the risk of pancreatic cancer. Cancer Epidemiol Biomarkers Prev. 2005;14:1470–6.
14. Wang L, Miao X, Tan W, Lu X, Zhao P, Zhao X, et al. Genetic polymorphisms in methylenetetrahydrofolate reductase and thymidylate synthase and risk of pancreatic cancer. Clin Gastroenterol Hepatol. 2005;3:743–51.
15. Suzuki T, Matsuo K, Sawaki A, Mizuno N, Hiraki A, Kawase T, et al. Alcohol drinking and one-carbon metabolism-related gene polymorphisms on pancreatic cancer risk. Cancer Epidemiol Biomarkers Prev. 2008;17:2742–7.
16. Matsubayashi H, Skinner HG, Iacobuzio-Donahue C, Abe T, Sato N, Riall TS, et al. Pancreaticobiliary cancers with deficient methylenetetrahydrofolate reductase genotypes. Clin Gastroenterol Hepatol. 2005;3:752–60.
17. Ohnami S, Sato Y, Yoshimura K, Ohnami S, Sakamoto H, Aoki K, et al. His595Tyr polymorphism in the methionine synthase reductase (MTRR) gene is associated with pancreatic cancer risk. Gastroenterology. 2008;135:477–88.
18. Ulrich CM, Robien K, McLeod HL. Cancer pharmacogenetics: polymorphisms, pathways and beyond. Nat Rev Cancer. 2003;3:912–20.
19. Lin Y, Ueda J, Yagyu K, Ishii H, Ueno M, Egawa N, et al. Association between variations in the fat mass and obesity-associated gene and pancreatic cancer risk: a case-control study in Japan. BMC Cancer. 2013;13:337.
20. Evans DM, Purcell S. Power calculations in genetic studies. Cold Spring Harb Protoc. 2012;6:664–74.
21. Tokudome Y, Goto C, Imaeda N, Hasegawa T, Kato R, Hirose K, et al. Relative validity of a short food frequency questionnaire for assessing nutrient intake versus three-day weighed diet records in middle-aged Japanese. J Epidemiol. 2005;15:135–45.
22. Tu YL, Wang SB, Tan XL. MTHFR gene polymorphisms are not involved in pancreatic cancer risk: a meta-analysis. Asian Pac J Cancer Prev. 2012;13:4627–30.
23. Leenders M, Bhattacharjee S, Vineis P, Stevens V, Bueno-de-Mesquita HB, Shu XO, et al. Polymorphisms in genes related to one-carbon metabolism are not related to pancreatic cancer in PanScan and PanC4. Cancer Causes Control. 2013;24:595–602.
24. Hunter DJ. Gene-environment interactions in human diseases. Nat Rev Genet. 2005;6:287–98.
25. Sharp L, Little J. Polymorphisms in genes involved in folate metabolism and colorectal neoplasia: a HuGE review. Am J Epidemiol. 2004;159:423–43.

4

Endoscopic ultrasonography with fine-needle aspiration for histological diagnosis of solid pancreatic masses

Omar Banafea[1], Fabian Pius Mghanga[2], Jinfang Zhao[1], Ruifeng Zhao[1] and Liangru Zhu[1*]

Abstract

Background: Previous studies have demonstrated that endoscopic ultrasound-fine needle aspiration (EUS-FNA) is a reliable tool for diagnosing pancreatic lesions; however, the reported sensitivity and specificity vary greatly across studies. The aim of this study was to pool the existing literature and assess the overall performance of EUS-FNA in the diagnosis of solid pancreatic lesions.

Methods: A systematic search of MEDLINE, Cochrane Database for Systematic Reviews, and EMBASE was performed to identify original and review articles published between January 1995 and January 2014 that reported the accuracy of EUS-FNA in the diagnosis of pancreatic masses. Quality of the included studies was assessed using the quality assessment of diagnosis accuracy studies score tool. Meta-DiSc software was used to calculate the pooled sensitivity and specificity, positive and negative likelihood ratios, and to construct the summary receiver operating characteristics curve.

Results: Twenty studies involving a total of 2,761 patients were included in the study. The pooled sensitivity and specificity of EUS-FNA in the diagnosis of solid pancreatic lesions were 90.8 % [95 % confidence interval (CI), 89.4–92 %] and 96.5 % (95 % CI, 94.8–97.7 %), respectively. The positive and negative likelihood ratios were 14.8 (95 % CI, 8.0–27.3) and 0.12 (95 % CI, 0.09–0.16), respectively. The overall diagnostic accuracy was 91.0 %.

Conclusions: Our findings suggest that EUS-FNA has high sensitivity and specificity in the diagnosis of solid pancreatic lesions.

Keywords: Endoscopic ultrasound, Fine needle aspiration, Pancreatic mass

Abbreviations: AUC, Area under the curve; CT, Computed tomography; DOR, Diagnostic odd ratio; ERCP, Endoscopic retrograde chlolaniopancreatography; EUS, Endoscopic ultrasound; EUS-FNA, Endoscopic ultrasound with fine needle aspiration; FN, False negative; FP, False positive; MRI, Magnetic resonance imaging; NLRs, Negative likelihood ratio; PC, Pancreatic cancer; PLRs, Positive likelihood ratio; ROC, Receiver operating characteristic curve; ROSE, Rapid on-site evaluation; SROC, Summary receiver operating characteristic curve; TN, True negative; TP, True positive

* Correspondence: zhuliangru05@126.com
[1]Division of Gastroenterology, Union Hospital, Tongji Medical College, Huazhong University of Science and Technology, No. 1277 Jiefang Avenue, Wuhan 430022, Hubei Province, China
Full list of author information is available at the end of the article

Table 1 The characteristics of included studies in current meta-analysis

Study name	QUADAS score (14)	Study design	Study center	On site Cyto.
Giovannini et al. 1995 [8]	12	R	S	No
Cahn et al. 1996 [9]	8	R	M	No
Bhutani et al. 1997 [10]	10	p	S	Yes
Faigel et al. 1997 [11]	12	P	S	Yes
Chang et al. 1997 [23]	11	P	S	No
Bentz et al. 1998 [24]	13	P	S	Yes
Voss et al. 2000 [12]	12	P	S	No
Gress et al. 2001 [13]	11	p	S	No
Ylagan et al. 2002 [14]	10	R	S	No
Harewood 2002 [15]	13	P	M	Yes
Raut et al. 2003 [16]	13	P	S	No
Afify et al. 2003 [17]	11	R	S	Yes
Agarwal et al. 2004 [18]	11	R	S	No
Ryozawa et al. 2005 [19]	9	R	M	Yes
Eloubeidi et al. 2007 [20]	13	P	S	No
Fisher et al. 2009 [25]	13	P	S	No
Krishna et al. 2009 [21]	12	P	S	Yes
Touchefeu et al. 2009 [22]	13	P	S	No
Cherian et al. 2010 [7]	10	P	S	No
Uehara et al. 2011 [26]	9	R	S	No

P Prospective, *R* Retrospective, *M* Multiple centers, *S* Single center

Background

Pancreatic cancer is the tenth most common type of cancer, and the fourth leading cause of cancer-related deaths among men and women, accounting for 6 % of all cancer-related deaths worldwide [1]. Pancreatic cancer is difficult to diagnose in its early stages, and nearly 26 % of all diagnosed cases have regional spread, with 52 % of cases reported to have metastatic disease at the time of diagnosis [2]. Studies have shown that one-year survival rate for pancreatic cancer is 24 %, and the overall 5-year survival rate is 5 % [2]. Since curative resection is currently the only potential cure for patients with pancreatic cancer, early diagnosis has an important impact on prognosis.

Pancreatic lesions encompass a variety of benign and malignant conditions, and the diagnosis of pancreatic cancer is complicated by indistinct detection of pancreatic masses either clinically or by imaging. Clinically, the diagnosis of a regional pancreatic mass may be confused with that of a primary pancreatic tumor, as in pancreatic adenocarcinoma, while focal chronic pancreatitis may be confused with pancreatic metastasis from a distant primary tumor [3]. Thus, accurate preoperative diagnosis is essential for selecting an appropriate treatment for these lesions [4].

Currently, there are many laboratory tests and imaging techniques that may be useful in discriminating pancreatic lesions [5, 6]. Among them, cytological examination of pancreatic masses by fine needle aspiration (FNA) can assist greatly in differentiating a pancreatic tumor from other malignancies. Endoscopic ultrasound (EUS), due to its high resolution, can provide easy visualization of the pancreas, common bile duct and adjacent anatomic structures, and has been the most important imaging modality for the diagnosis of pancreatic tumors [7]. EUS combined with FNA (EUS-FNA) has been demonstrated to be more accurate in diagnosing solid pancreatic lesions and has gained wide acceptance [7]. However, the reported sensitivity and specificity of EUS-FNA vary greatly across studies (sensitivity: 73.20–96.50 %; specificity: 71.40–100 %) [7–26]. In addition, the majority of previous studies were dependent on single-center trials. Since there is a learning curve for FNA, its diagnostic accuracy is greatly influenced by operator experience [22]. In addition, the performance of FNA may be related to the size and location of pancreatic lesions and the presence of an on-site cytopathologist [7, 26]. At present, there has been no systematic approach to estimate the accuracy of EUS-FNA in diagnosing solid pancreatic lesions.

The current meta-analysis aimed at reviewing the existing literature and evaluating the overall performance of EUS-FNA in diagnosing solid pancreatic lesions.

Methods

Identification of studies

A systematic search of PubMed (including MEDLINE compiled by the United States National Library of Medicine, Bethesda, Maryland, USA), EMBASE (Elsevier, Amsterdam, Netherlands), and the Cochrane Database for Systematic Reviews (The Cochrane Collaboration, Oxford, UK) was performed to identify published original and review articles reporting the accuracy of EUS-FNA in the diagnosis of pancreatic masses. The electronic search was supplemented by a manual search of the listed references. Searches were limited to studies conducted from January 1995 to January 2014. We used the keywords ["pancreatic mass" or "pancreatic lesion" or "pancreatic tumor"] and ["endoscopic ultrasound" or "endoscopic ultrasound fine needle aspiration" or "EUS-FNA" or "EUS-FNA in pancreatic lesions")] and ["sensitivity" or "specificity" or "diagnostic accuracy"].

We identified 285 studies through this search strategy. We also hand-searched several imaging and oncology journals for the specified period to ensure that the electronic search did not miss reports of eligible studies; no additional study was identified using this strategy.

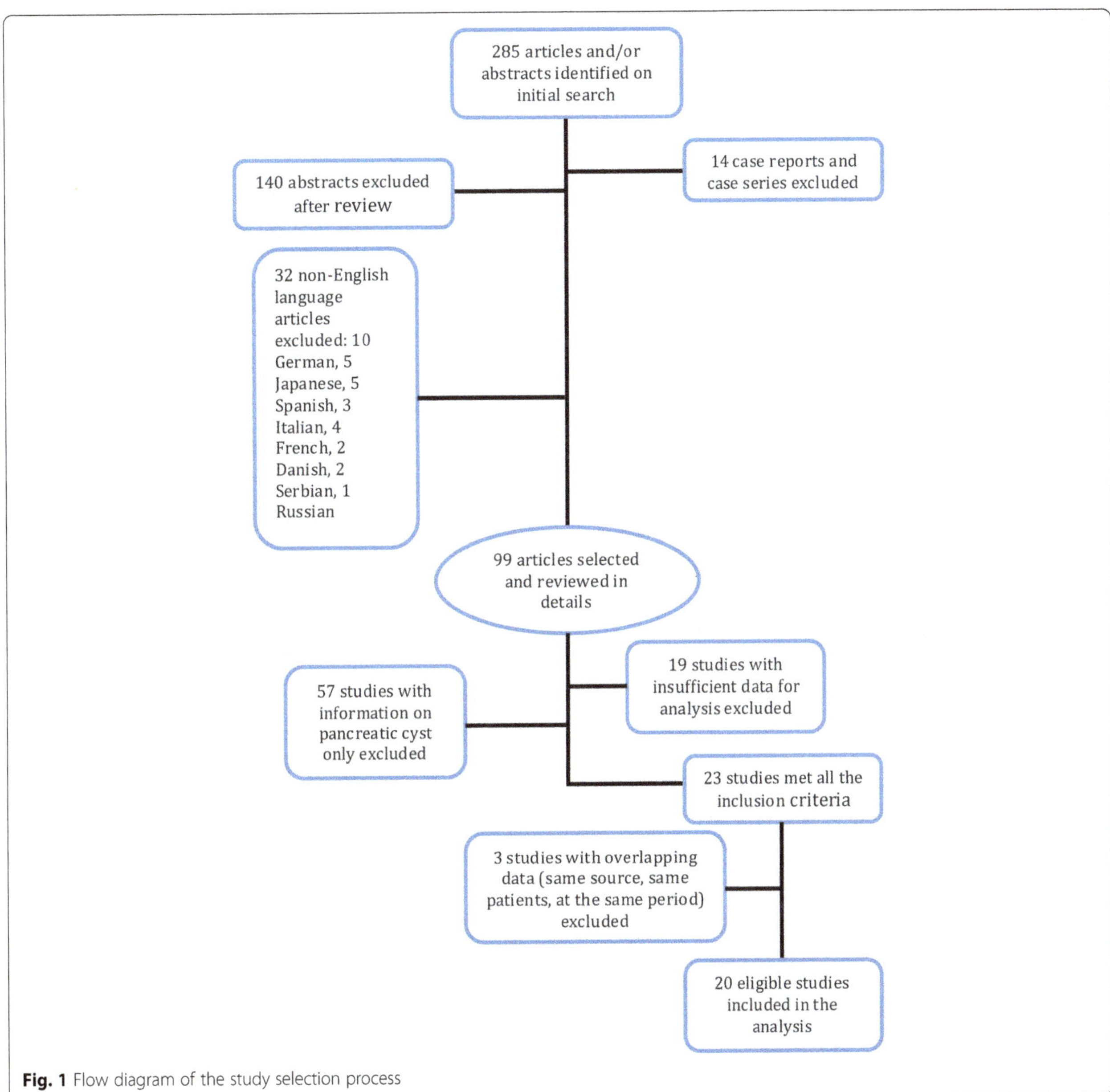

Fig. 1 Flow diagram of the study selection process

The reference list of the retrieved studies was searched for any additional publications, and none of the articles was found in this approach. We restricted searching to studies that were published in English only and included more than 10 patients.

Eligibility criteria

Studies were eligible for inclusion if they fulfilled the following criteria: (i) articles were published in English; (ii) appropriate data were presented to enable computation of true positive (TP), false negative (FN), false positive (FP) and true negative (TN) results of EUS-FNA in the diagnosis of solid pancreatic lesions; (iii) at least 10 patients and/or lesions were included; (iv) a final diagnosis was obtained by surgical biopsy or histological examination of surgically resected specimen; (v) the population had a suspected solid pancreatic mass based on imaging modalities such as ultrasound, EUS, computed tomography (CT) and magnetic resonance imaging (MRI), and only patients who had a solid pancreatic mass (in case of mixed lesions, separate results were reported for solid and cystic lesions) were included in the study; (vi) studies were retrospective and/or prospective, and had results of EUS-FNA based on surgical cytological/ histological specimens, or a follow-up period of at least 6 months; and (vii) articles were published from January1995 to January 2014.

Table 2 Complications of EUS-FNA reported in the included studies

Study	Number	Percent	Post-procedural complications
Giovannini et al. 1995 [8]	0	0	No complications reported
Cahn et al. 1996 [9]	Unknown	-	-
Bhutani et al. 1997 [10]	1/47	2	Infection (*n* = 1)
Faigel et al. 1997 [11]	0/45	0	No complications reported
Chang et al. 1997 [23]	1/44	2	Fever (*n* = 1)
Bentz et al. 1998 [24]	Unknown	-	-
Voss et al. 2000 [12]	5/90	5	Bleeding (*n* = 4), abdominal pain (*n* = 1)
Gress et al. 2001 [13]	3/102	2.9	Gastric mucosal bleeding (*n* = 2), pancreatitis (*n* = 1)
Ylagan et al. 2002 [14]	1/91	1	Acute pancreatitis (*n* = 1).
Harewood 2002 [15]	1/185	0.5	Mild pancreatitis (*n* = 1).
Raut et al. 2003 [16]	4/233	2	Duodenal perforation (*n* = 2), abdominal pain (*n* = 1), pancreatitis (*n* = 1)
Afify et al. 2003 [17]	Unknown	-	-
Agarwal et al. 2004 [18]	2/81	2.5	Abdominal pain (*n* = 2)
Ryozawa et al. 2005 [19]	0	0	No complications reported
Eloubeidi et al. 2007 [20]	11/547	2	Acute pancreatitis (*n* = 5), abdominal pain (*n* = 3), fever (*n* = 2), the use of reversal medication (*n* = 1)
Fisher et al. 2009 [25]	2/100	2	Mucosal bleeding (*n* = 1), abdominal pain (*n* = 1)
Krishna et al. 2009 [21]	Unknown	-	-
Touchefeu et al. 2009 [22]	2/90	2.2	Fever (*n* = 1), abdominal pain (*n* = 1)
Cherian et al. 2010 [7]	Unknown	-	-
Uehara et al. 2011 [26]	2/120	1.6	Mild pancreatitis (*n* = 2)

We excluded: (i) case reports and abstracts; (ii) studies that did not report sufficient data to construct a diagnostic 2 × 2 contingency table to calculate statistics including TP, FP, TN and FN; and (iii) studies involving patients with a cystic lesion or other malignancy like cholangiocarcinoma, duodenal adenocarcinoma, and periampullary adenocarcinoma and studies that involved other FNA procedures like CT-guided FNA or MRI-guided FNA. We excluded cystic lesions from the current analysis, because their diagnosis and management were different from those of solid pancreatic lesions [27].

Study quality assessment

We used the quality assessment of diagnosis accuracy studies (QUADAS) tool [28] to assess the methodological quality of the included studies. The tool had 14 questions with responses denoted as "yes," "no," or "unavailable." A score of 1 was given to a "yes" response, and a score of zero was given if the response was "no" or "unavailable". An article was deemed of adequate quality for inclusion if it scored a minimum of 8 of 14 points in the "QUADAS" checklist as in Table 1.

Data extraction

Data from all eligible studies were extracted independently by two of the authors (O.B and F.P.M). Information extracted included the first author's name, journal, year of publication, study design, sample size and clinical indication. We also extracted demographic characteristics including mean or median age, patient gender, number of lesions and lesion size. Other extracted information included needle manufacturing company, frequency of EUS, needle size and number of needles that passed through the lesion during procedure. In cases of any differences between the two authors, a consensus was reached by discussion.

Statistical analysis

For each included study, we constructed a 2 × 2 table to calculate the TP, FN, FP and TN values. The data were then analyzed using Meta-DiSc software (version 1.4; Unit of Clinical Biostatistics Team of the Romany Cajal Hospital, Madrid, Spain) to compute sensitivity, specificity, positive likelihood ratio, negative likelihood ratio, positive predictive value (PPV), negative predictive value (NPV) and diagnostic odds ratio (DOR) for each study. As per the DerSimonian-Liard random effects model, we pooled all results and using the same model, we constructed a summary receiver operating characteristic curve (SROC). By numeric integration of the SROC using the trapezoidal equation, the software was used to compute the area under the curve (AUC). A preferred test has an AUC close to 1, and

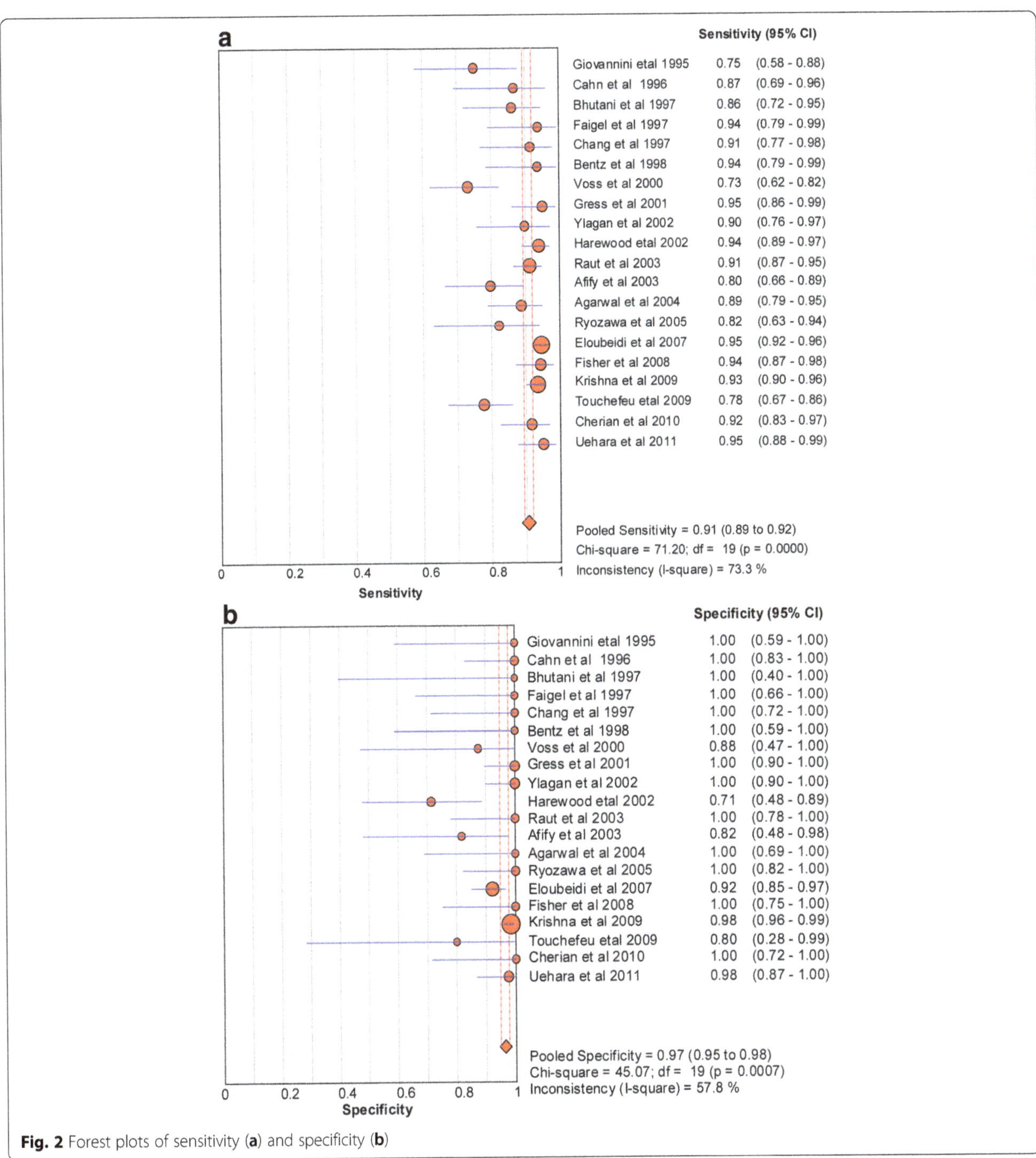

Fig. 2 Forest plots of sensitivity (**a**) and specificity (**b**)

an AUC close to 0.5 is considered a poor test. NPV and FP rate (i.e., 1 − specificity) were also calculated. Q*, the maximum joint specificity and sensitivity, was calculated from the SROC. This is the point on the SROC curve where sensitivity is equal to specificity. A chi-square test was used to test for the occurrence of heterogeneity among studies, and sources of heterogeneity were explored using meta-regression analysis. *P*-values < 0.05 were considered statistically significant.

Results

Eligible studies

Our searches yielded a total of 285 titles and abstracts. Of these, 140 abstracts and 32 studies published in languages other than English (10 in German, 5 in Japanese, 5 in Spanish, 4 in French, 3 in Italian, 2 in Danish, 2 in Serbian and 1 in Russian) were excluded. Upon further review of the studies, 14 case reports and case series with a sample size less than 10 patients were excluded. We also excluded 57 studies with information on

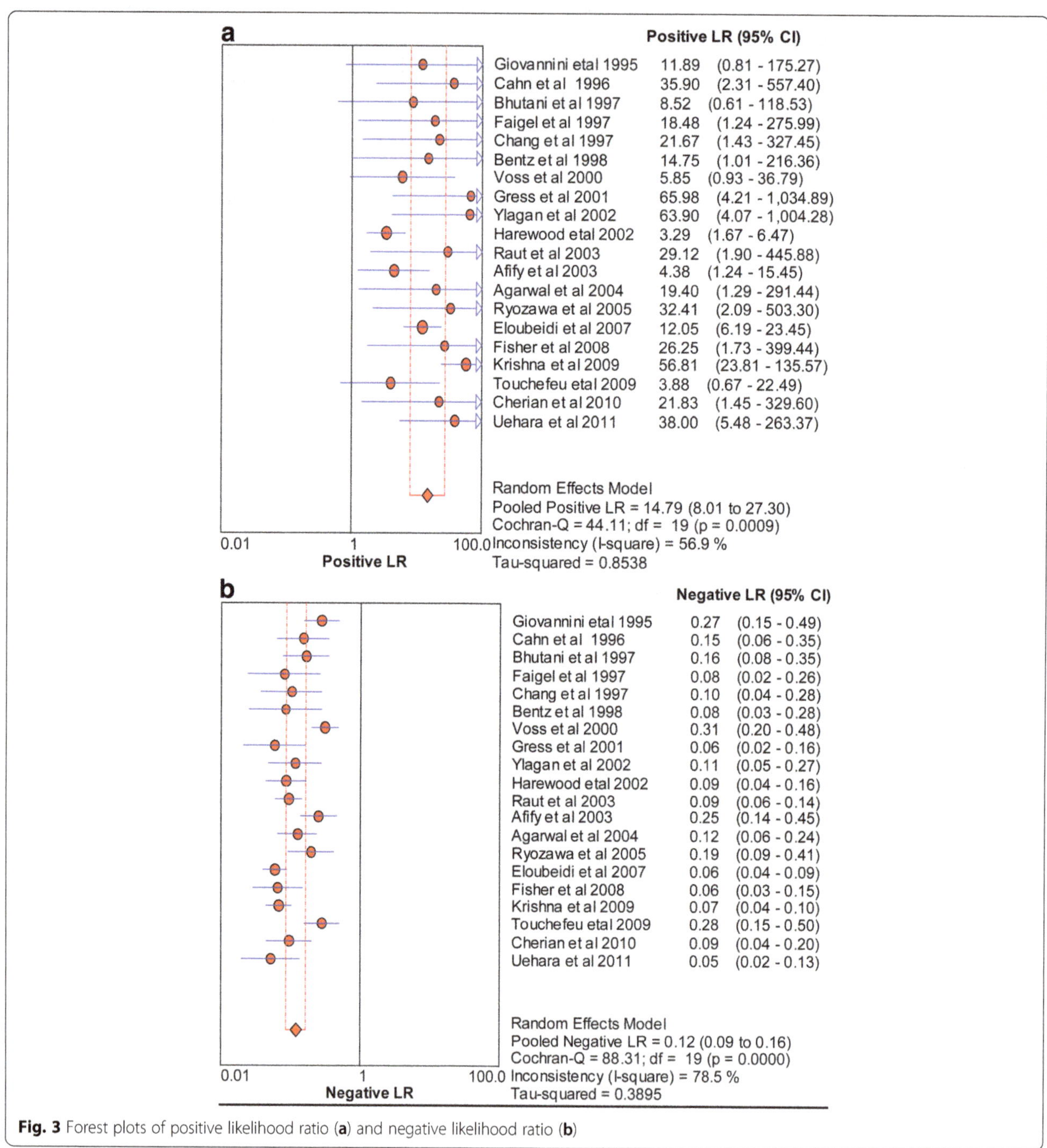

Fig. 3 Forest plots of positive likelihood ratio (**a**) and negative likelihood ratio (**b**)

pancreatic cyst only and 19 studies with insufficient data. Five duplicate studies, three in one batch and two in the other, had the same sources of data, so we excluded the 3 studies from the duplicated studies and included the 2 studies that had included data from the same database (Table 3). Finally, a total of 20 studies [7–26] were eligible for analysis based on the inclusion and exclusion criteria. Figure 1 shows the flow chart of study selection.

Study description and patient characteristics

Of the 20 studies included, 13 were prospective [7, 10–13, 15, 16, 19, 20–25] and 7 were retrospective [8, 9, 14, 17–19, 26] (Table 1). The studies involved a total of 2,761 patients with a total of 2,776 pancreatic lesions. The median age of the subjects was reported in 15 articles, and 5 did not mention the age of the patients. The male/female ratio of the study subjects was 1.3:1.

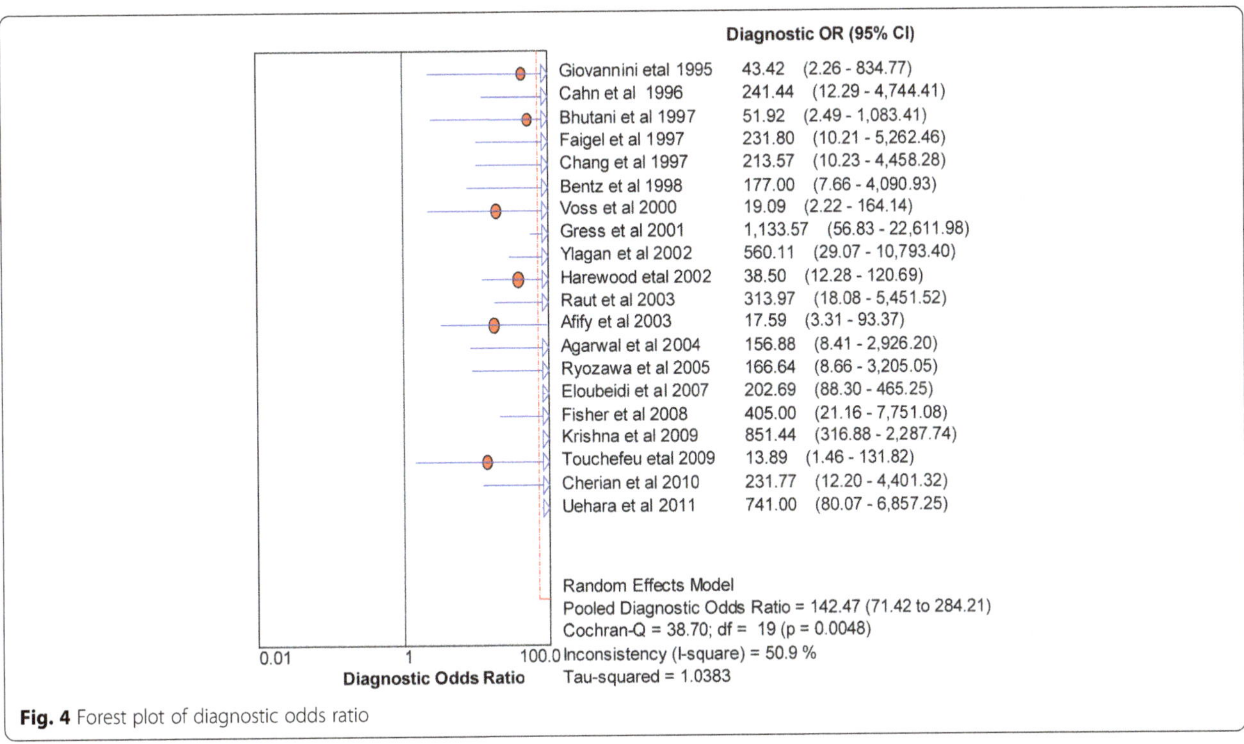

Fig. 4 Forest plot of diagnostic odds ratio

EUS-FNA techniques

The majority of studies used 22-gauge needles in EUS-FNA procedures [7, 11, 13–22, 24–26], although some of these needles were made by different manufacturers. Other sizes used were 19-gauge (Wilson cook, Winston Salem, North Carolina NC) [10, 13] and 25-gauge (manufacturing company not mentioned) needles [8].

Fifteen of the 20 included studies mentioned pancreatic mass size which varied between 0.6 and 14 cm whereas the rest 5 studies did not mention the size of

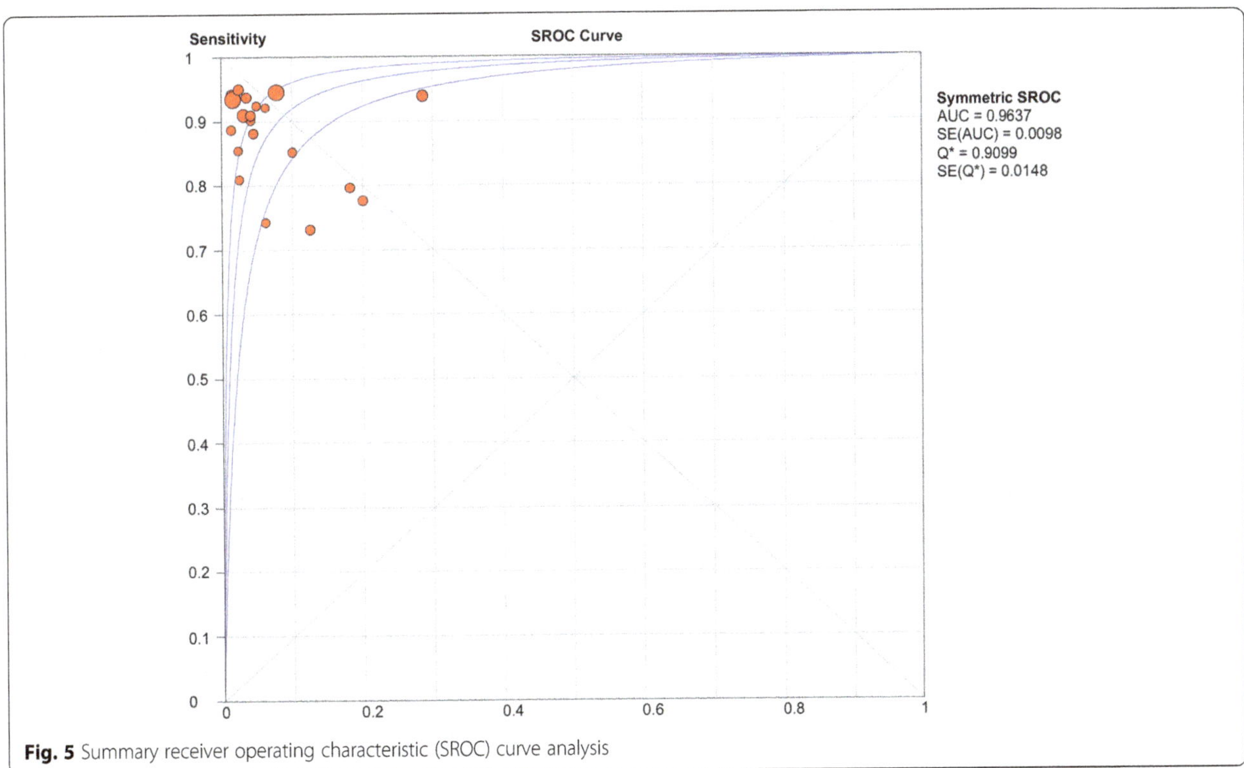

Fig. 5 Summary receiver operating characteristic (SROC) curve analysis

Table 3 Summary of diagnostic performance of endoscopic ultrasonography with fine-needle aspiration for solid pancreatic lesions

Study	Year	TP	FP	FN	TN	Sensitivity	Specificity	LR+	LR-	DOR
Giovannini	1995	27	0	9	7	75 (58–88)	100 (59–100)	11.9 (0.81–175)	0.3 (0.15–0.49)	43 (2–835)
Cahn	1996	26	0	4	20	87 (69–96)	100 (83–100)	35.9 (2.3–557)	0.15 (0.06–0.4)	241 (12–4744)
Bhutani	1997	37	0	6	4	86 (72–94)	100 (40–100)	8.5 (0.6–118.5)	0.16 (0.08–0.35)	52 (2.5–1083)
Faigel	1997	30	0	2	9	94 (79–99)	100 (66–100)	18.5(1.2–276)	0.08 (0.02–0.27)	232(10–5263)
Chang	1997	32	0	3	11	91 (77–98)	100 (72–100)	21.7 (1.4–327.5)	0.1 (0.04–0.28)	214(10–4458)
Bentz	1998	29	0	2	7	94 (79–99)	100 (59–100)	14.8 (1–216.4)	0.08 (0.025–0.28)	177(8–4090)
Voss	2000	60	1	22	7	73 (62–82)	88 (47–99.7)	5.8 (0.9–36.8)	0.3 (0.2–0.48)	19 (2.2–164)
Gress	2001	57	0	3	34	95 (86–99)	100 (90–100)	66 (4.2–1035)	0.06 (0.02–0.16)	1134 (56.828–22612)
Ylagan	2002	35	0	4	35	90 (76–97)	100 (90–100)	63.9 (4.1–1004)	0.11 (0.048–0.27)	560(29–10793)
Harewood	2002	154	6	10	15	94 (89–97)	71 (48–89)	3.3 (1.7–6.5)	0.09 (0.044–0.17)	39(12–121)
Raut	2003	197	0	19	15	91 (87–95)	100 (78–100)	29 (1.9–446)	0.09 (0.06–0.14)	314(18.083–5451.5)
Afify	2003	43	2	11	9	80 (67–89)	82 (48–98)	4.4 (1.2–15.5)	0.25 (0.14–0.45)	18 (3–93)
Agarwal	2004	63	0	8	10	89 (79–95)	100 (69–100)	19 (1.3–291)	0.12 (0.07–0.24)	157 (8–2926.2)
Ryozawa	2005	23	0	5	19	82 (63–94)	100 (82–100)	32.4 (2.1–503)	0.2 (0.09–0.414)	166 (9–3205)
Eloubeidi	2007	414	8	24	94	95 (92–97)	92 (85–97)	12.1 (6.2–23.5)	0.06 (0.04–0.09)	202.69 88.302–465.25
Fisher	2009	82	0	3	13	97 (90–99)	100 (75–100)	26.3 (1.7–399)	0.07 (0.03–0.15)	405 (21.2–7751)
Krishna	2009	299	5	21	299	93 (90–96)	98 (96–99.5)	57 (24–136)	0.07 (0.044–0.1)	851 (317–2288
Touchefeu	2009	66	1	19	4	78 (67–86)	80 (28–99.5)	3.9 (0.7–22.5)	0.28 (0.16–0.5]	13.9 (1.5–132)
Cherian	2010	65	0	6	11	92 (83–97)	100 (72–100)	22 (2–330)	0.09 (0.05–0.2)	232 (12–4401)
Uehara	2011	76	1	4	39	95 (88–99)	98 (87–100)	38 (6–263)	0.05 (0.02–0.13]	741 (80–6857)

TP true positive, *FP* false positive, *FN* false negative, *TN* true negative, *LR+* positive likely ratio, *LR-* negative likely ratio, *DOR* Diagnostic Odds Ratio

masses [7, 9–13, 15, 18–20, 22–26]. The mean tumor size was 3.4 cm, with a range of 0.6–14 cm. The median number of needle passes through each pancreatic lesion was 3.4, ranging between 1 and 5.

Safety of EUS-FNA

As shown in Table 2, actual complications of EUS-FNA procedures occurred in 35 of 1,760 patients in 15 studies that mentioned complications [7, 8, 10–13, 15, 16, 19, 20, 22, 23, 25, 26], mainly abdominal pain, pancreatitis, hematoma, bleeding at needle sites and fever (not accompanied by other symptoms). There were two cases of major complication (duodenal perforations, which were immediately managed by laparotomy).

Pooled results

The sensitivity and specificity of EUS-FNA in the diagnosis of solid pancreatic masses were found to range from 73.20 to 96.50 % and 71.40 to 100 %, respectively. The median sensitivity and specificity were 91.30 % and 100 %, respectively. The pooled sensitivity and specificity were 90.80 % [95 % confidence interval (CI): 89.40–92.00 %] and 96.5 % (95%CI: 94.8–7.7 %), respectively (Fig. 2). The positive and negative likelihood ratios were 14.80 (95%CI, 8.00–27.30) and 0.12 (95%CI, 0.09–0.16), respectively (Fig. 3). The diagnostic odds ratio is 142.47 (71.42–284.21) (Fig. 4).

ROC analysis

The AUC was used to summarize the overall diagnostic accuracy of EUS-FNA. From the curve, the maximum joint sensitivity and specificity, denoted as Q* (the point at which the sensitivity and specificity of a diagnostic tool are equal), was found to be 91.0 % (Fig. 5). This finding suggests a relatively high overall diagnostic performance of EUS-FNA in the diagnosis of solid pancreatic lesions.

Sources of heterogeneity

To explore potential sources of heterogeneity, a meta-regression analysis was performed. A multivariable regression model with a backward stepwise algorithm was used. The possible sources of heterogeneity in our study included publication bias, study design and methodological quality. None of the analyzed variables showed statistical significance (Table 3), e.g., higher quality studies (QUADAS score ≥ 10) and lower quality studies (QUADAS score <10) were not significantly different.

Discussion

Many previous studies have demonstrated that EUS-FNA is a reliable tool for the diagnosis of pancreatic masses; however, the reported sensitivity and specificity varied greatly among these different studies [7–26]. In this study, we conducted a meta-analysis to pool the

Table 4 Diagnostic accuracy of all 20 included studies

	No. of studies	Sensitivity	Specificity	LR(+)	LR(-)	DOR
All of 20 studies		90.80	96.5	14.80	0.12	142.47
	20					
P		0	.0007	0.0009	0.000	0.0048
Study design:						
Prospective	13	91.4	94.3	10.928	0.110	122.14
P						
		0	0.006	0.130	0	0.348
Study design:						
Retrospective	7	89.5	97.9	19.004	0.128	162.38
P		0.001	0.076	0.009	0	0.001
QUADAS score ≥10		90.8	96.2	13.162	0.116	127.44
P	17					
		0	0	0.001	0	0.002
QUADAS score <10		90.6	98.7	36.008	0.119	370.78
	3					
P		0.103	0.503	0.996	0.076	0.687
With on-site cytology.		91.5	96.5	12.136	0.120	108.83
	7					
P		0.024	0	0	0.002	0
Without on-site cytology.		904	96.5	14.365	0.114	170.05
	13					
P		0	0.097	0.757	0	0.263

existing literature and assess the overall performance of EUS-FNA in the diagnosis of solid pancreatic lesions. We found that the pooled sensitivity and specificity were as high as 90.8 % and 96.5 %, respectively. The SROC analysis revealed that the Q* value, which represents the maximum joint sensitivity and specificity, was 91 %. These findings suggest that EUS-FNA has a high accuracy in diagnosing solid pancreatic lesions.

The wide variation of the reported sensitivity and specificity of EUS-FNA may be due to a combination of several factors. Operator experience has been proposed as one of the most significant factors that affect the accuracy of EUS-FNA [7, 26, 29], which is a demonstrated significant predictor of diagnostic accuracy in pancreatic lesions in the multivariable model [30]. Since the majority of previous studies depended on the results of one center and the operators had greatly varied experience, the diagnostic performance of EUS-FNA may have been overestimated or underestimated. Thus, an important strength of our meta-analysis is that it included studies performed by operators with different expertise from different centers in different countries. The level of operators' experience should be reported in future studies. In addition, the diagnostic accuracy of EUS-FNA for pancreatic lesions may also be affected by tumor size and location, needle size, and the presence of an on-site cytopathologist [26, 31], although some studies reported that the diagnostic accuracy of EUS-FNA is irrespective of these parameters [26]. Future studies should carefully resolve these problems.

Low NPV has been suggested to be a major drawback of EUS-FNA, and this may limit its clinical utility in patients with suspected pancreatic cancer because early resectable tumors may be missed [21]. An NLR < 0.1 often suggests that the predictive value of a given diagnostic tool is valid or rather convincing. In the present study, the pooled NLR was 0.118 (95%CI: 0.086–0.163), which is near 0.1. Considering that we calculated all inadequate biopsies and technical failures in the included studies as FNs, the pooled NLR may have been underestimated. In this regard, the predictive value of EUS-FNA for solid pancreatic lesions is acceptable.

The FN results of EUS-FNA in the diagnosis of pancreatic masses are often caused by a high frequency of inadequate specimens due to several reasons. First, comparative studies of EUS-FNA have demonstrated that larger needles were associated with inferior accuracy rates because of their disadvantage in placement precision in pancreatic lesions located in difficult anatomical positions [32–35]. Second, the number of needle passes through the lesion may affect the collection of adequate specimens [35], and a recent report recommended that seven needle passes would be necessary to ensure a highly accurate diagnosis of solid pancreatic lesions by EUS-FNA [36]. Finally, the absence of on-site cytology in the procedure may also reduce the aspiration of adequate sample, although some studies indicated that the unavailability of a cytopathologist did not significantly affect the diagnostic yield [26, 37]. The current study indicated that the absence of on-site cytology has no significant impact on the diagnostic yield (Table 4).

Studies have indicated that EUS-guided FNA biopsy of pancreatic masses is as accurate as CT/US-guided and surgical biopsies [38]. However, EUS-FNA has many advantages over other techniques [39]: (i) the capability to get a sample from a tiny lesion; (ii) the capability to get a sample of the lesion through a part of the intestinal wall and decrease the risk of needle tract seeding; and (iii) the capability to supply extra information about staging of the disease. In particular, EUS-guided FNA can be carried out in the entire pancreas (the hook and tail included) [16, 17], even for difficult or unreachable regions via the percutaneous access or when the percutaneous route is not indicated [12].

Although many diagnostic modalities are currently available for the diagnosis of pancreatic lesions, some are associated with a higher incidence of complications. For example, the rate of complications of CT/US-guided FNA is as high as about 5 %, with pancreatitis being the most common complication [39]. In the present study, only 2.2 % (39/1760) of cases developed complications, and the majority of complications were mild, self-limited and seldom required transfusion, except that two cases had duodenal perforations that were successfully treated by surgery. These finding suggest that EUS-FNA is a safe technique for the diagnosis of solid pancreatic lesions.

Ultimately in considering to tumor size of pancreatic malignancy was diagnosed by Endoscopic Ultrasound-guided FNA with high accuracy regardless of their tumor size, or location. So we can get initial diagnosis of malignant lesion was obtained by EUS-guided FNA in all adenocarcinoma ≤ 10 mm but unfortunately most of studies included in this study mentioned only the range or median of the tumors size that included sizes < 2 cm which means that the small size (<2 cm) can be detected by EUS-FNA even if it cannot be detected by CT or US guided FNA.

Conclusion

This meta-analysis indicates that EUS-FNA for pancreatic masses has a high overall sensitivity (91 %) and specificity (96.5 %). Compared with other diagnostic modalities, EUS-FNA may be safer and probably provides advantages over other modalities, such as the ability to detect a tiny lesion and obtain much more diagnostic information.

Acknowledgements
Not applicable.

Funding
Not applicable.

Authors' contributions
OB—data collection, organization, analysis and writing; FPM–statastics; JZ–help OB collect data; RZ–help OB collect data; LZ– project design,progress guidance and responsible for the whole project. All authors read and approved the final manuscript.

Competing interests
The authors declare that they have no competing interests.

Consent for publication
Not applicable.

Author details
[1]Division of Gastroenterology, Union Hospital, Tongji Medical College, Huazhong University of Science and Technology, No. 1277 Jiefang Avenue, Wuhan 430022, Hubei Province, China. [2]Department of Nuclear Medicine, Union Hospital, Tongji Medical College, Huazhong University of Science and Technology, Hubei Province Key Laboratory of Molecular Imaging, Wuhan 430022, China.

References

1. Jemal A, Murray T, Ward E, Samuels A, Tiwari RC, Ghafoor A, et al. Cancer statistics, 2005. CA Cancer J Clin. 2005;55(1):10–30.
2. Figures CFa. American Cancer Society. Available at http://www.cancer.org/acs/groups/content/@nho/documents/document/500809webpdf.pdf. Accessed 5 Feb 2009.
3. Warshaw AL, Fernandez-del CC. Pancreatic carcinoma. N Engl J Med. 1992; 326(7):455–65. doi:10.1056/nejm199202133260706.
4. Erickson RA, Garza AA. Impact of endoscopic ultrasound on the management and outcome of pancreatic carcinoma. Am J Gastroenterol. 2000;95(9):2248–54. doi:10.1111/j.1572-0241.2000.02310.x.
5. Podolsky DK, McPhee MS, Alpert E, Warshaw AL, Isselbacher KJ. Galactosyltransferase isoenzyme II in the detection of pancreatic cancer: comparison with radiologic, endoscopic, and serologic tests. N Engl J Med. 1981;304(22):1313–8. doi:10.1056/nejm198105283042201.
6. Neff CC, Simeone JF, Wittenberg J, Mueller PR, Ferrucci Jr JT. Inflammatory pancreatic masses. Problems in differentiating focal pancreatitis from carcinoma. Radiology. 1984;150(1):35–8. doi:10.1148/radiology.150.1.6689784.
7. Cherian PT, Mohan P, Douiri A, Taniere P, Hejmadi RK, Mahon BS. Role of endoscopic ultrasound-guided fine-needle aspiration in the diagnosis of solid pancreatic and peripancreatic lesions: is onsite cytopathology necessary? HPB. 2010;12(6):389–95. doi:10.1111/j.1477-2574.2010.00180.x.
8. Giovannini M, Seitz JF, Monges G, Perrier H, Rabbia I. Fine-needle aspiration cytology guided by endoscopic ultrasonography: results in 141 patients. Endoscopy. 1995;27(2):171–7. doi:10.1055/s-2007-1005657.
9. Cahn M, Chang K, Nguyen P, Butler J. Impact of endoscopic ultrasound with fine-needle aspiration on the surgical management of pancreatic cancer. Am J Surg. 1996;172(5):470–2. doi:10.1016/s0002-9610(96)00222-x.
10. Bhutani MS, Hawes RH, Baron PL, Sanders-Cliette A, van Velse A, Osborne JF, et al. Endoscopic ultrasound guided fine needle aspiration of malignant pancreatic lesions. Endoscopy. 1997;29(9):854–8. doi:10.1055/s-2007-1004321.

11. Faigel DO, Ginsberg GG, Bentz JS, Gupta PK, Smith DB, Kochman ML. Endoscopic ultrasound-guided real-time fine-needle aspiration biopsy of the pancreas in cancer patients with pancreatic lesions. J Clin Oncol. 1997;15(4): 1439–43.
12. Voss M, Hammel P, Molas G, Palazzo L, Dancour A, O'Toole D, et al. Value of endoscopic ultrasound guided fine needle aspiration biopsy in the diagnosis of solid pancreatic masses. Gut. 2000;46(2):244–9.
13. Gress F, Gottlieb K, Sherman S, Lehman G. Endoscopic ultrasonography-guided fine-needle aspiration biopsy of suspected pancreatic cancer. Ann Intern Med. 2001;134(6):459–64.
14. Ylagan LR, Edmundowicz S, Kasal K, Walsh D, Lu DW. Endoscopic ultrasound guided fine-needle aspiration cytology of pancreatic carcinoma: a 3-year experience and review of the literature. Cancer. 2002;96(6):362–9. doi:10.1002/cncr.10759.
15. Harewood GC, Wiersema MJ. Endosonography-guided fine needle aspiration biopsy in the evaluation of pancreatic masses. Am J Gastroenterol. 2002;97(6):1386–91. doi:10.1111/j.1572-0241.2002.05777.x.
16. Raut CP, Grau AM, Staerkel GA, Kaw M, Tamm EP, Wolff RA, et al. Diagnostic accuracy of endoscopic ultrasound-guided fine-needle aspiration in patients with presumed pancreatic cancer. J Gastrointest Surg. 2003;7(1):118–26. discussion 27-8.
17. Afify AM, al-Khafaji BM, Kim B, Scheiman JM. Endoscopic ultrasound-guided fine needle aspiration of the pancreas. Diagnostic utility and accuracy. Acta Cytol. 2003;47(3):341–8.
18. Agarwal B, Abu-Hamda E, Molke KL, Correa AM, Ho L. Endoscopic ultrasound-guided fine needle aspiration and multidetector spiral CT in the diagnosis of pancreatic cancer. Am J Gastroenterol. 2004;99(5):844–50. doi: 10.1111/j.1572-0241.2004.04177.x.
19. Ryozawa S, Kitoh H, Gondo T, Urayama N, Yamashita H, Ozawa H, et al. Usefulness of endoscopic ultrasound-guided fine-needle aspiration biopsy for the diagnosis of pancreatic cancer. J Gastroenterol. 2005;40(9):907–11. doi:10.1007/s00535-005-1652-6.
20. Eloubeidi MA, Varadarajulu S, Desai S, Shirley R, Heslin MJ, Mehra M, et al. A prospective evaluation of an algorithm incorporating routine preoperative endoscopic ultrasound-guided fine needle aspiration in suspected pancreatic cancer. J Gastrointest Surg. 2007;11(7):813–9. doi:10.1007/s11605-007-0151-x.
21. Krishna NB, Mehra M, Reddy AV, Agarwal B. EUS/EUS-FNA for suspected pancreatic cancer: influence of chronic pancreatitis and clinical presentation with or without obstructive jaundice on performance characteristics. Gastrointest Endosc. 2009;70(1):70–9. doi:10.1016/j.gie.2008.10.030.
22. Touchefeu Y, Le Rhun M, Coron E, Alamdari A, Heymann MF, Mosnier JF, et al. Endoscopic ultrasound-guided fine-needle aspiration for the diagnosis of solid pancreatic masses: the impact on patient-management strategy. Aliment Pharmacol Ther. 2009;30(10):1070–7. doi:10.1111/j.1365-2036.2009.04138.x.
23. Chang KJ, Nguyen P, Erickson RA, Durbin TE, Katz KD. The clinical utility of endoscopic ultrasound-guided fine-needle aspiration in the diagnosis and staging of pancreatic carcinoma. Gastrointest Endosc. 1997;45(5):387–93.
24. Bentz JS, Kochman ML, Faigel DO, Ginsberg GG, Smith DB, Gupta PK. Endoscopic ultrasound-guided real-time fine-needle aspiration: clinicopathologic features of 60 patients. Diagn Cytopathol. 1998;18(2):98–109.
25. Fisher L, Segarajasingam DS, Stewart C, Deboer WB, Yusoff IF. Endoscopic ultrasound guided fine needle aspiration of solid pancreatic lesions: Performance and outcomes. J Gastroenterol Hepatol. 2009;24(1):90–6. doi: 10.1111/j.1440-1746.2008.05569.x.
26. Uehara H, Ikezawa K, Kawada N, Fukutake N, Katayama K, Takakura R, et al. Diagnostic accuracy of endoscopic ultrasound-guided fine needle aspiration for suspected pancreatic malignancy in relation to the size of lesions. J Gastroenterol Hepatol. 2011;26(8):1256–61. doi:10.1111/j.1440-1746.2011.06747.x.
27. Thosani N, Thosani S, Qiao W, Fleming JB, Bhutani MS, Guha S. Role of EUS-FNA-based cytology in the diagnosis of mucinous pancreatic cystic lesions: a systematic review and meta-analysis. Dig Dis Sci. 2010;55(10):2756–66. doi: 10.1007/s10620-010-1361-8.
28. Whiting P, Rutjes AW, Reitsma JB, Bossuyt PM, Kleijnen J. The development of QUADAS: a tool for the quality assessment of studies of diagnostic accuracy included in systematic reviews. BMC Med Res Methodol. 2003;3:25. doi:10.1186/1471-2288-3-25.
29. Wiersema MJ, Vilmann P, Giovannini M, Chang KJ, Wiersema LM. Endosonography-guided fine-needle aspiration biopsy: diagnostic accuracy and complication assessment. Gastroenterology. 1997;112(4):1087–95.
30. Harewood GC, Wiersema LM, Halling AC, Keeney GL, Salamao DR, Wiersema MJ. Influence of EUS training and pathology interpretation on accuracy of EUS-guided fine needle aspiration of pancreatic masses. Gastrointest Endosc. 2002;55(6):669–73.
31. Hwang CY, Lee SS, Song TJ, Moon SH, Lee D, Park Do H, et al. Endoscopic ultrasound guided fine needle aspiration biopsy in diagnosis of pancreatic and peripancreatic lesions: a single center experience in Korea. Gut Liver. 2009;3(2):116–21. doi:10.5009/gnl.2009.3.2.116.
32. Itoi T, Itokawa F, Sofuni A, Nakamura K, Tsuchida A, Yamao K, et al. Puncture of solid pancreatic tumors guided by endoscopic ultrasonography: a pilot study series comparing Trucut and 19-gauge and 22-gauge aspiration needles. Endoscopy. 2005;37(4):362–6. doi:10.1055/s-2004-826156.
33. Levy MJ, Jondal ML, Clain J, Wiersema MJ. Preliminary experience with an EUS-guided trucut biopsy needle compared with EUS-guided FNA. Gastrointest Endosc. 2003;57(1):101–6. doi:10.1067/mge.2003.49.
34. Larghi A, Verna EC, Stavropoulos SN, Rotterdam H, Lightdale CJ, Stevens PD. EUS-guided trucut needle biopsies in patients with solid pancreatic masses: a prospective study. Gastrointest Endosc. 2004;59(2):185–90.
35. Varadarajulu S, Fraig M, Schmulewitz N, Roberts S, Wildi S, Hawes RH, et al. Comparison of EUS-guided 19-gauge Trucut needle biopsy with EUS-guided fine-needle aspiration. Endoscopy. 2004;36(5):397–401. doi:10.1055/s-2004-814316.
36. LeBlanc JK, Ciaccia D, Al-Assi MT, McGrath K, Imperiale T, Tao LC, et al. Optimal number of EUS-guided fine needle passes needed to obtain a correct diagnosis. Gastrointest Endosc. 2004;59(4):475–81.
37. Hikichi T, Irisawa A, Bhutani MS, Takagi T, Shibukawa G, Yamamoto G, et al. Endoscopic ultrasound-guided fine-needle aspiration of solid pancreatic masses with rapid on-site cytological evaluation by endosonographers without attendance of cytopathologists. J Gastroenterol. 2009;44(4):322–8. doi:10.1007/s00535-009-0001-6.
38. Mallery JS, Centeno BA, Hahn PF, Chang Y, Warshaw AL, Brugge WR. Pancreatic tissue sampling guided by EUS, CT/US, and surgery: a comparison of sensitivity and specificity. Gastrointest Endosc. 2002;56(2): 218–24.
39. Iwashita T, Yasuda I, Doi S, Nakashima M, Tsurumi H, Hirose Y, et al. Endoscopic ultrasound-guided fine-needle aspiration in patients with lymphadenopathy suspected of recurrent malignancy after curative treatment. J Gastroenterol. 2009;44(3):190–6. doi:10.1007/s00535-008-2302-6.

5

Effect of mobile phone reminder messages on adherence of stent removal or exchange in patients with benign pancreaticobiliary diseases

Yong Gu[1,2†], Limei Wang[3†], Lina Zhao[4†], Zhiguo Liu[3], Hui Luo[3], Qin Tao[3], Rongchun Zhang[3], Shuixiang He[1], Xiangping Wang[3], Rui Huang[3], Linhui Zhang[3], Yanglin Pan[3*] and Xuegang Guo[3*]

Abstract

Background: Plastic and covered metal stents need to be removed or exchanged within appropriate time in case of undesirable complications. However, it is not uncommon that patients do not follow the recommendation for further stent management after Endoscopic Retrograde Cholangiopancreatography (ERCP). The effect of short message service (SMS) intervention monthly on the stent removal/exchange adherence in patients after ERCP is unknown at this time.

Methods: A prospective, randomized controlled study was conducted. After receiving regular instructions, patients were randomly assigned to receive SMS reminding monthly (SMS group) for stent removal/exchange or not (control group). The primary outcome was stent removal/exchange adherence within appropriate time (4 months for plastic stent or 7 months for covered stent). Multivariate analysis was performed to assess factors associated with stent removal/exchange adherence within appropriate time. Intention-to-treat analysis was used.

Results: A total of 48 patients were randomized, 23 to the SMS group and 25 to the control. Adherence to stent removal/exchange was reported in 78.2 % (18/23) of patients receiving the SMS intervention compared with 40 % (10/25) in the control group (RR 1.98, 95 % CI 1.16–3.31; $p = 0 \cdot 010$). Among patients with plastic stent insertion, the median interval time from stent implantation to stent removal/exchange were 90 days in the SMS group and 136 days in the control respectively (HR 0.36, 95 % CI 0.16–0.84, $p = 0.018$). No difference was found between the two groups regarding late-stage stent-related complications. The rate of recurrent abdominal pain tended to be lower in SMS group without significant difference (8.7 vs 28 %, $p = 0.144$). Multivariate logistic regression analyses revealed that SMS reminding was the only factor associated with adherence of stent removal/exchange (OR 6.73, 95 % CI 1.64–27.54, $p = 0.008$).

Conclusion: This first effectiveness trial demonstrated that SMS reminding monthly could significantly increase the patient adherence to stent removal/exchange after ERCP.

(Continued on next page)

* Correspondence: panyanglin@gmail.com; xuegangguo@gmail.com
†Equal contributors
[3]Xijing Hospital of Digestive Diseases, Fourth Military Medical University, Xi'an, Shannxi, China
Full list of author information is available at the end of the article

(Continued from previous page)

Keywords: Short message service, Adherence, Stent exchange, ERCP, Biliary stricture

Abbreviation: CI, Confident interval; CT, Computed tomography; ERCP, Endoscopic retrograde cholangiopancreatography; FCSEMS, Fully covered self-expandable metal stent.; HR, hazard ratio; ITT, Intention-to-treat; MRCP, Magnetic resonance cholangiopancreatography; OR, Odd ratio; PD, Pancreatic duct; PSC, Primary sclerosing cholangitis; RR, Relative risk; SMS, Short message service

Background

Endoscopic implantation of plastic or covered metal stents is widely used in a variety of benign pancreaticobiliary diseases, including duct stricture, large or difficult stones, bile or pancreatic duct leak, etc. [1–4]. There are some complications after stent insertion, such as stent occlusion, proximal or distal migration, secondary duct injury and even the failure of stent removal [5–8]. For plastic stents, occlusion is the main disadvantage, limiting their patency to around 3 months. For fully covered metal stents, stent migration, occlusion and even the failure of stent removal may happen after long-term implantation [8, 9]. The longer the stents areplaced, more likely the complications may happen.

Although the optimal time of stent placement has not been well established, it has been recommended that plastic stent should be removed/exchanged within 3–4 months and covered metal stent be removed within 6 months [10]. However, it is not uncommon that patients with stent implantation do not follow the recommendation of further stent management [11]. With the stents left in biliary or pancreatic duct for a long-term period, stone formation, acute duct inflammation and even chronic pancreatitis and secondary sclerosing cholangitis can happen. Occasionally, breakage of the stent can be also found [12]. Some patients in this situation may need emergent endoscopic management or even surgery. In addition, endoscopic management may thus be technically challenging, and the treatment cost can be increased.

Many methods have been used to improve the adherence of patients in medical service [13–15]. With the advance of mobile technology and popular use of mobile phones, it is believed that the patient-centered outcome (e.g. suppressed viral loads due to antivirus treatment) can be improved by mobile telecommunication with the timely support of a patient by a health professional [13]. Here we hypothesize that mobile technology, reminding the patients the necessity of stent management in time by short message service (SMS), may increase the patient adherence. The purpose of this prospectively randomized, controlled study is to evaluate the effect of SMS intervention monthly on the stent removal/exchange adherence in patients with benign pancreaticobiliary diseases after ERCP.

Methods

Patients

This is a prospective, randomized, controlled study with consecutive patients with benign pancreaticobiliary diseases undergoing endoscopic stent insertion at Endoscopy Center of Xijing Hospital of Digestive Diseases in China. The study protocol and informed consent form were approved by Institutional Review Board of Xijing Hospital (protocol number: 20160707–1). The study was respectively registered on July 10 in 2016 at ClinicalTrials.gov (NCT02831127). The informed consent was obtained from all patients. Patients more than 18 years old with plastic or covered stent implantation for the drainage of bile or pancreatic juice were eligible for participation in the study. Patients should be able to communicate via SMS by mobile phones of themselves or relatives living together. Exclusion criteria included: 1. primary or secondary sclerosing cholangitis (PSC), 2. malignant or suspected malignant stricture of biliary or pancreatic duct, 3.implantation of pancreatic duct (PD) stent for prevention of post-ERCP pancreatitis, 4.expected survival time less than 6 months, 5. plan of surgery within 6 months, 6. pregnant or lactating women, 7. patients who could not give informed consent.

Written informed consent was obtained from all the patients. Patients were randomized (1:1) to either the SMS intervention (SMS group) or standard care (control group) after stent insertion by opening an opaque and sealed envelope. The envelopes were randomized by using computer-generated random numbers generated by one of the investigators (HR) who kept the randomization key under lock until the inclusion of the last patient. At least two telephone numbers of all patients or their relatives living together were recorded in case of failed connection later. In the beginning of the enrollment, all patients were instructed not to tell doctors, nurses and investigators whether they received SMS reminding or not. The investigator (ZLN) performing data analysis was blinded to the allocation until the final analysis was finished.

Endoscopic treatment

The diagnosis of all the patients was primarily based on symptoms, surgical history, chemical test and imaging modalities (contrast-enhanced CT or ultrasound). All patients underwent MRCP for determination of etiology and the site of stricture. Only the patients with benign stricture of CBD or PD were considered eligible for this study. During ERCP, tissue samples were obtained with brush and/or forceps to confirm the benign nature of the stricture when clinically indicated. Single or multiple plastic stents (8.5Fr, Advanix, Boston Scientific, Natick, MA) or a fully covered self-expandable metal stent (FCSEMS) (Wallflex, Boston Scientific, Natick, MA) was inserted across the site of obstruction. The length of the stent varied depending on the anatomic location of the stricture. No covered metal stent was placed in PD. The number and type of the stents was determined based on the characteristics of stricture or diseases, which was determined at the discretion of the attending endoscopists.

Intervention

After stent implantation, all patients received oral and written instructions about further management. If single or multiple plastic stents were inserted, patients were informed to come back to the hospital at 3 months for stent removal/exchange; if FCSEMS was inserted, they were informed to come back to the hospital at 6 months after ERCP. Patients in SMS group received additional reminding by SMS messages from an investigator (TQ) blinded to further clinical data collection. Each month after stent implantation, the investigator sent a text message by SMS to inform patients the necessity of regular stent removal/exchange and the disadvantage of delayed management, and to remind them the appropriate date to come back to the hospital for stent management. Patients were requested to respond by SMS and were encouraged to contact the investigator if they had any questions about stent management. Patients in control group were not contacted after ERCP. At the end of the study, all the patients who did not come back to the hospital were called and informed again to return for further stent management. Follow-up was at least 6 months for all patients.

Outcome measurement

The primary outcome was stent removal/exchange adherence within appropriate time (4 months for plastic stent or 7 months for covered stent). Secondary outcomes were stent-related complications, including cholangitis, stent migration and abdominal pain.

Statistical analysis

At the beginning of the study, a sample size calculation was performed. Based on our previous experience, only 1/3 of patients in common practice will readmit for stent removal/exchange within appropriate time. The adherence in SMS group was estimated to be 80 %. To detect the difference with a significance level (α) of .05 and a power of 80 % with a 2-tailed test, we calculated that at least 42 patients were needed. However, about 10 % of patients might be lost during follow up. Thus, we estimated that totally 48 patients would be enough for the detection of a significant difference in the primary outcome.

Intention-to-treat (ITT) analysis was used to assess primary outcome from all evaluable patients. Relative risk (RR) was reported for adherence, with an RR more than 1 suggesting better outcome for SMS intervention group. Since only a small group of patients would be included, categorical variables, such as adherence rate of stent exchange/removal and complication rates, were analyzed using Fisher's exact test. Continuous variables

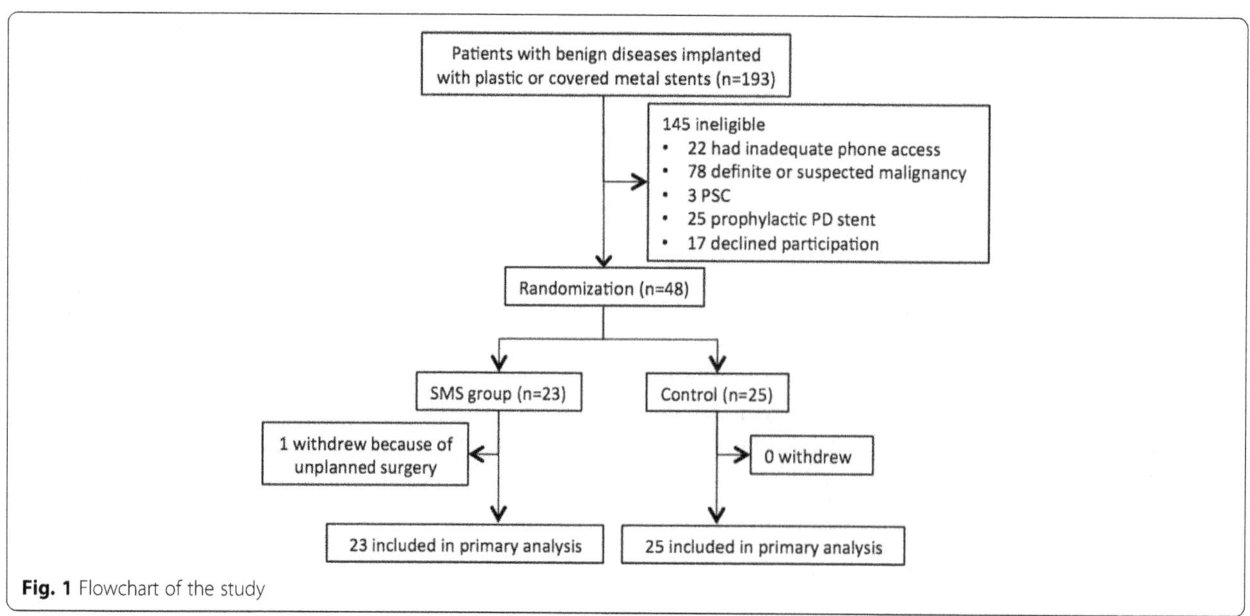

Fig. 1 Flowchart of the study

were expressed as means with standard deviations and analyzed with student's t-test. Cumulative proportion of patients readmitting with plastic stent implanted during follow up was determined by the Kaplan-Meier method, and the difference was assessed using the log-rank test.

To assess factors associated with stent removal/exchange adherence, multivariate logistic analysis was performed using variables with p values of <0.1 in the univariate logistic analysis. Forward stepwise method was used in the multivariate model. Analyses were performed with SPSS software version 19.0 for Windows (SPSS Inc, IBM Company). A p value <0.05 was considered statistically significant.

Results

From Feb in 2012 to Oct in 2013, 193 consecutive patients were enrolled. After screening, 145 patients were excluded, including 22 with inadequate phone access, 78 with definite or suspected malignancy, 3 with PSC, 25 with prophylactic PD stent implanted and 17 with declined participation. Finally, 48 patients were randomly assigned to the SMS group ($n = 23$) or to control group ($n = 25$). After randomization, all the patients in SMS group responded by SMS or phone call. However, 1 subject with distal stricture of CBD in SMS group underwent unplanned surgery because of pancreatic cancer. The subject flow is detailed in Fig. 1. All baseline characteristics but alkaline phosphatase (336.5 ± 324.2 U/L in SMS group vs. 125.8 ± 76.2 U/L in control, $p = 0.003$) between the two groups were well balanced (Table 1).

In ITT analysis, adherence to stent removal/exchange was reported in 78.2 % (18/23) of patients receiving the SMS intervention compared with 40 % (10/25) in the control group (relative risk [RR] 1.98, 95 % CI 1.16–3.31; $p = 0 \cdot 010$) (Table 2). Among patients undergoing insertion of plastic stent ($n = 39$), adherence to stent removal/exchange was 77.8 % in SMS group and 33.3 % in control ($p = 0.010$). The cumulative proportions of patients coming back to the hospital during follow up are shown in Fig. 2. The mean interval time between stent implantation and stent removal/exchange was 90 days in SMS group and 136 days in the control group respectively (hazard ratio [HR] 0.36, 95 % CI 0.16–0.84, $p = 0.018$).As shown in Table 2, no difference was found regarding FCSEMS removal adherence between the two groups (80 vs. 75 %, $p = 1.000$). There were also no differences between the two groups with regard to stent-related complications, such as cholangitis (9 vs 8 %, $p = 1.000$), stent migration (13 vs. 8 %, $p = 0.653$) and recurrent abdominal pain (9 vs. 28 %, $p = 0.144$). However, the rate of recurrent abdominal pain tended to be lower in SMS group (8.7 vs 28 %, $p = 0.144$).

Multivariate logistic regression analyses were performed to identify any significant factors for stent removal or

Table 1 Baseline of the characteristics of patients

	SMS group ($n = 23$)	Control ($n = 25$)	P value
Age	54.4 ± 15.0	52.2 ± 19.5	0.672
Male (%)	14 (60.9 %)	11 (44 %)	0.265
Smoking	7	3	0.162
Drinking	4	6	0.727
Education			1.000
Elementary school or less	5	6	
High school or higher	18	19	
Payment			0.610
By insurance	22	22	
By self	1	3	
Previous Stenting			0.511
Yes	7	5	
No	16	20	
Previous surgery			0.818
Cholecystectomy	8	7	
Liver transplantation	0	1	
Other	3	2	
Main symptom			0.467
Jaundice	7	4	
Fever	1	2	
Abdominal pain	13	16	
Chemical test before ERCP			
White blood cell (×10^9)	5.8 ± 1.3	5.6 ± 2.8	0.714
Total bilirubin (mg/dL)	60.6 ± 93.3	30.0 ± 65.9	0.193
Alkaline phosphatase (U/L)	336.5 ± 324.2	125.8 ± 76.2	0.003
Stricture site			0.849
Proximal CBD	6	7	
Distal CBD	11	10	
PD	6	8	
Reason for stenting			0.501
Biliary benign stricture	10	12	
Pancreatic benign stricture	10	8	
Other	3	5	
Stent type			0.719
Plastic stent (average number of stents)	18 (1.39)	21 (1.43)	
FCSEMS	5	4	
ERCP complication			1.000
Pancreatitis	1	1	
Biliary infection	2	1	

CBD common bile duct, *PD* pancreatic duct, *FCSEMS* fully covered self-expanded metal stent

Table 2 Outcomes of SMS reminding compared with standard care

	SMS group (*n* = 23)	Control (*n* = 25)	*P* value
Stent removal/exchange adherence, n (%)	18/23 (78 %)	10/25 (40 %)	0.010
Plastic stent (<4 month)	14/18 (78 %)	7/21 (33 %)	0.010
FCSEMS (<7 month)	4/5 (80 %)	3/4 (75 %)	1.000
Stent-related complications, n (%)			
Cholangitis	2 (9 %)	2 (8 %)	1.000
Stent migration	3 (13 %)	2 (8 %)	0.653
Recurrent pain	2 (9 %)	7 (28 %)	0.144

FCSEMS, fully covered self-expanded metal stent

Table 3 Multivariate logistic regression analysis of the association between patient characteristics and stent removal/exchange adherence

Variable		Adherence		*p* value
		OR	95 % CI	
SMS reminding	No	1		
	Yes	6.73	1.64–27.54	0.008
Surgery history	No	1		
	Yes	3.20	0.74–13.80	0.119
Stent type	Plastic	1		
	Metal	2.34	0.33–16.71	0.398
Stent number	Single	1		
	Multiple	2.10	0.51–8.73	0.306

exchange adherence. The factors analyzed were age, gender, history of surgery, education level, pre-ERCP total bilirubin level, location of stenosis, stent type, stent number, reasons for stenting, post-ERCP complications and SMS reminding or not. As shown in Table 3, only SMS reminding were significantly associated with adherence of stent removal/exchange (OR 6.73, 95 % CI 1.64–27.54, $p = 0.008$).

Among patients coming back to the hospital finally (19 in SMS group vs 18 in the control, $p = 0.297$), 11 in the SMS group and 9 in the control group underwent plastic stent exchange ($p = 0.746$). The remaining patients in both groups needed no further management after stent removal and clearance of biliary or pancreatic duct.

Discussion

Plastic stents and covered metal stent are commonly used for the drainage and relief of benign stricture of biliary and pancreatic ducts [1–4]. It is suggested that

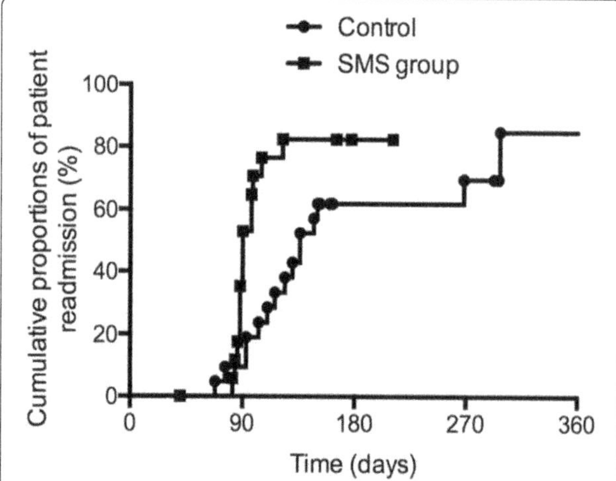

Fig. 2 Kaplan-Meier survival analysis of proportions of patients with plastic stent implanted undergoing stent removal/exchange later in SMS group ($n = 17$) and control ($n = 21$). $p = 0.018$ by log-rank test

these stents should be removed or exchanged within 3–6 months to prevent late complications [7, 8]. Although patients are usually instructed the details of further stent management, some of them may be not compliant with the recommendation. The reasons may include: 1, the unawareness of the necessity of regular stent removal/exchange; 2, the unawareness of the possible complications of delayed stent management; 3, forgetting the appropriate date to come back to the hospital for stent management; 4, financial consideration. Here we found that SMS reminding monthly could significantly increase the patient adherence to stent removal/exchange. This is, to our knowledge, the first effectiveness trial assessing the ability of a mobile health technology intervention to influence the stent removal/exchange adherence.

Patients' forgetfulness is considered one of the main reasons for missed appointments. There are many modes of communicating reminders for appointments to patients, such as face-to-face communication, postal messages, phone calls and SMS [16]. The later represent a convenient, less time-consuming and inexpensive delivery medium for improving the adherence of healthcare appointments. Studies that compare the outcomes of SMS reminding versus other methods for the patients with removable stents is of interest.

With the better adherence to stent removal or exchange, it could be expected that the stent-related complications due to long-term placement of plastic or cover metal stents might be reduced [7, 8, 17, 18]. However, the late-stage complications between the two groups in this study were not significantly different, although the rate of recurrent abdominal pain tended to be lower after SMS reminding. The reason may be due to small numbers of patients enrolled in each subgroup. The power of the study may be insufficient to detect the differences of stent-related complications and identify more predictive factors related to stent removal/exchange adherence.

There are some other limitations of this study. Firstly, the follow up time of this study is relatively short. It has been recommended that multiple plastic stents should be placed and exchanged for at least one year for long-term stricture of biliary stricture [19]. With better adherence to plastic stent exchange, it will be interesting to further evaluate the long-term resolution rate of biliary stricture after SMS reminding. Secondly, although patients with plastic stents in SMS group had better adherence to stent removal or exchange, no difference was found regarding the adherence to covered metal stent management. It is necessary to enroll more patients with covered metal stent to investigate whether they will be also benefit from SMS reminding. Thirdly, although number of patients undergoing placement of covered metal stent was similar between the two group, whether patients received metal stent were determined at the discretion of the attending endoscopists. The possible bias of patient selection may have impacts on the adherence in metal group. Last but not the least, the present study was performed in one tertiary center in a less developed area in China. The adherence rate without interference seems to be quite low (40 %). The beneficial effect of SMS on adherence of stent removal/exchange needs to be further investigated in other settings, especially in centers with higher adherence of stent removal/exchange.

Conclusions

In conclusion, our study demonstrated that SMS reminding could improve the patient adherence to stent removal/exchange within appropriate time for the first time. SMS reminding could shorten the mean interval time between stent implantation and stent removal/exchange. Patients with stent implantation might be benefit from SMS reminding strategy.

Acknowledgement

We are grateful to the doctors and nurses working in Xijing Hospital of digestive diseases for the help in conducting of this study.

Funding

This work was supported in part by the National Natural Science Foundation of China to Yanglin Pan (No. 81172288 and 81372388).

Authors' contributions

Study concept and design: PYL, GY; acquisition of data: WLM,; analysis and interpretation of data: ZLN, LH,; drafting of the manuscript: GY PYL, HSX; critical revision of the manuscript for important intellectual content: ZRC, GXG, LZG; statistical analysis: HR, WXP, ZLH; administrative and material support: GXG. All authors read and approved the final manuscript.

Competing interests

The authors declare that they have no competing interests.

Consent for publication

Not applicable.

Author details

[1]Department of Gastroenterology, the first affiliated hospital of Xi'an Jiao Tong university, Xi'an, China. [2]Digestive System Department, Shaanxi Provincial Crops Hospital of Chinese People's Armed Police Force, Xi'an, China. [3]Xijing Hospital of Digestive Diseases, Fourth Military Medical University, Xi'an, Shannxi, China. [4]Department of Radiotherapy, Xijing Hospital, Xian, China.

References

1. Tuvignon N, Liguory C, Ponchon T, et al. Long-term follow-up after biliary stent placement for postcholecystectomy bile duct strictures: a multicenter study. Endoscopy. 2011;43:208–16.
2. Tabibian JH, Asham EH, Han S, et al. Endoscopic treatment of postorthotopic liver transplantation anastomotic biliary strictures with maximal stent therapy. Gastrointest Endosc. 2010;71:505–12.
3. Mahajan A, Ho H, Sauer B, et al. Temporary placement of fully covered self-expandable metal stents in benign biliary strictures: midterm evaluation. Gastrointest Endosc. 2009;70:303–9.
4. Jong EA, Moelker A, Leertouwer T, et al. Percutaneous transhepatic biliary drainage in patients with postsurgical bile leakage and nondilated intrahepatic bile ducts. Dig Surg. 2013;30:444–50.
5. ASGE Technology Assessment Committee, Pfau PR, Pleskow DK, et al. Pancreatic and biliary stents. Gastrointest Endosc. 2013;77:319–27.
6. Khashab MA, Kim K, Hutfless S, et al. Predictors of early stent occlusion among plastic biliary stents. Dig Dis Sci. 2012;57:2446–50.
7. Slattery E, Kale V, Anwar W, et al. Role of long-term biliary stenting in choledocholithiasis. Dig Endosc. 2013;25:440–3.
8. Balmadrid B, Kozarek R. Prevention and management of adverse events of endoscopic retrograde cholangiopancreatography. Gastrointest Endosc Clin N Am. 2013;23:385–403.
9. Baron TH. Covered self-expandable metal stents for benign biliary tract diseases. Curr Opin Gastroenterol. 2011;27:262–7.
10. Kasher JA, Corasanti JG, Tarnasky PR, et al. Amulticenter analysis of safety and outcome of removal of a fully coveredself-expandable metal stent during ERCP. Gastrointest Endosc. 2011;73:1292–7.
11. Lawrence C, Romagnuolo J, Payne KM, et al. Low symptomatic premature stent occlusion of multiple plastic stents for benign biliary strictures: comparing standard and prolonged stent change intervals. Gastrointest Endosc. 2010;72:558–63.
12. Haapamäki C, Kylänpää L, Udd M, et al. Randomized multicenter study of multiple plastic stents vs covered self-expandable metallic stent in the treatment of biliary stricture in chronic pancreatitis. Endoscopy. 2015;47:605–10.
13. Lester RT, Ritvo P, Mills EJ, et al. Effects of a mobile phone short message service on antiretroviral treatment adherence in Kenya (WelTel Kenya1): a randomised trial. Lancet. 2010;376:1838–45.
14. Margolis KL, Asche SE, Bergdall AR, et al. Effect of home blood pressure telemonitoring and pharmacist management on blood pressure control: a cluster randomized clinical trial. JAMA. 2013;310:46–56.
15. Liu X, Luo H, Zhang L, et al. Telephone-based re-education on the day before colonoscopy improves the quality of bowel preparation and the polyp detection rate: a prospective, colonoscopist-blinded, randomised, controlled study. Gut. 2014;63:125–30.
16. Gurol-Urganci I, de Jongh T, Vodopivec-Jamsek V, et al. Mobile phone messaging reminders for attendance at healthcare appointments. Cochrane Database Syst Rev. 2013;12:CD007458.
17. Romagnuolo J, Cotton PB. Recording ERCP fluoroscopy metrics using a multinational quality network: establishing benchmarks and examining time-related improvements. Am J Gastroenterol. 2013;108:1224–30.
18. Kachaamy TA, Faigel DO. Improving ERCP quality and decreasing risk to patients and providers. Expert Rev Gastroenterol Hepatol. 2013;7:531–40.
19. Coté GA, Slivka A, Tarnasky P, et al. Effect of covered metallic stents compared with plastic stents on benign biliary stricture resolution: a randomized clinical trial. JAMA. 2016;315:1250–7.

6

Analysis of risk factors related to gastrointestinal fistula in patients with severe acute pancreatitis: a retrospective study of 344 cases in a single Chinese center

Zhipeng Hua[1], Yongjie Su[1], Xuefeng Huang[1], Kang Zhang[2], Zhengyu Yin[1,2], Xiaoming Wang[1,2] and Pingguo Liu[1,2*]

Abstract

Background: Gastrointestinal fistula (GIF) in severe acute pancreatitis (SAP) is considered as a sparse episode and studied sporadically in the literature. There is paucity of data on the prediction of the effect on risk of GIF in patient with SAP. This study was aimed to investigate risk factors related to GIF in the development of SAP.

Methods: The clinical data of 344 patients with SAP from 2011 to 2016 were reviewed retrospectively. All patients were divided into the GIF group and the non-GIF group, and their data analyzed with respect to 15 parameters were applied to explore potential risk factors for GIF in patients with SAP.

Results: Of the 344 eligible patients, 52 (15.12%) progressed to GIF. Only occurrence of infected pancreatic and extra-pancreatic necrosis (IPN) ($P = 0.004$, OR = 3.012) and modified CT severity index (MCTSI) ($P = 0.033$, OR = 1.183) were proved to be independent risk factors for GIF in patients with SAP, and blood type B ($P = 0.048$, OR = 2.096, 95% CI: 0.748–3.562) indicated weaker association of risk factor for GIF. The early (48–72 h after admission) enteral nutrition (EEN) ($P = 0.016$, OR = 0.267) acted as a protective factor.

Conclusions: Occurrence of IPN and high MCTSI are independent risk factors for the development of GIF in patients with SAP, blood type B reveals a potential correlation with GIF in patients with SAP. EEN is helpful to prevent the progression of GIF secondary to SAP.

Keywords: Severe acute pancreatitis, Gastrointestinal fistula, Risk factor, Infected pancreatic necrosis, MCTSI, EEN, Blood type B

Background

Severe acute pancreatitis (SAP) is a devastating disease that is characterized by a high mortality rate (ranging from 15% to as high as 85%) due to the development of pancreatic and extra-pancreatic necrosis infection, and multi-system organ failure (MOF) [1, 2]. The management of SAP is complicated because of the incomplete understanding of the pathogenesis and multi-causation of the disease, uncertainties in predicting outcome and limited effective treatment modalities [2, 3]. Gastrointestinal fistula (GIF) is a well-recognized complication secondary to SAP, although the incidence of GIF in SAP is low and sporadically reported in the literature. As previously reported, GIF is one of the most fatal and intractable complications after SAP, and associated with other major complications and serious clinical consequences, such as hemorrhage and exacerbation of infection which can lead to a fatal outcome [4–7]. The etiology and pathogenesis of GIF in patients with SAP involve complex processes, which are far from fully understood. Indeed, the management of GIF in SAP is complicated and controversial,

* Correspondence: 1900508954@qq.com
[1]Department of Hepatobiliary Surgery, Zhongshan Hospital of Xiamen University, Hubing South Road, Xiamen, Fujian, China
[2]Fujian Provincial Key Laboratory of Chronic Liver Disease and Hepatocellular Carcinoma (Xiamen University Affiliated ZhongShan Hospital), Xiamen, China

which could lead to a prolonged hospital course, and significant morbidity and mortality [8, 9]. The sites of fistula may involve the stomach, duodenum, jejunum, ileum, and colon, either in localization or diffusion. GIF may result from direct erosion from digestive enzymes excreted by the inflamed pancreas on the adjacent gastrointestinal (GI) tract, or it could occur as a consequence of intestinal necrosis due to vascular thrombosis in an area of inflammation and infection. In addition, GIF may be associated with iatrogenic intervention [10–12].

It has been reported that GIF may cause none of additional symptoms in some cases, which are usually detected incidentally on radiologic imaging or during surgical intervention [10, 13–15]. The resulting events of GIF we observed also confused us frequently, which led to either further complications or spontaneous resolution. Interestingly, more of GIF often tended to relatively facile resolution rather than thorny complications, especially serious GIF, such as the case of multiple or diffuse. Little data exists regarding the risk factors for this complication, and few publications provide precise and adequate predictions of the risk for GIF in patients with SAP. Therefore, the early prediction of GIF and specific targeted interventions are imperative to reduce GIF-related mortality [16, 17]. In this retrospective study we analyzed the data from patients with SAP to determine the risk factors for developing GIF. Moreover, we also studied the different clinical characteristics and outcomes of GIF in the setting of SAP.

Methods

Patient enrollment

From January 2011 to January 2016, patients with a primary diagnosis of SAP admitted to Departments of Emergency, Hepatopancreatobiliary Surgery, Gastroenterology, Surgical Intensive Care Units of Zhongshan Hospital (Xiamen, China) within 72 h from the onset of the disease were screened for enrollment, and including some critical patients confirmed SAP who transferred from other facilities. Demographic and clinical characteristics of patients were collected at the time of admission.

Our criteria are consistent with that recommended in the Revised Atlanta Classification (RAC-2013) [18] and the revised guidelines of the Italian Association for the Study of the Pancreas (AISP-2014) [9]. To ensure the inclusion of only eligible patients with SAP, only those with an acute inflammatory process of the pancreas associated with variable severity were included, such as the presence of organ failure and local/systemic complications. Patients who met the following criteria were excluded: (1) patients developed GIF after iatrogenic intervention or surgical management;(2) younger than 18 years old age; (3) previous diagnosis of chronic liver and gastrointestinal disease; (4) pregnancy or severe immune system disorders; (5) end-stage chronic disease; (6) patients with incomplete data (e.g., deceased within 24 h after admission, missing computed tomography (CT) diagnosis, or termination of treatment on halfway); (7) patients with chronic pancreatitis, known malignancy were excluded.

Diagnosis and classification of SAP

According to RAC-2013 and AISP-2014, the diagnosis of SAP requires clinical course, laboratory parameters and imaging evaluation such as contrast-enhanced CT (CECT), ultrasonography (US) and/or magnetic resonance imaging (MRI), Endoscopic ultrasound (EUS) [19–21]. The severity of SAP is stratified moderately severe (MSAP) and severe (SAP). MSAP is defined as the presence of transient organ failure (<48 h), local complications or exacerbation of co-morbid disease. SAP is defined as persistent organ failure (> 48 h) affecting respiration, renal function or the cardiovascular system. The SAP diagnosis requires at least one of the following criteria: (a) Acute Physiology and Chronic Health Evaluation II (APACHE II) score 8; (b) Ranson score 3; (c) organ failure (i.e., transient and persistent); and (d) local complications (i.e., necrosis, abscess or pseudocyst) [22]. The presence of organ failure was defined by Modified Marshall Scoring System [18, 23]. Local complications have been defined in RAC-2013, include acute pancreatic or peripancreatic fluid collection (APFC), acute necrotic collection (ANC), and walled-off necrosis (WON), pancreatic pseudocysts. IPN is defined as the presence of infection in the development of ANCs and WONs. Other local complications include pancreatic fistula, gastric outlet dysfunction, splenic and portal vein thrombosis, gastrointestinal necrosis and fistula, hemorrhage etc [24–26]. Systemic complications are involved as exacerbation of preexisting conditions like systemic inflammatory response syndrome (SIRS), coronary artery disease, congestive cardiac failure, chronic obstructive pulmonary disease, diabetes, and chronic liver disease, precipitated by acute pancreatitis [27]. GIF is defined as pathological communications that connect any portion of GI tract with the necrotic cavity, the peritoneal space, the retroperitoneal areas, or another internal organ. For overlapped with clinical manifestations of pancreatitis, diagnosis of GIF is often based on fistulography, digestive endoscopy, or operative findings [28].

Etiologies

The etiology was considered to be of biliary origin when biliary tract stones were detected by US, CT or magnetic resonance cholangiopancreatography (MRCP), endoscopic retrograde cholangiopancreatography (ERCP). Alcohol was considered to be secondly etiological factor. For pancreatitis due to hypertriglyceridemia (HTG), a serum triglyceride (TG) level of more than 1000 mg/dL or 500–1000 mg/dL with a history of HTG was necessary, in addition to exclusion of other triggers. Lacking any of the above evidence or other direct causes, any unexplained pancreatitis, such as sphincter of Oddi dysfunction, pregnancy associated, ampullary obstruction, hyper-calcemia, drugs related and autoimmune, were defined as idiopathic AP in this study [29].

Clinical management protocol

Immediately after admission, all patients administrated individualized conservative therapy for SAP that included intensive monitoring, fluid resuscitation, oxygen administration, fasting, analgesia and suppression of pancreatic exocrine function by pharmacological agents, such as somatostatin. Nasoduodenal feeding tubes were placed, and feeding was initiated 48-120 h after admission. EEN was defined as feeding within 48-72 h after admission. Additionally, antibiotic therapies were guided by the results of culture and sensitivity. Rather than preventing infection, antibiotics were prescribed in these often critical patients with established infected necrosis or the presence of other infections (e.g., biliary tract, urinary tract, pulmonary, etc.). CECT was performed routinely for all patients within 72 h after admission or earlier when warranted by diagnostic dilemmas. IPN was diagnosed according to the positive gram stain and culture results of pancreatic or peripancreatitic necrotic tissue obtained by means of CT guided fine needle aspiration, or from the first percutaneous drainage or operation. IPN, WON and pseudocyst with complications were managed with a minimally invasive based step-up approach firstly, next step was performed if there was no clinical improvement. Nonsurgical procedures included percutaneous drainage and continuous negative pressure irrigation. Once GIF in patients with SAP was confirmed, which in most cases were already at least 2 weeks after initiating EEN. Enteral nutrition (EN) was deprived conditionally, and intra or extra-luminal drainage (applicable for the localized GIF), or enterostomy (applicable for the diffuse GIF) might be performed if necessary by the rationale of minimally invasive procedure, as well as interventional management with a step-up approach for SAP.

Data collection

Data pertaining to clinical characteristics, including laboratory parameters, imaging record, phase and location of GIF, intervention for GIF, and outcomes were recorded. The metrics analyzed in the present investigation included demographic characteristics like age, gender, cause of illness, and clinical parameters such as MCTSI, APACHE II score, C-reactive protein (CRP) level, intra-abdominal pressure (IAP), blood type and occurrence of IPN. All the laboratory results were obtained at the Central Laboratory of Zhongshan Hospital according to the standard protocols. IAP was measured with a catheter inserted into the bladder, and patients underwent EEN were also documented.

Statistical analysis

SPSS 22.0 software (IBM SPSS Statistics; IBM Corporation; Armonk, NY) was used for data analysis. The distributions of quantitative variables were tested. Normally and non-normally distributed quantitative variables were presented as the median (interquartile range), respectively. Continuous variables were compared between the groups using an unpaired *t*-test and a paired *t*-test within each group. Categorical variables were compared using the Chi-square test. For small samples, analysis of variance and Fisher's exact test were used to analyze continuous and categorical variables as appropriate. Statistical significance was set at $P < 0.05$.

To identify risk factors for GIF, several series of univariate logistics regression analyses were performed involving 15 indices above mentioned. Variables that showed statistical significance were tested in further multiple logistic regression analyses with the stepwise method.

Results

During the observational period, 344 patients were enrolled in the analyses. The demographic data and clinical characteristics of both GIF and non-GIF groups are shown in Table 1. Of the 344 patients, GIF developed in 52 patients (15.12%) and most of the GIF cases were confirmed clinically 4-8 weeks after onset of the disease. Table 2 shows the results of the univariate regression analysis of GIF in SAP. Hyperlipidemia, MCTSI, APACHE II score, EEN, B blood type and WON showed significant difference between patients with or without GIF. The results of our study correlate well with the statistical results shown in Table 1, which also suggests differences in respect of these six parameters between GIF and non-GIF patients. Taking these significant variables by univariate analysis together into the multiple logistic regression model as showing in Table 3, Only occurrence of IPN ($P = 0.004$, OR = 3.012) and MCTSI ($P = 0.033$, OR = 1.183) were proved to be independent risk factors for GIF in SAP. EEN ($P = 0.016$, OR = 0.267) confirmed as a protective factor for GIF in patients with SAP. Unfortunately, blood type B ($P = 0.048$), although just marginal statistical significance was reached, but the 95% confidence interval (0.748–3.562) observed in the multivariate logistic regression are paradoxical. Table 4 demonstrates the general characteristics and outcome data of SAP with GIF. Most of GIF (92.3%) occurred beyond the phase of APFC, and diffuse GIF was rarely found in WON. All localized GIF were managed using non-surgical procedures. Forty of 52 fistulas closed spontaneously over time after drainage and the source of infection was controlled. Eight of 40

Table 1 Demographic data and clinical characteristics of the patients with SAP

Characteristic	GIF (n =52)	Non-GIF(n =292)	Total(n = 344)	P value
Age, years(range)	51 (34–77)	49(27–70)	50(27–77)	0.572
Gender, M/F	32/20	160/132	192/152	0.047
Etiology				
Biliary	29	156	185	
Alcohol	7	35	42	
Hyperlipidemia	5	37	42	
Idiopathic	11	64	75	
BMI (kg/m2)	22.84(16.25–25.72)	24.13(16.93–28.32)	23.05(16.20–28.42)	0.053
EEN	10	204	214	0.001
APACHE II score	16(11–19)	10(8–15)	10(8–16)	0.035
MCTSI	8(6–10)	6(6–8)	6(6–10)	0.039
CRP level(mg/dl)	143.0(85.0–186.0)	124.6(50.6–184.3)	128.0(64.5–187.0)	0.027
Albumin	10(8–20)	14(11–24)	13(10–28)	0.046
B blood type	16	55	71	0.022
IAP(mmHg)	10.50(9–12.48)	8.50(6.35–11.50)	9.20(6.54–11.75)	0.093
ascites	30	152	182	0.419
thrombosis	9	38	47	0.181
IPN	43	137	180	0.032
death	14	62	75	0.754

M male, *F* female, *APACHE* Acute Physiology and Chronic Health Evaluation, *BMI* body mass index, *EEN* the early enteral nutrition, *CRP* C-reactive protein, *IAP* intra-abdominal pressure, *MCTSI* modified CT severity index, *IPN* infected pancreatic and extra-pancreatic necrosis

Table 2 Univariate logistic regression analysis of GIF

Variable	OR	95% CI		*P* value
		Lower	Upper	
Age	1.406	0.972	1.732	0.937
Gender	1.031	0.948	1.431	0.873
Alcohol	1.370	0.253	0.724	0.284
Hyperlipidemia	2.471	0.542	2.797	0.029
BMI	1.151	1.017	1.314	0.056
APACHE II score	1.632	0.951	3.118	0.044
MCTSI	4.233	1.026	4.965	0.025
CRP level	1.973	0.927	2.531	0.172
EEN	0.346	0.253	0.764	0.004
Albumin	2.427	0.862	2.253	0.122
B blood type	2.994	1.181	6.137	0.036
IAP	1.038	0.929	1.287	0.087
ascites	1.279	0.764	3.249	0.126
thrombosis	1.878	0.912	3.104	0.201
IPN	3.174	1.783	11.902	0.002

APACHE Acute Physiology and Chronic Health Evaluation, BMI body mass index, *EEN* the early enteral nutrition, *CRP* C-reactive protein, *IAP* intra-abdominal pressure, *MCTSI* modified CT severity index, *IPN* infected pancreatic and extra-pancreatic necrosis

fistulas closed spontaneously with nothing but conservative supportive management. Seven of 40 patients (17.5%) failed to survive due to MOF or septic shock. For 10 of 12 diffuse GIF, ileostomy or colostomy was performed. Two of them were managed by percutaneous drainage procedure because the patients could not tolerate surgery. Five of fistulas survived and seven (58.3%) died of MOF or other serious complications. The overall mortality was 14 of 52 (26.9%).

Discussion

GIF is a well-recognized complication that occurs in the late phase of AP. However, the clinical relevance of GIF in patients with AP has been rarely studied by investigators, and the reported incidence ranges from 3 to 12% in

Table 3 Independent risk factors in a multivariate logistic regression analysis of GIF

Variable	OR	95% CI		*P* value
		Lower	Upper	
Occurrence of IPN	3.012	1.693	15.026	0.004
EEN	0.267	0.182	0.738	0.016
MCTSI	1.183	1.096	2.547	0.037
B blood type	1.006	0.748	3.562	0.048

IPN infected pancreatic and extra-pancreatic necrosis, *EEN* the early enteral nutrition, *MCTSI* modified CT severity index

Table 4 General characteristics data of SAP with GIF

GIF style	Phase			Management			Death
	APFC	INP	WON	operation	drainage	Selfhealing	
Localization	2	12	26	0	32	8	7/40
diffusion	2	10	0	10	2	0	7/12
total	4	22	26	10	34	8	14/52

APFC acute pancreatic or peripancreatic fluid collection, *WON* walled-off necrosis, *IPN* infected pancreatic or peripancreatic necrosis

different studies [28–30]. In the present retrospective study, GIF developed in 52 of 344 patients (15.12%), which was relatively higher than previously reported. The higher incidence should be mainly due to screening only SAP patients for enrollment in our study, and in addition, some critical patients admitted to our center who were transferred from other facilities.

We evaluated 15 potential risk factors for GIF in SAP patients and demonstrated the occurrence of IPN resulting from ANC or WON and high MCTSI to be independent risk factors ($P = 0.004$, OR = 3.012; $P = 0.037$, OR = 1.183). EEN acted as a protective factor for GIF with SAP ($P = 0.0001$, OR = 1.006). Unfortunately, our data suggested that blood type B was also correlated with GIF ($P = 0.048$, OR = 1.006), not only less strongly, but the 95% confidence interval (0.748-3.562) was paradoxical based on multivariate logistic regression.

Previous studies have confirmed infection of pancreatic necrosis can be observed in 25-70% of patients with necrotizing disease [31]. Occurrence of pancreatic and peripancreatic necrosis and formation of WON serve as nidus for bacterial superinfection are prone to develop infections which thought to be involved in the pathogenesis of GIF. The microbial pathogens that cause IPN in necrotizing pancreatitis are predominantly gut-derived [32]. A transition from a pro-inflammatory to an anti-inflammatory response occurs within the first 1-2 weeks, the patient is at risk for the translocation of intestinal flora as a result of intestinal barrier failure followed by the development of consequent IPN and fluid collections, which is thought to be associated with severe local inflammatory response and may erode the blood vessel directly, stimulate vessel spasm, enhance thrombosis, and reduce capillary perfusion, especially, when secondary infection occurs [33]. Inflammation or infected necrosis and enzyme-rich fluid can exacerbate the condition of gastrointestinal (GI) tract, which facilitate the formation of oedema, thrombosis, ischemia, necrosis and resulting in formation of fistula eventually [11]. With respect to the time of occurrence of GIF during the course of SAP, 85% patients had GIF beyond 4-8 weeks [34], which suggests that the development of GIF is associated with the long-term effects of the pancreatic or peripancreatic inflammation and infection. The finding is in agreement with our results, as patients with IPN had a higher risk of GIF. Hence, due to the anatomical characteristics of GI tract and the nature of pancreatic necrosis, the region of GIF was local or diffuse, but the underlying pathogenesis of both were same. Timely drainage of infected necrotizing collection could significantly decrease the risk of GIF.

For preventing infections in patients with SAP, recent studies have universally supported the optimal strategy of fluid resuscitation, which involves aggressive fluid administration during the first 24h of admission, highlight optimal targeting of individualized fluid requirements, and utilizing lactated Ringer's as the fluid type of preferred choice [35–37]. Additionally, routine antibiotic or probiotic prophylaxis is recommended for patients with SAP. Antibiotic therapy should be initiated while the source of the infection is suspected or investigated [38].

Reliable evidence from several randomized controlled trials and meta-analyses comparing the outcomes of EN to parenteral nutrition (PN) in patients with AP has clearly shown the superiority of EN in decreasing the infectious complication rate, MOF, mortality, and length of hospitalization [39]. Our data suggest that EEN, in contrast to the maximum IPN and maximum WON level, acts as a protective factor for GIF secondary to SAP ($P = 0.016$, OR = 0.267). EN starting in the early phase (48-72h after admission) of SAP is superior to later EN (72 h after admission) and PN. Some studies have demonstrated that EEN can timely deliver nutritional support, while it preserves gut mucosal integrity, inhibits bacterial overgrowth and translocation, supports splanchnic metabolism, and mitigates the systemic inflammation and risk of infection [40, 41]. The results of a well-designed multicentric randomized clinical trial did not show positive effects of EEN (within 24 h after admission) against on-demand nutrition (48 h since admission), with the incidence of IPN as an endpoint. Conversely, feeding within the first 24 h might act as a burden, which might be of no benefit to prevent gut-derived infectious complications. Accordingly, it is not recommended to initiate feeding within first 24 h, rather feeding initiated 48 h after admission is more beneficial [42, 43]. However, SAP is always accompanied with delayed gastric emptying and intestinal ileus that lead to anorexia, nausea, and vomiting that prevent the patient from tolerating oral fluids and diet. And ventilator support executing sedation in the ICU preclude oral feeding in patients with SAP. So EN need to be supplied via nasogastric (NG), nasoduodenal, or nasojejunal (NJ) feeding. In patients who have gastric outlet obstruction from pancreatic inflammation or fluid collection related duodenal compression, a nasogastrojejunal (NGJ) tubing system, a double lumen tube with proximal gastric decompression, and distal jejunal feeding ports can be used to meet both the purposes without the need for two separate tubes [44, 45]. In our center, nasoduodenal feeding tubes as the primary method of enteral feeding were placed by endoscopists or radiologists, NJ and NGJ were managed secondarily if necessary, and fluid feeding was initiated after 48–120 h after admission.

It was confirmed in the present study that patients with SAP and high MCTSI scores were at a higher risk for GIF. The MCTSI is one of the most preferred modality for severity assessment of acute pancreatitis by incorporating extra-pancreatic complications. CECT is considered the non-invasive reference standard for diagnosing AP, and is highly accurate in assessing IPN and its complications when performed 72–96 h after symptom onset [24, 46]. MCTSI is credited with IPN and involvement of pleural effusion, ascites, vascular or gastrointestinal complications, and as expected, has the greatest accuracy for predicting SAP, which correlates more closely with patient outcome in terms of duration of hospital stay and development of organ failure [47, 48]. Because MCTSI is intrinsically implicated with gastrointestinal complications, which involves the potential opportunity for occurrence of GIF. MCTSI is inevitably as a sensitive risk factor for GIF in patients with SAP.

Previous reports have suggested that blood type B may be a genetic eliciting factor for chronic autoimmune pancreatitis [49]. Unfortunately, our results revealed a slight correlation between blood type B and the development of GIF in patients with SAP. For blood type B ($P = 0.048$,OR = 1.006), marginal statistical significance was reached, but there was an ambiguity with respect to the paradoxical 95% confidence interval (0.748–3.562) observed in the multivariate logistic regression, which indicated a weaker association of risk factor for GIF or implied a relatively limited sample size in our study. How the intrinsic relationship between these observed factors is confusedly unclear. Even though our data have shown an association between the development of GIF in patients with SAP and blood type B, previous analyses should not be regarded as an outcome of our study, and further investigation is warranted.

The clinical outcomes, as illustrated in Table 4 suggest that patients with SAP in combination with diffuse GIF have much longer hospital stays, more severe complications, extremely poor prognosis, and require more invasive treatments than localized counterparts, which might cause none of additional symptoms and are even detected incidentally [4, 50]. In our study, only 12 of 52 fistulas (23.1%) were shown to be diffuse GIF, and 40 of 52 fistulas (76.9%) were in localized GIF.

It was easy to neglect GIF because its symptom always overlap with clinical manifestations of SAP, and visible air pockets within the necrotic area on the imaging of CECT are frequently confused with infection of necrosis [51, 52]. Even diffuse GIF might not be observed timely unless persistent deterioration aroused attention. Nevertheless, the morbidity associated with localized GIF is significantly higher than diffuse GIF. Thus, it is not difficult to explain why there is no remarkably discrepancy in mortality (26.92% vs. 21.23%; $P = 0.754$) related to the SAP between patients with and without GIF, as shown in Table 1. This consistency may be mainly attributed to the following: First, the occurrence of severe intestinal edema, ischemia, necrosis and fistula caused by erosion and necrosis of enzyme-rich fluid and infected necrotic tissue is most localized in the retroperitoneal space and diffusion is limited. Therefore, most GIF of upper GI tract can usually close spontaneously with time if the infected source can be well controlled [12, 14]. Second, GIF can potentially benefit the patient by draining IPN into GI tract, especially when IPN, WON, or pseudocyst communicate with the gut [4, 53]. Third, advances in technology, a sufficient nutrition supply, effective anti-infective treatment, and timely surgical intervention have also played extremely important roles [54].

There were two primary advantages in the present study. First, we observed originally that blood type B is an independent risk factor for GIF in patients with SAP, albeit the relatively small sample of the present study might have reduced the statistical power. Second, we attempted to identify specific, routinely tested and reproducible baseline clinical parameters that predict the risk factors which are associated with GIF secondary to SAP. There were also several limitations to our study. First, this was a retrospective study with a relatively limited sample size. The actual incidence of GIF might be lower than our report because some patients transferred to our center were critical and most had been treated in other facilities for a long time. The non-parametric test applied may bring some uncertainty to the conclusions. Second, the guidelines that some experts recommended (the prophylactic administration of antibiotics and some pharmacologic agents are not necessary in all patients with acute pancreatitis) [55–58] were also not implemented in the present study owing to lacking of uniform experimental assessments. Third, as a relative contra-indication of EN, SAP was associated with delayed gastric emptying and intestinal ileus. EEN might be executed unsuccessfully due to subjective bias of the individual administrator. Finally, by introducing the updated classification of SAP, it was inevitable to make selection bias by ruling in or out patients who were over-or-underestimated due to the seemingly homologous definition. Whether or not these aspects could affect the incidence and analysis of GIF in patients with SAP is uncertain.

Conclusion

We conclude that occurrence of IPN and higher MCTSI are independent significant risk factors for the development of GIF in patients with SAP. EN in 48–72 h after admission is conformed to be an independent significant protective factor of GIF secondary to SAP. Also the patient with blood type B is predisposed to develop GIF in the patient with SAP, perhaps which need more support.

Abbreviations

ANC: Acute necrotic collection; APFC: Acute pancreatic or peripancreatic fluid collection; EEN: Early enteral nutrition; GIF: Gastrointestinal fistula; IPN: Defined when the presence of the ANCs and WONs development of infection; MCTSI: Modified CT severity index; SAP: Severe acute pancreatitis; WON: and walled-off necrosis

Acknowledgements

We want to thank the staff of Department of Hepatobiliary Surgery of Zhongshan Hospital of Xiamen University, Xiamen, China. We also are grateful for the support received from Jianming Wang Pro. Department of Biliary-Pancreatic Surgery, Affiliated Tongji Hospital, Tongji Medical College, Huazhong University of Science and Technology, Wuhan, China.

Funding

The retrospective study design, the preparation of research, the analysis and the interpretation of results data for this research was mainly supported by Science and Technology Bureau of Xiamen for the Promotion of Healthy Grants-in-aid for Scientific Research (3502Z20154021).

Authors' contributions

Each author had participated sufficiently to take public responsibility for its content. PGL designed the research; ZPH, YJS, ZYY performed the research; XFH, KZ, XMW provided new agents and analytic tools; and ZPH, YJS, XFH, KZ drafted the paper. PGL, ZYY, XMW were involved in revising the manuscript critically for important intellectual content. All authors read and approved the final manuscript.

Competing interests

The authors declare that they have no competing interests.

Consent for publication

Not applicable.

References

1. Petrov MS, Shanbhag S, Chakraborty M, Phillips AR, Windsor JA. Organ failure and infection of pancreatic necrosis as determinants of mortality in patients with acute pancreatitis. Gastroenterology. 2010;139:813–20.
2. Buter A, Imrie CW, Carter CR, Evans S, McKay CJ. Dynamic nature of early organ dysfunction determines outcome in acute pancreatitis. Br J Surg. 2002;89:298–302.
3. Petrov MS. Predicting the severity of acute pancreatitis: choose the right horse before hitching the cart. Dig Dis Sci. 2011;56:3402–4.
4. Kochhar R, Jain K, Gupta V, et al. Fistulization in the GI tract in acute pancreatitis. Gastrointest Endosc. 2012;75:436–40.
5. Talukdar R, Nechutova H, Clemens M, Vege SS. Could rising BUN predict the future development of infected pancreatic necrosis? Pancreatology. 2013;13:355–9.
6. van Baal MC, van Santvoort HC, Bollen TL, Bakker OJ, Besselink MG, Gooszen HG. Systematic review of percutaneous catheter drainage as primary treatment for necrotizing pancreatitis. Br J Surg. 2011;98:18–27.
7. Flati G, Andrén-Sandberg A, La Pinta M, Porowska B, Carboni M. Potentially fatal bleeding in acute pancreatitis: pathophysiology, prevention, and treatment. Pancreas. 2003;26:8–14.
8. Beger HG, Rau BM. Severe acute pancreatitis: Clinical course and management. World J Gastroenterol. 2007;13:5043–51.
9. Pezzilli R, Zerbi A, Campra D, Capurso G, Golfieri R, Arcidiacono PG, et al. Consensus guidelines on severe acute pancreatitis. Dig Liver Dis. 2015;47(7):532–43.
10. Doberneck RC. Intestinal fistula complicating necrotizing pancreatitis. Am J Surg. 1989;158:581–4.
11. Tsiotos GG, Smith CD, Sarr MG. Incidence and management of pancreatic and enteric fistulas after surgical management of severe necrotizing pancreatitis. Arch Surg. 1995;130:48–52.
12. Mohamed SR, Siriwardena AK. Understanding the colonic complications of pancreatitis. Pancreatology. 2008;8(2):153–8.
13. Suzuki A, Suzuki S, Sakaguchi T, et al. Colonic fistula associated with severe acute pancreatitis: report of two cases. Surg Today. 2008;38:178–83.
14. Van Minnen LP, Besselink MG, Bosscha K, van Leeuwen MS, Schipper ME, Gooszen HG. Colonic involvement in acute pancreatitis. A retrospective study of 16 patients. Dig Surg. 2004;21:33–8.
15. Yeom HJ, Yi SY. Spontaneous resolution of pancreatic gastric fistula. Dig Dis Sci. 2007;52:561–4.
16. Sun B, Li HL, Gao Y, Xu J, Jiang HC. Factors predisposing to severe acute pancreatitis: evaluation and prevention. World J Gastroenterol. 2003;9:1102–5.
17. Sun B, Li HL, Gao Y, Xu J, Jiang HC. Analysis and prevention of factors predisposing to infections associated with severe acute pancreatitis. Hepatobiliary Pancreat Dis Int. 2003;2:303–7.
18. Banks PA, Bolen TL, Dervenis C, Gooszen HG, Johnson CD, Sarr MG, et al. Classifi cation of acute pancreatitis-2102: revision of the Atlanta classifi cation and defi nitions by international consensus. Gut. 2013;62(1):102–11.
19. Bollen TL. Imaging of acute pancreatitis: update of the revised Atlanta classifi cation. Radiol Clin North Am. 2012;50(3):429–45.
20. Thoeni RF. The revised Atlanta classifi cation of acute pancreatitis: its importance for the radiologist and its effect on treatment. Radiology. 2012;262(3):751–64.
21. Banks PA, Freeman ML. Practice parameters committee of the American college of gastroenterology. Practice guidelines in acute pancreatitis. Am J Gastroenterol. 2006;101(10):2379–400.
22. Papachristou GI, Muddana V, Yadav D, O'Connell M, Sanders MK, Slivka A, et al. Comparison of BISAP, Ranson's, APACHE-II, and CTSI scores in predicting organ failure, complications, and mortality in acute pancreatitis. Am J Gastroenterol. 2010;105:435–41.
23. Marshall JC, Cook DJ, Christou NV, Bernard GR, Sprung CL, Sibbald WJ. Multiple organ dysfunction score: a reliable descriptor of a complex clinical outcome. Crit Care Med. 1995;23:1638–52.
24. Balthazar EJ, Robinson DL, Megibow AJ, Ranson JH. Acute pancreatitis: value of CT in establishing prognosis. Radiology. 1990;174:331–6.
25. Lenhart DK, Balthazar EJ. MDCT of acute mild (nonnecrotizing pancreatitis): abdominal complications and fate of fl uid collections. Am J Roentgenol. 2008;190:643–9.
26. Pelaez-Luna M, Vege SS, Petersen BT, Chari ST, Clain JE, Levy MJ, et al. Disconnected pancreatic duct syndrome in severe acute pancreatitis: clinical and imaging characteristics and outcomes in a cohort of 31 cases. Gastrointest Endosc. 2008;68:91–7.
27. Salomone T, Tosi P, Palareti G, et al. Coagulative disorders in human acute pancreatitis: role for the D-dimer. Pancreas. 2003;26:111–6.
28. Falconi M, Pederzoli P. The relevance of gastrointestinal fistulae in clinical practice: a review. Gut. 2001;49 Suppl 4:iv2–iv10.

29. Forsmark CE. The clinical problem of biliary acute necrotizing pancreatitis: epidemiology, pathophysiology, and diagnosis of biliary necrotizing pancreatitis. J Gastrointest Surg. 2001;5:235–9.
30. Urakami A, Tsunoda T, Hayashi J, et al. Spontaneous fistulization of a pancreatic pseudocyst into the colon and duodenum. Gastrointest Endosc. 2002;55:949–51.
31. Singh RK, Poddar B, Baronia AK, Azim A, Gurjar M, Singhal S, et al. Audit of patients with severe acute pancreatitis admitted to an intensive care unit. Indian J Gastroenterol. 2012;31(5):243–52.
32. Besselink MG, van Santvoort HC, Boermeester MA, et al. Timing and impact of infections in acute pancreatitis. Br J Surg. 2009;96:267–73.
33. Noor MT, Radhakrishna Y, Kocchar R, Kocchar R, Wig JD, Sinha SK, et al. Bacteriology of infection in severe acute pancreatitis. JOP. 2011;12:19–25.
34. Dellinger EP, Tollado JM, Soto NE, Ashley SW, Barie PS, Dugernier T, et al. Early antibiotic treatment for severe acute necrotizing pancreatitis: a randomized, double-blind, placebo-controlled study. Ann Surg. 2007;245:674–83.
35. Working Group IAP/APA Acute Pancreatitis Guidelines. IAP/APA evidence-based guidelines for the management of acute pancreatitis. Pancreatology. 2013;13(4 Suppl 2):e1–15.
36. Hartman H, Sippola T, Kupcinskas J, Lindström O, Johnson C, Regnér S. Raised intestinal fatty acid binding protein correlates to severe acute pancreatitis. Abstract presented at the 45th annual meeting of the European Pancreatic Club, June 26–29, 2013, Zurich, Switzerland. Pancreatology. 2013;13(3):S68.
37. Rahman SH, Ammori BJ, Holmfi eld J, Larvin M, McMahon MJ. Intestinal hypoperfusion contributes to gut barrier failure in severe acute pancreatitis. J Gastrointest Surg. 2003;7(1):26–35.
38. Pezzilli R. Pharmacotherapy for acute pancreatitis. Expert Opin Pharmacother. 2009;10(18):2999–3014.
39. Singh N, Sharma B, Sharma M, Sachdev V, Bhardwaj P, Mani K, Joshi YK, Saraya A. Evaluation of early enteral feeding through nasogastric and nasojejunal tube in severe acute pancreatitis: a noninferiority randomized controlled trial. Pancreas. 2012;41:153Y159.
40. Marik PE, Zaloga GP. Meta-analysis of parenteral nutrition versus enteral nutrition in patients with acute pancreatitis. BMJ. 2004;328(7453):2.
41. Al-Omran M, Albalawi ZH, Tashkandi MF, Al-Ansary LA. Enteral versus parenteral nutrition for acute pancreatitis. Cochrane Database Syst Rev. 2010;20(10):CD002837.
42. Petrov MS, van Santvoort HC, Besselink MG, van der Heijden GJ, Windsor JA, Gooszen HG. Enteral nutrition and the risk of mortality and infectious complications in patients with severe acute pancreatitis:a meta-analysis of randomized trials. Arch Surg. 2008;143(11):1111–7.
43. McClave SA, Heyland DK. The physiologic response and associated clinical benefi ts from provision of early enteral nutrition. Nutr Clin Pract. 2009;24(3):305–15.
44. O'Keefe S, Rolniak S, Raina A, Graham T, Hegazi R, Centa-Wagner P. Enteral feeding patients with gastric outlet obstruction. Nutr Clin Pract. 2012;27(1):76–81.
45. Kumar A, Singh N, Prakash S, Saraya A, Joshi YK. Early enteral nutrition in severe acute pancreatitis: a prospective randomized controlled trial comparing nasojejunal and nasogastric routes. J Clin Gastroenterol. 2006;40(5):431–4.
46. De Waele JJ, Delrue L, Hoste EA, De Vos M, Duyck P, Colardyn FA. Extrapancreatic infl ammation on abdominal computed tomography as an early predictor of disease severity in acute pancreatitis: evaluation of a new scoring system. Pancreas. 2007;34:185–90.
47. Bollen TL, Singh VK, Maurer R, Repas K, van Es HW, Banks PA, et al. A comparative evaluation of radiologic and clinical scoring systems in the early prediction of severity in acute pancreatitis. Am J Gastroenterol. 2012;107:612–9.
48. Mortele KJ, Wiesner W, Intriere L, Shankar S, Zou KH, Kalantari BN, et al. A modifi ed CT severity index for evaluating acute pancreatitis: improved correlation with patient outcome. AJR Am J Roentgenol. 2004;183:1261–5.
49. Weiss FU, Schurmann C, Teumer A, Mayerle J, Simon P, Völzke H, Greinacher A, Kuehn JP, Zenker M, Völker U, et al. ABO blood type B and fucosyltransferase 2 non-secretor status as genetic risk factors for chronic pancreatitis. Gut. 2016;65(2):353–4. Epub 2015 Apr 28.
50. Gardner A, Gardner G, Feller E. Severe colonic complications of pancreatic disease. J Clin Gastroenterol. 2003;37(3):258–62.
51. Van Baal MC, Bollen TL, Bakker OJ, van Goor H, Boermeester MA, Dejong CH, et al. The role of routine fi ne-needle aspiration in the diagnosis of infect ed necrotizing pancreatitis. Surgery. 2014;155(3):442–8.
52. Balthazar EJ. Complications of acute pancreatitis: clinical and CT evaluation. Radiol Clin North Am. 2002;40:1211–27.
53. Levy I, Ariche A. Complete recovery after spontaneous drainage of pancreatic abscess into the stomach. Scand J Gastroenterol. 1999;34:939–41.
54. van Santvoort HC, Bakker OJ, Bollen TL, Besselink MG, Ahmen Ali U, Schrijver AM, et al. A conservative and minimally invasive approach to necrotizing pancreatitis improves outcome. Gastroenterology. 2011;141:1254–63.
55. Delcenserie R, Yzet T, Ducroix JP. Prophylactic antibiotics in treatment of severe acute alcoholic pancreatitis. Pancreas. 1996;13:198–201.
56. Sharma VK, Howden CW. Prophylactic antibiotic administration reduces sepsis and mortality in acute necrotizing pancreatitis: a meta-analysis. Pancreas. 2001;22:28–31.
57. Takeda K, Yamauchi J, Shibuya K, Sunamura M, Mikami Y, Matsuno S. Benefit of continuous regional arterial infusion of protease inhibitor and antibiotic in the management of acute necrotizing pancreatitis. Pancreatology. 2001;1:668–73.
58. Griesbacher T. Kallikrein-kinin system in acute pancreatitis: potential of B(2)-bradykinin antagonists and kallikrein inhibitors. Pharmacology. 2000;60:113–20.

7

How to select patients and timing for rectal indomethacin to prevent post-ERCP pancreatitis

Jianhua Wan[†], Yuping Ren[†], Zhenhua Zhu, Liang Xia[*] and Nonghua Lu[†]

Abstract

Background: Acute pancreatitis is a severe complication of endoscopic retrograde cholangiopancreatography (ERCP). Previous meta-analyses have shown that indomethacin effectively prevents this complication; however, the data are limited. We performed a systematic review and meta-analysis to clarify the applications for rectal indomethacin.

Methods: A systematic search was performed in June 2016. Human prospective, randomized, placebo-controlled trials that compared rectally administered indomethacin with a placebo for the prevention of post-ERCP pancreatitis (PEP) were included. A meta-analysis was performed using a random-effects model to assess the outcomes (PEP) using Review Manager 5.0.

Results: Seven randomized controlled trials met the inclusion criteria ($n = 3013$). The overall incidence of PEP was significantly lower after prophylactic administration of rectal indomethacin than after administration of the placebo (RR, 0.58, 95% CI, 0.40–0.83; $P = 0.004$). A subgroup analysis was performed for rectal indomethacin administration compared to a placebo in high-risk patients (RR, 0.46; 95% CI, 0.32–0.65; $P < 0.00001$) and average-risk patients (RR, 0.75; 95% CI, 0.46–1.22; $P = 0.25$) and for administration before ERCP (RR, 0.56; 95% CI, 0.39–0.79; $P = 0.001$) and after the procedure (RR, 0.61; 95% CI, 0.26–1.44; $P = 0.26$).

Conclusions: This meta-analysis indicated that prophylactic rectal indomethacin is not suitable for all patients undergoing ERCP but it is safe and effective to prevent PEP in high-risk patients. In addition, rectal indomethacin administration before ERCP is superior to its administration after ERCP for the prevention of PEP.

Keywords: Indomethacin, Pancreatitis, ERCP, Meta-analysis

Background

Acute pancreatitis is the most common complication after post-endoscopic retrograde cholangiopancreatography (ERCP). The incidence rate of post-ERCP pancreatitis (PEP) ranges between 1.6 and 15.7%, with an overall average of 3.5% [1]. While most cases of PEP are mild, 10-20% of patients may develop severe acute pancreatitis with adverse outcomes and many intractable complications. Therefore, the social and financial burdens caused by PEP need to be addressed. One study noted that the possible pathogenesis of PEP includes both increased pressure and radiocontrast exposure, which contribute to injury in the PEP model [2]. However, the detailed pathogenesis of PEP remains unknown, and no specific or effective treatment for pancreatitis has been developed. Numerous factors have been found to be correlated with the development of PEP, including patient-related factors, such as an age of less than 50 years, female sex, pancreas divisum, sphincter of Oddi dysfunction (SOD), a history of recurrent pancreatitis (≥2 episodes) or history of PEP, and

* Correspondence: xialiang79@163.com
[†]Equal contributors
Department of Gastroenterology, The First Affiliated Hospital of Nanchang University, 17 Yongwaizheng Street, Nanchang, Jiangxi 330006, People's Republic of China

procedure-related factors, such as pancreatic sphincterotomy, precut sphincterotomy, difficult cannulation, pancreatic duct injection or endoscopist experience [3].

Over the past two decades, many methods have been used to prevent PEP, including pharmacologic prevention and mechanical-related interventions. Treatment has been unsatisfactory with the exception of the use of rectal nonsteroidal anti-inflammatory drugs (NSAIDs) and prophylactic pancreatic stents. A network meta-analysis based on existing randomized controlled trials (RCTs) showed that rectal NSAIDs are one of the most efficacious agents for preventing PEP [4]. However, prophylactic stent placement is not cost-effective in patients at average risk for the development of PEP [5]. NSAIDs, especially indomethacin, are potent inhibitors of phospholipase A2 activity, which can regulate proinflammatory mediators such as prostaglandins, leukotrienes and platelet-activating factors in the initial inflammatory cascade of acute pancreatitis [6]. Therefore, prophylactic rectal indomethacin administration to prevent PEP is biologically plausible. A meta-analysis by Rustagi et al.[7] showed that only the rectal route resulted in a significant benefit for the prevention of PEP compared to non-rectal administration of indomethacin. Compared to other methods, rectal indomethacin is less expensive and easily administered, leading to potential beneficial effects in PEP.

Recent clinical trials and a large number of meta-analyses have suggested the promising outcomes of indomethacin use. The European Society of Gastrointestinal Endoscopy and the Japanese Society of Hepato-Biliary-Pancreatic Surgery guidelines recommended routine rectal administration of indomethacin in unselected (both high-risk and average-risk) patients to prevent PEP [8, 9]. However, recent high quality RCTs have revealed that prophylactic rectal indomethacin did not reduce the incidence or severity of PEP in consecutive patients undergoing ERCP [10]. It is necessary to reconsider the selection of suitable patients for prophylactic rectal indomethacin after ERCP. A survey from 29 countries reported using NSAIDs for PEP prophylaxis was not widely accepted by endoscopists performing ERCP due to the lack of convincing scientific evidence [11]. Therefore, a larger sample meta-analysis should examine the benefits of rectal indomethacin for PEP.

Methods

Literature search

We followed standard criteria for performing and reporting a meta-analysis of RCT studies [12]. A systematic search of PubMed, EMBASE and the Cochrane library (including CENTRAL) was performed to identify potentially relevant publications (through June 2016). Keywords included indomethacin, pancreatitis and ERCP. The search was restricted to human studies, and no language restrictions were set. In addition, the reference lists of all retrieved articles, as well as reviews and abstracts from recent conferences, were manually searched. When the same or similar patient studies were included in several publications, only the most recent or informative report was selected for analysis.

Study selection

Studies were initially selected based on their titles and abstracts. Two reviewers (JH.W. and YP.R.) independently screened all abstracts to determine whether the studies met the inclusion criteria. Differences were resolved by a third investigator (L.X.). Studies were considered eligible if they met the following criteria: (1) studies that examined the efficacy and safety of prophylactic rectal indomethacin use for PEP; (2) studies that were prospective and randomized; (3) studies in humans; and (4) data that were not duplicated in another article. Studies were excluded if (1) the study design was retrospective or the study was not an RCT or (2) unadjusted estimates were reported.

Data abstraction and quality assessment

To ensure homogeneity in data gathering and entry, the data extraction was conducted by two experienced investigators working independently (JH.W. and YP.R.). A third investigator (L.X.) was called upon to resolve any differences so that complete consensus was reached for all of the main variables to be assessed in the analysis. Data were recorded as follows: the first author's last name (year of publication), country, setting, study design, size of the trial, outcomes, intervention, inclusion criteria, exclusion criteria, definition of PEP, complications and study quality (recorded in Table 1). The quality of the included studies was assessed independently by two reviewers (JH.W. and YP.R.) using the Cochrane Collaboration tool for assessing the risk of bias [13] (Additional file 1 Figure S1). The grading system contains the following criteria: random sequence generation, allocation concealment, blinding of participants and personnel, blinding of outcome assessment, incomplete outcome data, selective reporting and other bias. Each trial was given an overall summary assessment of low, unclear, or high-risk of bias.

Statistical analysis

Statistical analysis of the Relative Risk (RR) with the 95% confidence interval (CI) was used as a common measure of the association between rectal indomethacin and PEP across studies. Taking both within-study and between-study variabilities into account, we used a random-effects model, which is more conservative than a fixed-effects model, to aggregate data and obtain the overall effect size

Table 1 Characteristics of Studies Included in Meta-analysis

Study	Year	Location	Indomethacin (n)	Placebo (n)	Number of PEPs (n)	Intervention	Definition of PEP
Montaño Loza *et al.*	2007	Mexico	75	75	16	100 mg indomethacin 2 h before ERCP	Pain, Amylase > 3 times
Sotoudehmane sh *et al.*	2007	Iran-Single centre	245	245	22	100 mg indomethacin immediately before ERCP	Pain, Amylase > 3 times admission
Elmunzer *et al.*	2012	US-Multicentre	295	307	79	two 50-mg indomethacin after ERCP	Pain, Amylase > 3 times admission > 2 nigh
döbrönte *et al.*	2014	Hungary-Multicentre	347	318	42	100 mg indomethacin 10–15 min before ERCP	Pain, Amylase > 3 times a prolognation of admission, CT/MRI
Andrade-Dávila *et al.*	2015	Mexico	82	84	21	100 mg indomenthacin after ERCP	Pain, Amylase > 3 times admission > 2 nigh
Patai *et al.*	2015	USA-Single centre	270	296	55	100 mg indomethacin within 1 before ERCP	Pain, Amylase > 3 times
Levenick *et al.*	2016	USA-Single centre	223	226	27	two 50-mg indomethacin during ERCP	Pain, Amylase > 3 times admission > 2 nigh

and 95% CI. Heterogeneity across studies was assessed by performing X^2 tests (assessing the P value) and calculating I^2, which is a quantitative measure of inconsistency across studies. Studies with an I^2 of 25 to 50% were considered to have low heterogeneity; studies with an I^2 of 50to 75% were considered to have moderate heterogeneity; and studies with an $I^2 > 75\%$ were considered to have high heterogeneity. If $I^2 > 50\%$, potential sources of heterogeneity were identified by sensitivity analyses conducted by omitting one study at a time and investigating the influence of a single study on the overall pooled estimate. Publication bias was examined by Egger's test and Begg's test. All calculations were conducted with Review Manager V 5.0 software (provided by the Cochrane Collaboration, Oxford, UK) and Stata version 12.0 (Stata Corporation, College Station, TX, USA). All P values were two-sided, and the significance level was 0.05.

Results

Identification of eligible studies

Based on our search criteria, we identified 332 papers from MEDLINE/PubMed, EMBASE and the Cochrane Central Register of Controlled Trials in the Cochrane

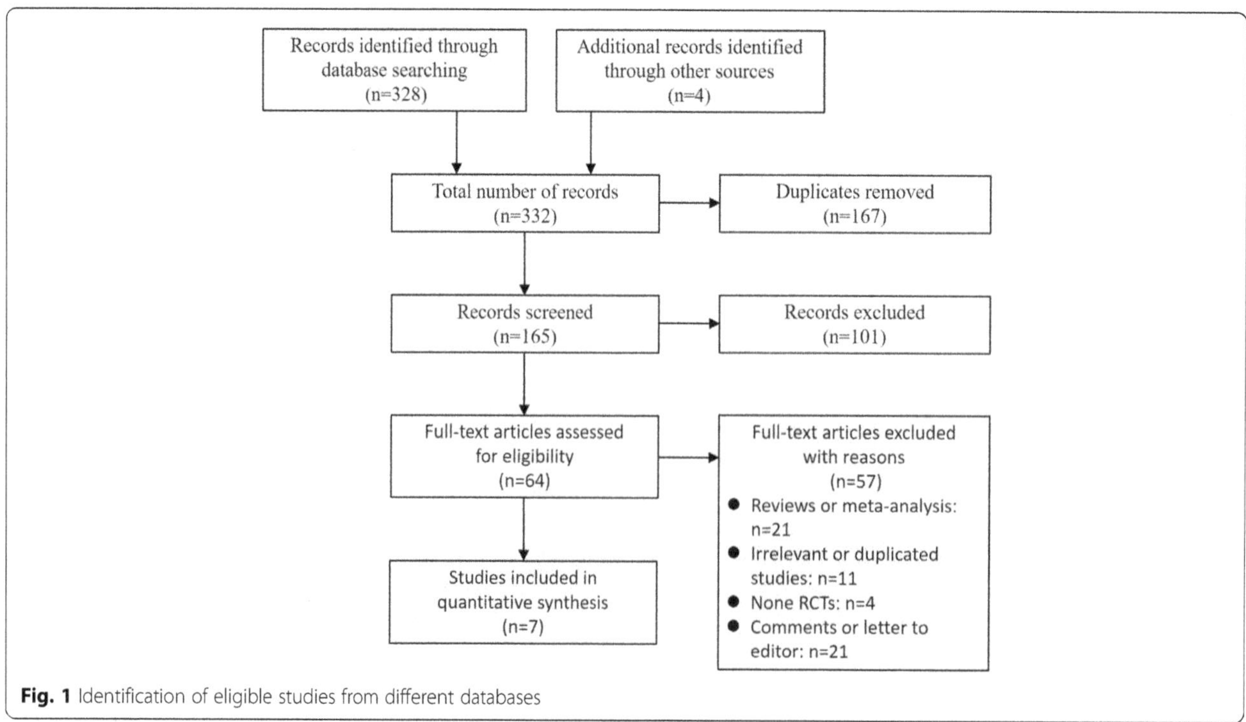

Fig. 1 Identification of eligible studies from different databases

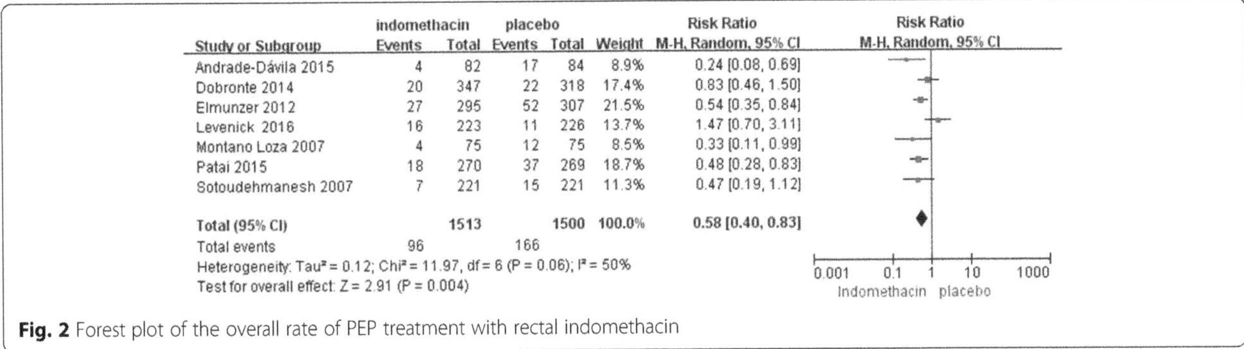

Fig. 2 Forest plot of the overall rate of PEP treatment with rectal indomethacin

Library. Of these articles, 167 duplicate articles were removed. Of those articles, the majority were excluded after reviewing titles and abstracts, mainly because they were reviews, letters, comments, retrospective studies or not relevant to our analysis, leaving 64 papers that appeared to meet our selection criteria. Of those papers, 21 were excluded because they were reviews or meta-analyses; 11 were excluded for irrelevance or were duplicate studies; 4 studies were excluded because they were non-RCTs and 21 papers were excluded because they were comments or letters to the editor. Finally, a total of 7 RCTs with 3013 participants were included in the meta-analysis [10, 14–19]. A detailed flowchart of the selection process is shown in Fig. 1.

Study characteristics

The main characteristics of the studies in the meta-analysis are presented in Table 1. These studies were published between 2007 and 2016. Among the 7 studies, 3 were conducted in America [10, 15, 16], 2 studies were conducted in Mexico [14, 19] and the remaining 2 studies were conducted in Hungary [18] and Iran [17]. All studies were published in English language journals. All studies used a total dose of 100 mg of rectal indomethacin, but included pre-ERCP and post-ERCP administration. Two studies selected patients with an elevated baseline risk of PEP.

Main results

As the primary outcome, the incidence of PEP was measured in all 7 studies. The RR was evaluated between rectal indomethacin and a placebo for the prevention of PEP. The Mantel-Haenszel pooled RR for PEP after prophylactic administration of rectal indomethacin compared to the placebo was 0.58 (95% CI, 0.40–0.83; P = 0.004; Fig. 2), corresponding to an absolute risk reduction of 4.8 percentage points (number needed to treat [NNT] to prevent one episode of post-ERCP pancreatitis was 21) and a relative risk reduction of 43%. Statistically, heterogeneity was observed ($I^2 = 50\%$; $P = 0.06$), which may have occurred due to the following three factors: two studies selected patients with an elevated baseline risk of PEP, two studies used the prophylactic placement of pancreatic stents for most of the patients, and the timing of administration of rectal indomethacin differed among the studies. Therefore, the random effects model was used.

Subgroup analyses

In our subgroup analysis by severity of PEP, 7 studies ($n = 3013$; weight, 74.5%) using rectal indomethacin for the prevention of mild PEP showed a significant difference (RR, 0.61; 95% CI, 0.40–0.93; $P = 0.02$), and similarly, 6 studies ($n = 3013$; weight, 25.5%) using rectal indomethacin for prevention of moderate-to-severe PEP showed a significant benefit (RR, 0.53; 95% CI, 0.31–0.88; $P = 0.01$) (Fig. 3 and 4). In

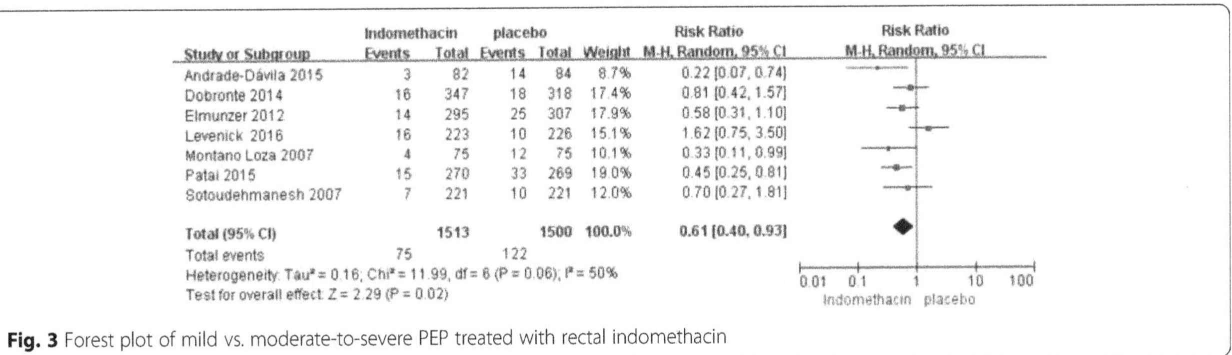

Fig. 3 Forest plot of mild vs. moderate-to-severe PEP treated with rectal indomethacin

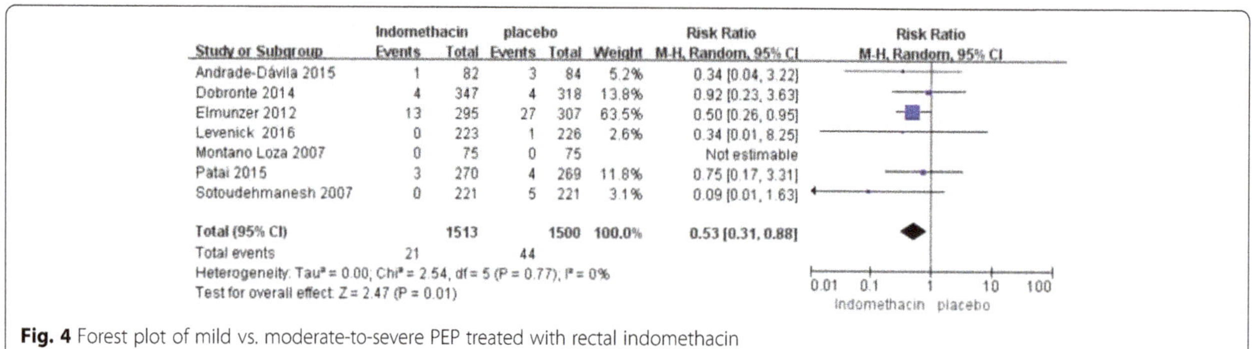

Fig. 4 Forest plot of mild vs. moderate-to-severe PEP treated with rectal indomethacin

summary, rectal indomethacin can reduce the incidence of mild and moderate-to-severe PEP.

When comparing patients at average risk and high risk for PEP, rectal indomethacin showed a significant overall reduction in the incidence of PEP only in the high-risk patients (3 studies with 1161 patients; weight, 45.3%) (RR, 0.46; 95% CI, 0.32–0.65; $P <$ 0.00001), whereas pooled data from 5 studies ($n =$ 1852; weight, 54.7%) involving patients at average risk for PEP showed that rectal indomethacin had no significant benefit (RR, 0.75; 95% CI, 0.46–1.22; $P = 0.25$) (Fig. 5). The NNT to prevent 1 episode of PEP in the high-risk patient group was 10.

In the subgroup analysis of the timing of administration of rectal indomethacin, pooled data from 4 studies ($n = 1796$; weight, 55.8%) in which rectal indomethacin was administered before ERCP showed a statistically significant difference in the occurrence of PEP related to this timing (RR, 0.56; 95% CI, 0.39–0.79; $P = 0.001$). However, 3 studies (n =1217; weight, 44.2%) in which rectal indomethacin was administered after the procedure showed no significant benefit (RR, 0.61; 95% CI, 0.26–1.44; $P = 0.26$) for PEP prophylaxis (Fig. 6).

Only four studies reported bleeding as an adverse event that was potentially related to indomethacin. The results showed no statistical significance between the two groups (RR, 0.97; 95% CI, 0.44–2.12; $P = 0.94$) (Fig. 7).

Sensitivity Analysis

When a single study involved in the meta-analysis was deleted each time, the results of meta-analysis remained unchanged, indicating that the results of the present meta-analysis were stable.

Publication bias

A funnel plot showed that the studies were reasonably well scattered (Fig. 8). There was no statistical evidence of publication bias among studies by using both Egger's regression asymmetry test ($P = 0.61$) (Additional file 2 Figure S2) and the Begg's adjusted rank correlation ($P = 0.37$) (Additional file 3 Figure S3).

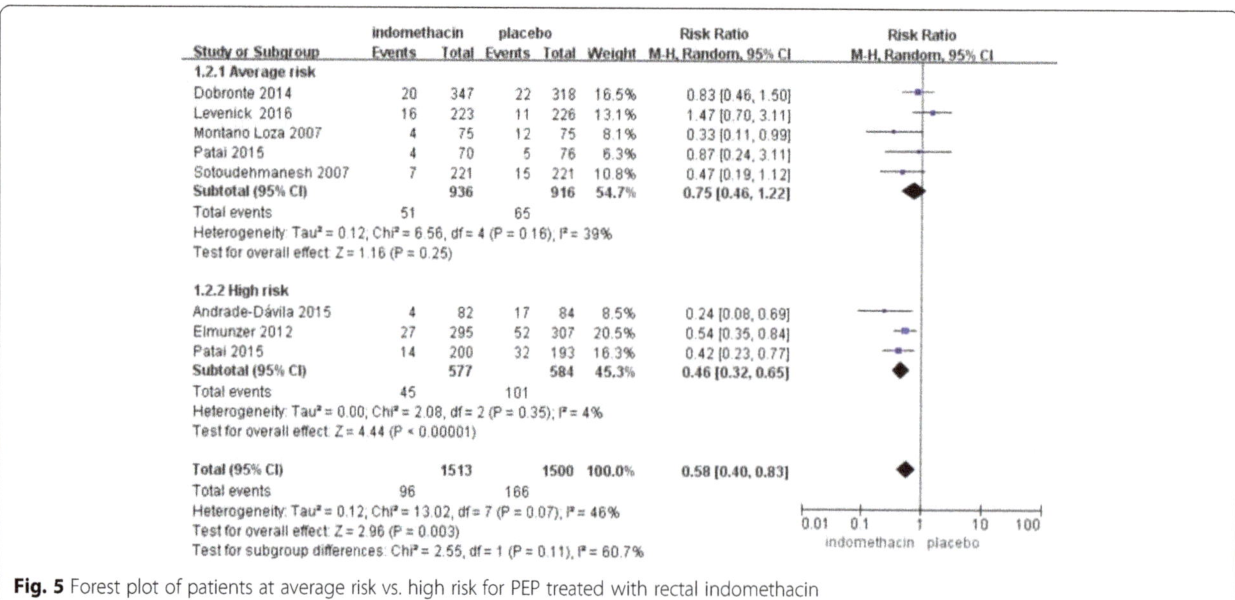

Fig. 5 Forest plot of patients at average risk vs. high risk for PEP treated with rectal indomethacin

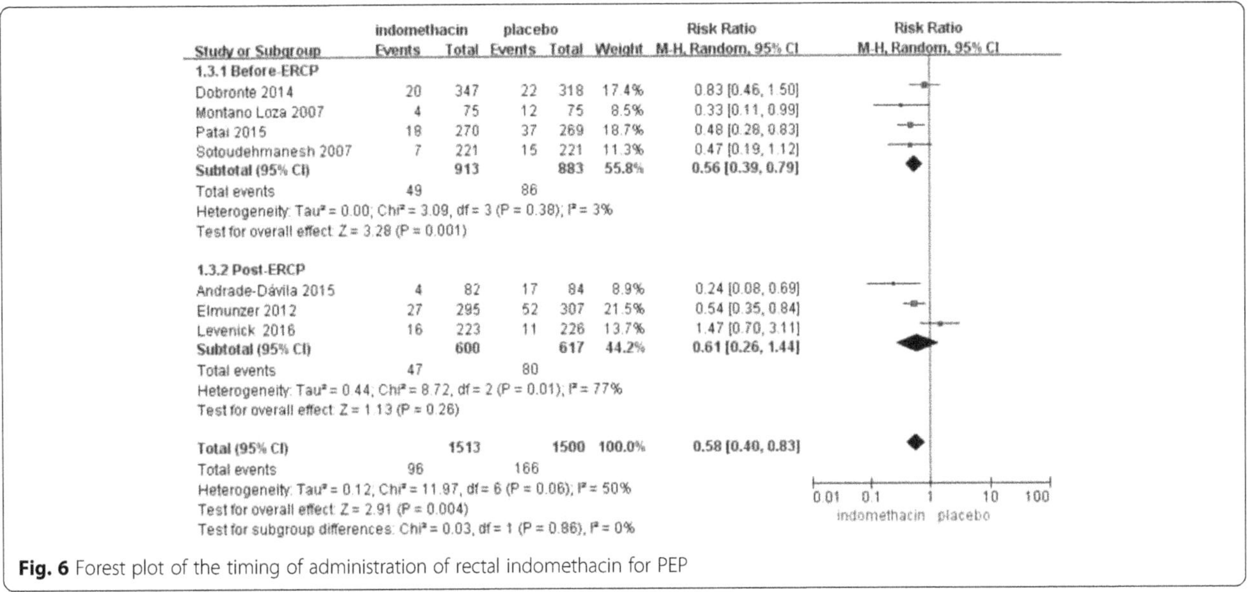

Fig. 6 Forest plot of the timing of administration of rectal indomethacin for PEP

Discussion

In this meta-analysis, we found that rectal indomethacin is generally more effective than a placebo for preventing PEP in patients undergoing ERCP. It reduces the incidence of PEP by nearly 43%, with an NNT of approximately 22 subjects. However, some studies included patients of different classification, leading to the presence of clinical heterogeneity. Therefore, this result is not very persuasive. Previous meta-analyses all concluded that rectal indomethacin was superior to a placebo for preventing PEP in both average- and high-risk patients undergoing ERCP [7, 20–28]. However, those meta-analyses included only a small number of patients who used indomethacin, which reduces the precision of the comparative results, and their conclusions were limited. Three of those meta-analyses included only 3 or 4 studies [20, 21, 23]. Another meta-analysis included indomethacin and other NSAIDs, such as diclofenac, or other routes of administration [7, 22, 24–28]. Compared to the results of previous meta-analyses, the results of the present meta-analysis included more recent RCTs that were different from the RCTs included in the previous analyses. In our subgroup analysis of average- and high-risk patients, rectal indomethacin was not effective in patients at average risk for PEP. Recently, an RCT from a single center showed that prophylactic rectal indomethacin did not reduce the incidence or severity of PEP in consecutive patients undergoing ERCP [10]. In this study, patients were deliberately not categorized into high- and low-risk groups for PEP. Hence, rectal indomethacin should be applied as the choice for patients at high risk for PEP, considering its effectiveness, economy and side effects. Similarly, Elmunzer et al. [15] showed that two 50-mg doses of rectal indomethacin significantly reduced the risk of PEP from 16.9% in those receiving the placebo to 9.2% in those receiving indomethacin for patients at high risk for PEP, including 82.3% of patients who had a clinical suspicion of SOD dysfunction. It should be noted that in this study, the authors placed a pancreatic stent in 246 patients in the indomethacin group (83.4%) and in 250 individuals in the placebo group (81.4%).

In our subgroup analysis of post-ERCP and pre-ERCP prophylactic administration, rectal indomethacin was

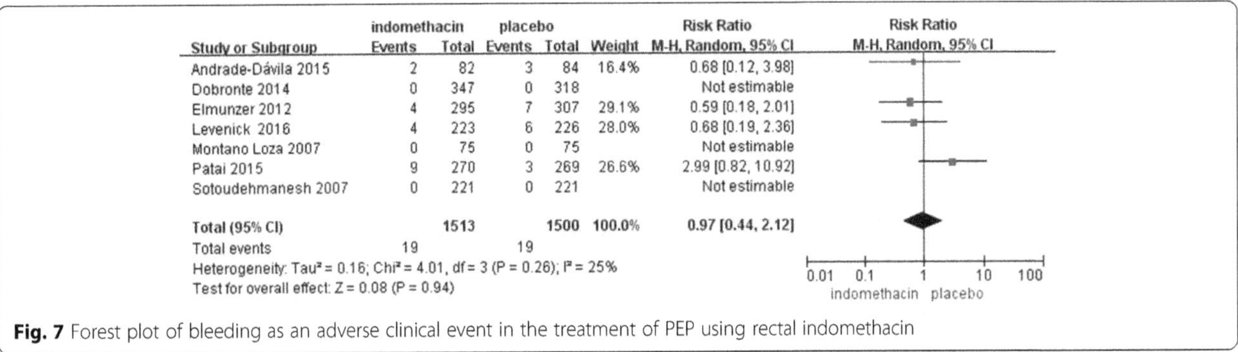

Fig. 7 Forest plot of bleeding as an adverse clinical event in the treatment of PEP using rectal indomethacin

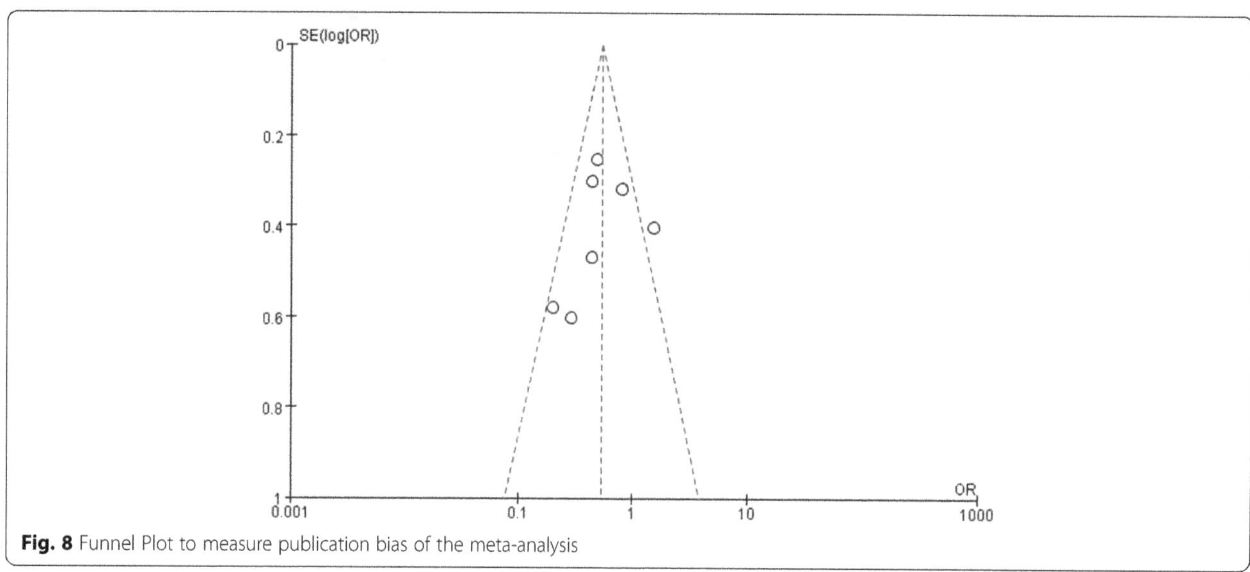

Fig. 8 Funnel Plot to measure publication bias of the meta-analysis

not effective in patients when administered post-ERCP. Previous research has found that the peak plasma concentration of indomethacin is reached 30 min after rectal administration, when bioavailability is complete [29]. The elimination half-life of indomethacin is 4.5 h. When the drug was used before ERCP, the peak level was achieved at the desirable time. Theoretically, therefore, rectal indomethacin may be more effective before the ERCP than after the procedure. A meta-analysis by Rustagi et al. [7] in 2014 found that NSAID administration before ERCP had a greater benefit than administration after the procedure. Recently, Luo et al. found that the strategy of prophylactic pre-ERCP administration of rectal indomethacin for all patients was superior to the strategy of purposeful rectal indomethacin after ERCP in only high-risk patients for reducing the risk of PEP [30]. Therefore, the timing of administration of rectal indomethacin should be before rather than after ERCP.

Of note, no differences in adverse events potentially attributable to rectal indomethacin treatment were observed, suggesting that indomethacin is a safe pharmacologic agent for the prevention of PEP. Four studies reported bleeding as an adverse event, but statistical significance was not achieved. Three patients died from severe PEP in 3 studies, all of which occurred in the placebo group. Other adverse events also occurred in these 3 studies.

The present meta-analysis has some limitations. First, low-quality and small number of studies were included. Second, this meta-analysis exhibits statistical homogeneity. Andrade-Dávila et al. [19] and Elmunzer et al. [15] enrolled only patients at high risk for PEP, whereas the other 5 studies enrolled average-risk patients. Third, studies differed in their definition of PEP and did not always adhere to the Cotton criteria. Lastly, this meta-analysis did not consider the influence of prophylactic pancreatic stents. Patients in 2 studies underwent prophylactic placement of pancreatic stents [10, 15].

In summary, this is the first meta-analysis to suggest that rectal indomethacin is not suitable for all patients undergoing ERCP and should be recommended for preventing PEP in high-risk patients before ERCP. In addition, larger multi-center RCTs are still needed to determine the role of rectal indomethacin in low-risk patients.

Conclusion

Although this meta-analysis indicates that prophylactic rectal indomethacin is not suitable for all patients undergoing ERCP, it is safe and effective for the prevention of PEP in high-risk patients. In addition, administration of rectal indomethacin before ERCP is superior to administration after ERCP for the prevention of PEP. In conclusion, it is necessary to recommend rectal indomethacin before ERCP for the prevention of PEP in high-risk patients.

Abbreviations

CI: Confidence interval; ERCP: Endoscopic retrograde cholangiopancreatography; NNT: Number needed to treat; NSAIDs: Nonsteroidal anti-inflammatory drugs; PEP: Post-ERCP pancreatitis; RCTs: Randomized controlled trials; RR: Relative Risk; SOD: Sphincter of Oddi dysfunction

Acknowledgments

Not applicable.

Funding
The cost of this meta-analysis in the design of the study and collection of data was supported by the National Natural Science Foundation of China (No: 81460130) and the Science and Technology Support Plan Grant (No.20141BBG70022) from Science and Technology Department of Jiangxi Province, China.

Authors' contributions
JHW and LX designed the study; JHW, YPR, ZHZ, LX and NHL coordinated the study; JHW, YPR, ZHZ, LX and NHL performed the study; JHW and YPR analyzed the data; ZHZ, LX and NHL helped to draft the manuscript; JHW and LX wrote the manuscript. All authors read and approved the final manuscript.

Competing interests
The authors declare that they have no competing interests.

Consent for publication
Not applicable.

References

1. Anderson MA, Fisher L, Jain R, Evans JA, Appalaneni V, Ben-Menachem T, Cash BD, Decker GA, Early DS, Fanelli RD, et al. Complications of ERCP. GASTROINTEST ENDOSC. 2012;75(3):467–73.
2. Jin S, Orabi AI, Le T, Javed TA, Sah S, Eisses JF, Bottino R, Molkentin JD, Husain SZ. Exposure to radiocontrast agents induces pancreatic inflammation by activation of nuclear factor-kappaB, calcium signaling, and calcineurin. GASTROENTEROLOGY. 2015;149(3):753–64.
3. Wang AY, Strand DS, Shami VM. Prevention of post-endoscopic retrograde cholangiopancreatography pancreatitis: medications and techniques. Clin Gastroenterol Hepatol. 2016;14:1521–32.
4. Akshintala VS, Hutfless SM, Colantuoni E, Kim KJ, Khashab MA, Li T, Elmunzer BJ, Puhan MA, Sinha A, Kamal A, et al. Systematic review with network meta-analysis: pharmacological prophylaxis against post-ERCP pancreatitis. Aliment Pharmacol Ther. 2013;38(11–12):1325–37.
5. Das A, Singh P, Sivak MJ, Chak A. Pancreatic-stent placement for prevention of post-ERCP pancreatitis: a cost-effectiveness analysis. GASTROINTEST ENDOSC. 2007;65(7):960–8.
6. Makela A, Kuusi T, Schroder T. Inhibition of serum phospholipase-A2 in acute pancreatitis by pharmacological agents in vitro. Scand J Clin Lab Invest. 1997;57(5):401–7.
7. Rustagi T, Njei B. Factors affecting the efficacy of Nonsteroidal anti-inflammatory drugs in preventing post-endoscopic retrograde cholangiopancreatography pancreatitis: a systematic review and meta-analysis. PANCREAS. 2015;44(6):859–67.
8. Dumonceau JM, Andriulli A, Elmunzer BJ, Mariani A, Meister T, Deviere J, Marek T, Baron TH, Hassan C, Testoni PA, et al. Prophylaxis of post-ERCP pancreatitis: european society of gastrointestinal endoscopy (ESGE) guideline - updated june 2014. ENDOSCOPY. 2014;46(9):799–815.
9. Yokoe M, Takada T, Mayumi T, Yoshida M, Isaji S, Wada K, Itoi T, Sata N, Gabata T, Igarashi H, et al. Japanese guidelines for the management of acute pancreatitis: Japanese guidelines 2015. J Hepatobiliary Pancreat Sci. 2015;22(6):405–32.
10. Levenick JM, Gordon SR, Fadden LL, Levy LC, Rockacy MJ, Hyder SM, Lacy BE, Bensen SP, Parr DD, Gardner TB. Rectal indomethacin does Not prevent post-ERCP pancreatitis in consecutive patients. GASTROENTEROLOGY. 2016; 150(4):911–7.
11. Dumonceau JM, Rigaux J, Kahaleh M, Gomez CM, Vandermeeren A, Deviere J. Prophylaxis of post-ERCP pancreatitis: a practice survey. GASTROINTEST ENDOSC. 2010;71(6):934–9. 931–939.
12. Liberati A, Altman DG, Tetzlaff J, Mulrow C, Gotzsche PC, Ioannidis JP, Clarke M, Devereaux PJ, Kleijnen J, Moher D. The PRISMA statement for reporting systematic reviews and meta-analyses of studies that evaluate health care interventions: explanation and elaboration. J CLIN EPIDEMIOL. 2009;62(10): e1–e34.
13. Higgins JP, Altman DG, Gotzsche PC, Juni P, Moher D, Oxman AD, Savovic J, Schulz KF, Weeks L, Sterne JA. The Cochrane Collaboration's tool for assessing risk of bias in randomised trials. BMJ. 2011;343:d5928.
14. Montano LA, Rodriguez LX, Garcia CJ, Davalos CC, Cervantes GG, Medrano MF, Fuentes OC, Gonzalez OA. [Effect of the administration of rectal indomethacin on amylase serum levels after endoscopic retrograde cholangiopancreatography, and its impact on the development of secondary pancreatitis episodes]. REV ESP ENFERM DIG. 2007;99(6):330–6.
15. Elmunzer BJ, Scheiman JM, Lehman GA, Chak A, Mosler P, Higgins PDR, Hayward RA, Romagnuolo J, Elta GH, Sherman S, et al. A randomized trial of rectal indomethacin to prevent post-ERCP pancreatitis. NEW ENGL J MED. 2012;366(15):1414–22.
16. Patai A, Solymosi N, Patai AV. Effect of rectal indomethacin for preventing post-ERCP pancreatitis depends on difficulties of cannulation: results from a randomized study with sequential biliary intubation. J CLIN GASTROENTEROL. 2015;49(5):429–37.
17. Sotoudehmanesh R, Khatibian M, Kolahdoozan S, Ainechi S, Malboosbaf R, Nouraie M. Indomethacin May reduce the incidence and severity of acute pancreatitis after ERCP. Am J Gastroenterol. 2007;102(5):978–83.
18. Döbrönte Z. Is rectal indomethacin effective in preventing of post-endoscopic retrograde cholangiopancreatography pancreatitis? WORLD J GASTROENTERO. 2014;20(29):10151.
19. Andrade-Davila VF, Chavez-Tostado M, Davalos-Cobian C, Garcia-Correa J, Montano-Loza A, Fuentes-Orozco C, Macias-Amezcua MD, Garcia-Renteria J, Rendon-Felix J, Cortes-Lares JA, et al. Rectal indomethacin versus placebo to reduce the incidence of pancreatitis after endoscopic retrograde cholangiopancreatography: results of a controlled clinical trial. BMC GASTROENTEROL. 2015;15:85.
20. Shi N, Deng L, Altaf K, Huang W, Xue P, Xia Q. Rectal indomethacin for the prevention of post-ERCP pancreatitis: a meta-analysis of randomized controlled trials. TURK J GASTROENTEROL. 2015;26(3):236–40.
21. Ahmad D, Lopez KT, Esmadi MA, Oroszi G, Matteson-Kome ML, Choudhary A, Bechtold ML. The effect of indomethacin in the prevention of post-endoscopic retrograde cholangiopancreatography pancreatitis: a meta-analysis. PANCREAS. 2014;43(3):338–42.
22. Sethi S, Sethi N, Wadhwa V, Garud S, Brown A. A meta-analysis on the role of rectal diclofenac and indomethacin in the prevention of post-endoscopic retrograde cholangiopancreatography pancreatitis. PANCREAS. 2014;43(2): 190–7.
23. Yaghoobi M, Rolland S, Waschke KA, McNabb-Baltar J, Martel M, Bijarchi R, Szego P, Barkun AN. Meta-analysis: rectal indomethacin for the prevention of post-ERCP pancreatitis. Aliment Pharmacol Ther. 2013;38(9):995–1001.
24. Puig I, Calvet X, Baylina M, Isava A, Sort P, Llao J, Porta F, Vida F. How and when should NSAIDs be used for preventing post-ERCP pancreatitis? a systematic review and meta-analysis. PLoS ONE. 2014;9(3):e92922.
25. Yuhara H, Ogawa M, Kawaguchi Y, Igarashi M, Shimosegawa T, Mine T. Pharmacologic prophylaxis of post-endoscopic retrograde cholangiopancreatography pancreatitis: protease inhibitors and NSAIDs in a meta-analysis. J GASTROENTEROL. 2014;49(3):388–99.
26. Sun HL, Han B, Zhai HP, Cheng XH, Ma K. Rectal NSAIDs for the prevention of post-ERCP pancreatitis: a meta-analysis of randomized controlled trials. Surgeon. 2014;12(3):141–7.
27. Zheng MH, Meng MB, Gu DN, Zhang L, Wu AM, Jiang Q, Chen YP. Effectiveness and tolerability of NSAIDs in the prophylaxis of pancreatitis after endoscopic retrograde cholangiopancreatography: A systematic review and meta-analysis. Curr Ther Res Clin Exp. 2009;70(4):323–34.
28. Elmunzer BJ, Waljee AK, Elta GH, Taylor JR, Fehmi SM, Higgins PD. A meta-analysis of rectal NSAIDs in the prevention of post-ERCP pancreatitis. Gut. 2008;57(9):1262–7.

8

Clinicopathological features and surgical outcomes of neuroendocrine tumors of ampulla of Vater

Kwangho Yang[1,2], Sung Pil Yun[3], Suk Kim[4], Nari Shin[5], Do Youn Park[6] and Hyung Il Seo[3*]

Abstract

Background: The study aims to investigate the clinicopathological features and surgical outcomes of neuroendocrine tumors of ampulla of Vater (NETAoVs) patients who underwent pancreaticoduodenectomy.

Methods: From January 2007 to December 2014, 45 patients underwent pancreaticoduodenectomy for malignant disease of the ampulla of Vater in our institution. Of those, 5 patients were diagnosed as neuroendocrine tumors. The data included age, sex, presenting symptoms, preoperative imaging, preoperative type of biopsy results, type of operation, pathologic findings and survival status.

Results: The patient's mean age was 55.2 ± 9.7 years. Endoscopic ultrasound guided biopsy was performed in 4 patients and gastroduodenoscopic biopsy was performed in one patient. All showed neuroendocrine tumor without mitosis. Mean tumor size was 1.9 ± 0.56 cm (range, 1.2–2.0 cm). Lymph node metastases were detected in two patients. All patients were synaptophysin-positive. Median periods of follow-up were 45 months (range, 43–78 months). Recurrence after operation occurred in two patients. 4 patients were alive at the last follow-up.

Conclusions: Radical resection for NETAoVs can provide the information of status of lymph node metastasis after surgery. However, correlation between lymph node metastasis and overall survival is uncertain to date.

Keywords: Neoplasms, Neuroendocrine tumors, Ampulla of Vater, Pancreaticoduodenectomy, Treatment outcome

Background

Neuroendocrine tumors of ampulla of Vater (NETAoVs) are uncommon. To date, only approximately 120 NETAoVs have been described in the literature, most in less 10 cases reports [1–5]. The incidence and prevalence of neuroendocrine tumor seems to have increased in recent years, most likely due to diagnostic technical improvements and endoscopic healthcare surveillance [6].

Computed tomography (CT), magnetic resonance imaging (MRI) and endoscopic ultrasound (EUS) guided biopsy are the main tools for preoperative examinations, but immunohistochemical staining assessment using biopsied specimen is important for diagnosis. There is no standard treatment for NETAoVs, because their natural history and prognostic factors remain unclear. In spite of long term survival has been reported after local excision, many surgeons favor pancreaticoduodenectomy due to the high incidence of lymph node metastasis [6, 7]. In this study, we report clinicopathological features and surgical outcomes of 5 NETAoVs patients who underwent pancreaticoduodenectomy.

Methods

From January 2007 to December 2014, 45 patients underwent pancreaticoduodenectomy for malignant disease of the ampulla of Vater in our institution. The surgeries were performed by the same operator. Of those, 5 patients were diagnosed as NETAoVs. The data included age, sex, presenting symptoms, preoperative imaging, preoperative type of biopsy results, type of operation, pathologic findings and survival status. CT and MRI were performed to assess the presence of locoregional lymph node metastases or distant metastases. The pathological data were assessed by the same pathologist,

* Correspondence: seohi71@hanmail.net
[3]Department of Surgery, Biomedical Research Institute, Pusan National University Hospital, 179, Gudeok-Ro, Seo-Gu, Busan 602-739, South Korea
Full list of author information is available at the end of the article

according to 2010 World Health Organization (WHO) classification, and 2006 European Neuroendocrine Tumour Society (ENETS) and the seventh edition International Union Against Cancer (UICC) staging systems [8–10] (Table 1). Immunohistochemical analysis included CD56, synaptophysin and chromogranin A expression, and the Ki67 index was assessed for histological grading. The study was reviewed and approved by the Pusan National University Hospital Institutional Review Board.

Table 1 Staging system for neuroendocrine tumor of the ampulla of Vater

WHO classification (2010)								
	Grade 1				<2 mitoses/10 HPF and <3% Ki–67			
	Grade 2				2–20 mitoses/10 HPF or 3–20% Ki–67			
	Grade 3				>20 mitoses/10 HPF or >20% Ki–67			
TNM staging system								
	ENETS (2006)				UICC (7th edition, 2009)			
T – primary tumor								
Tx	Primary tumour cannot be assessed							
T0	No evidence of primary tumour							
T1	Invasion of lamina propria or submucosa and size ≤ 1 cm				Limited to ampulla of Vater or sphincter of Oddi			
T2	Invasion of muscularis propria or size > 1 cm				Invasion of the duodenum wall			
T3	Invasion of the pancreas or retroperitoneum				Invasion of the pancreas			
T4	Invasion of the peritoneum or other organs				Invasion in peripancreatic soft tissues or other adjacent organs or structures			
N – regional lymph nodes								
Nx	Regional lymph nodes cannot be assessed							
N0	No regional lymph node metastasis							
N1	Regional lymph node metastasis present							
M – distant metastasis								
Mx	Distant metastasis cannot be assessed							
M0	No distant metastasis							
M1	Distant metastasis present							
Staging	Stage I	T1	N0	M0	Stage Ia	T1	N0	M0
	Stage IIa	T2	N0	M0	Stage Ib	T2	N0	M0
	Stage IIb	T3	N0	M0	Stage IIa	T3	N0	M0
	Stage IIIa	T4	N0	M0	Stage IIb	T1–3	N1	M0
	Stage IIIb	Any T	N1	M0	Stage III	T4	Any N	M0
	Stage IV	Any T	Any N	M1	Stage IV	Any T	Any N	M1

ENETS European Neuroendocrine Tumour Society staging system, *HPF* high power fields, *UICC* International Union Against Cancer staging system, *WHO* World Health Organisation classification

Results

Clinical findings and preoperative evaluation

The clinical features of the 5 patients are listed in Table 2. Mean age was 55.2 ± 9.7 years (range, 36–62 years) and the male to female ratio was 3:2. One patient presented with obstructive jaundice, which led to endoscopic retrograde cholangiopancreatography. In 4 patients, the tumor was discovered during gastroduodenoscopy as part of a regular medical check-up. No patient had specific neuroendocrine symptoms, and signs of Recklinghausen's disease or Zollinger-Ellison syndrome [11, 12]. EUS-guided biopsy was performed in 4 patients and gastroduodenoscopic biopsy was performed in one patient. Histologically, all cases displayed neuroendocrine tumor without mitosis.

CT scan using a hepatopancreatic protocol was performed in all patients and MRI was performed in 3 patients. The imaging procedures showed an enhanced mural or intramural mass. Only one patient showed dilatation of main pancreatic duct in imaging study. Liver metastases were not detected in any patient. Positron emission tomography-CT performed in 4 patients showed fluorodeoxyglucose uptake in all the patients (mean SUVmax 4.2, range; 2.5–7).

Treatment

Three patients underwent pylorus-preserving pancreaticoduodenectomy. The other two patients underwent conventional pancreaticoduodenectomy because severe adhesion between stomach and pancreas, and tumor invasion to duodenal first portion, respectively. Lymph node dissection was performed as standard extent for pancreas cancer. Duct-to-mucosa Pancreaticojejunostomy was performed in every case. There was no mortality. There were three minor complications (grade I or II according to Clavien-Dindo classification) including 2 delayed gastric emptying and a pancreas fistulae grade A. No patient was treated by radiological intervention or re-exploration. After surgery, adjuvant chemotherapy using etoposide-cisplatin intravenous administration with or without octreotide LAR intramuscular injection was done in 4 patients. Distant recurrence of NETAoVs occurred in 2 patients (case 2 and case 5). Case 2 suffered single liver metastasis at 10 months after surgery and underwent radiofrequency ablation for the lesion followed by chemotherapy with etoposide-cisplatin. However, multiple liver metastases still occurred and the patient expired at 67 months after surgery. Case 5 had multiple liver metastases at 11 months after surgery. This patient underwent chemotherapy with sunitinib and complete remission was achieved.

Table 2 Clinical features and outcomes of patients

Case	Sex	Age range	Symptom	L/N ratio	Biopsy result	Operation	Adjuvant CTx	Recurrence site	Treatment for recurrence	Survival outcome
1	Female	50–59	Incidental	62.1%	NET	PPPD	Yes	NED		78 months alive
2	Male	60–69	Jaundice	15.8%	NET	PPPD	Yes	Liver	RFA, CTx	67 months dead
3	Female	50–59	Incidental	40.9%	NET	PPPD	Yes	NED		45 months alive
4	Male	30–39	Incidental	52.7%	NET	PD	Yes	NED		44 months alive
5	Male	60–69	Incidental	23.4%	NET	PD	No	liver	CTx	43 months alive

CTx chemotherapy, *L/N ratio* lymphocyte/neutrophil ratio, *NED* no evidence of disease, *NET* neuroendocrine tumor, *PD* pancreaticoduodenectomy, *PPPD* pylorus preserving pancreaticoduodenectomy, *RFA* radiofrequency ablation

Pathology

All patients underwent R0 resection, which was defined as no residual tumor with negative surgical margin. The mean tumor size was 1.9 ± 0.56 cm (range, 1.2–2.0 cm). Lymph node metastases were detected in two patients. All patients were synaptophysin-positive, 2 were chromogranin-positive and 5 were CD56-positive. Lymphovascular invasion was observed in 3 patients and there was no perineural invasion in all patients. In case 2, the histological result was collision tumor accompanied with poorly differentiated neuroendocrine carcinoma at the deepest invasive portion and well differentiated adenocarcinoma at superficial portion (pT3). Neuroendocrine carcinoma accounted for 90% of the tumor mass, and adenocarcinoma 10% (Fig. 1). In this patient, liver metastases were confirmed as neuroendocrine tumor by needle biopsy 10 months after surgery. The immunohistochemical data of the 5 patients and tumor assessments according to the staging system are listed in Table 3.

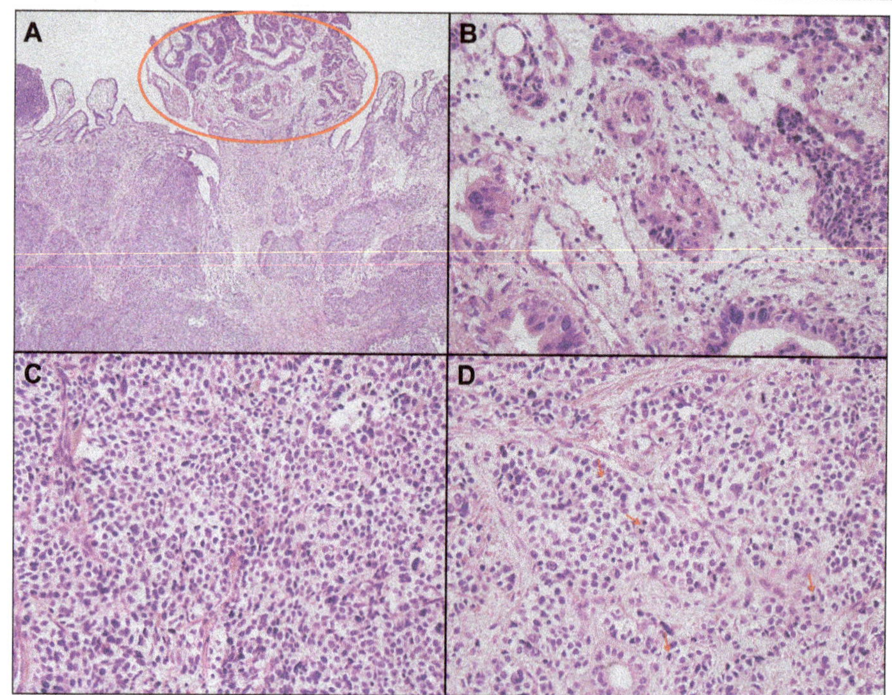

Fig. 1 Pathologic findings of collision tumor accompanied with neuroendocrine carcinoma and adenocarcinoma. **a** *Red circle*: adenocarcinoma, well-differentiated area. Tumor cells forming gland and showing infiltrative growth. Under area: solid tumor cell nest (H&E stain, ×40). **b** High power view of adenocarcinoma area (H&E stain, ×400). Atypical epithelial cells forming gland. **c** High power view of solid nest area (H&E stain, ×400). The tumor cell showing typical "salt and pepper" chromatin pattern which is compatible with neuroendocrine tumor cells. They are positive for neuroendocrine marker, synaptophysin and chromogranin in immunohistochemistry staining. **d** The neuroendocrine tumor area showing increased mitosis (*red arrow*), and increased Ki-67 index (about 70%) (H&E stain, ×400)

Table 3 Histopathological and immunohistochemical data and staging

Case	Size (cm)	Lymph node metastasis (n)	Mitosis (/10HPF)	Ki-67 (%)	Lymphovascular invasion	Perineural invasion	WHO	ENETS	UICC
1	2.2	No (0/12)	1	1	Yes	No	G1	IIA	IA
2	1.2	No (0/20)	102	70	Yes	No	G3	IIB	IIA
3	1.5	Yes (1/17)	5	3	No	No	G2	IIIB	IIB
4	2.6	Yes (4/20)	4	4	Yes	No	G2	IIIB	IIB
5	2.0	No (0/50)	1	5	No	No	G2	IIA	IB

ENETS European Neuroendocrine Tumour Society, *UICC* International Union Against Cancer, *WHO* World Health Organization

Survival

Median periods of follow-up were 45 months (range, 43–78 months), and complete follow-up data were available for all patients. Laboratory test and abdominal CT scan were performed every 3 months in the first 2 years after operation, and then every 6 months. Chest CT scan was performed once in a year to identify distant metastasis. 4 patients were alive at the last follow-up. Recurrence in the liver was observed in 2 patients. In these two patients, the Ki-67 index exceeded 5% and a low lymphocyte-neutrophil ratio was observed when compared to the other 3 patients (23.4% and 15.8% versus 52.7%, 40.9% and 62.1%).

Discussion

The small bowel is most common site of neuroendocrine tumor occur, however, neuroendocrine tumor very rarely occurs at the ampulla of Vater [13]. Neuroendocrine tumors originating in the duodenum represent merely 4% of all carcinoid tumors [14]. In the previous study of Randle et al., the proportion of neuroendocrine tumors from duodenum and ampulla of Vater were 92% and 8%, respectively [15]. The common clinical feature is jaundice, similar to other ampullary tumors. In some cases, patients complain of non-specific gastrointestinal symptoms [2, 5, 16]. In the latter, it is difficult to detect an ampulla of Vater tumor without performing endoscopy or other imaging studies. In the present study, these tumors were detecting during gastroduodenoscopy of medical check-up in 4 of 5 patients; the remaining patient had jaundice.

The diagnostic modalities for NETAoVs are same as those for ampullary adenocarcinoma. CT or MRI can reveal NETAoVs as a mural and intramural enhancing mass within the submucosal region [17]. For definite diagnosis, immunohistochemical staining is needed after tumor biopsy. Because of the finding of a submucosal tumor at the ampulla on endoscopy, the rate of preoperative histological diagnosis on endoscopic biopsy is low, ranging from 14 to 66% [2, 5, 13, 18]. In the present study, a correct diagnosis of NETAoVs without symptoms was confirmed preoperatively in 4 patients for a preoperative diagnostic accuracy of 100%; the excellent results reflected the use of EUS-guided biopsy. Therefore, EUS-guided biopsy is considered to be more useful than endoscopic biopsy alone in obtaining a preoperative accurate diagnosis [16]. However, mitosis count of biopsy specimen is an incorrect assessment at present, and requires refinement.

Previous studies reported that the incidence of lymph node metastases approaches 50%, which has led to the recommendation of pancreaticoduodenectomy as the procedure of choice for NETAoVs [5, 6, 13, 19–21]. Nodal involvement appears to be of lesser significance to long-term survival [5, 6, 16, 22, 23]. Because a more advanced stage does not predict a worse prognosis, the TNM and ENETS staging systems are limited in predicting prognosis. If lymph node metastasis is not a prognostic factor, endoscopic local resection or surgical ampullectomy might be available treatment options for selective patients with NETAoVs [2, 24, 25]. Although less radical operation may decrease postoperative complication rate and preserve pancreatic function, it has the risk of incomplete removal of metastatic lymph nodes [26]. Therefore, ampullectomy can be considered for the patients with well differentiated, slow-growing and small sized tumors, who cannot be tolerable for radical operation due to high surgical risk [5].

In this series, all the patients underwent pancreaticoduodenectomy. Lymph node metastasis occurred in 2 cases; both patients remain alive without recurrence. Under the WHO classification system, our cases consisted of one neuroendocrine tumor, 3 well differentiated neuroendocrine carcinomas and one poorly differentiated neuroendocrine carcinoma. Under the TNM staging system, we had two stage I, and three stage II. Under the ENETS system, we had three stage II, and two stage III. In this study, the Ki-67 index was 5 and 70% in two cases of liver metastases. Although it is difficult to downplay the importance of the Ki-67 index in neuroendocrine tumors, further research is needed for the prognostic significance of the Ki-67 index. Low lymphocyte/neutrophil ratio is a factor reducing disease-free survival [27]. In this study, low lymphocyte/neutrophil ratio appeared to be associated with early recurrence. However, due to the limited number of patients, statistical significance was doubtful.

There is no consensus regarding adjuvant treatment for NETAoVs. We have performed adjuvant chemotherapy for the patients who had lymphovascular invasion or lymph node. As a result, adjuvant chemotherapy was performed in 4 patients in this study. One patient among them and a patient without adjuvant chemotherapy experienced recurrence.

Conclusions

In conclusion, radical resection for NETAoVs can provide the information of status of lymph node metastasis after surgery. In present study, two of the five patients developed liver metastases within a year despite implementation of radical resection with lymph node dissection. This result suggests high aggressiveness of NETAoVs. However, correlation between lymph node metastasis and overall survival is uncertain to date due to lack of the number of NETAoVs. Regular medical check-up including gastroduodenoscopy may give a chance to detect and cure asymptomatic NETAoVs.

Abbreviations

CT: Computed tomography; EUS: Endoscopic ultrasound; MRI: Magnetic resonance imaging; NETAoV: Neuroendocrine tumors of ampulla of Vater

Acknowledgements

Not applicable.

Funding

This research received no specific grant.

Authors' contributions

KY performed data acquisition, analysis and interpretation of data, and drafted the manuscript; KY, SPY and HIS participated in the concept and design of the study; SK, NS and DYP supervised the manuscript for important intellectual content; KY and HIS critically revised the manuscript for important intellectual content. All authors read and approved the final manuscript.

Competing interests

The authors declare that they have no competing interests.

Consent for publication

Not applicable.

Author details

[1]Department of Surgery, Division of Hepato-Biliary-Pancreatic Surgery and Transplantation, Pusan National University Yangsan Hospital, 20, Geumo-ro, Mulgeum-eup, Yangsan, Gyeongsangnam-do 50612, South Korea. [2]Research Institute for Convergence of Biomedical Science and Technology, Pusan National University Yangsan Hospital, 20, Geumo-ro, Mulgeum-eup, Yangsan, Gyeongsangnam-do 50612, South Korea. [3]Department of Surgery, Biomedical Research Institute, Pusan National University Hospital, 179, Gudeok-Ro, Seo-Gu, Busan 602-739, South Korea. [4]Department of Radiology, Biomedical Research Institute, Pusan National University Hospital, 179, Gudeok-Ro, Seo-Gu, Busan 602-739, South Korea. [5]Department of Pathology, Pusan National University Yangsan Hospital, 20, Geumo-ro, Mulgeum-eup, Yangsan, Gyeongsangnam-do 50612, South Korea. [6]Department of Pathology, Biomedical Research Institute, Pusan National University Hospital, 179, Gudeok-Ro, Seo-Gu, Busan 602-739, South Korea.

References

1. Hatzitheoklitos E, Büchler MW, Friess H, Poch B, Ebert M, Mohr W, et al. Carcinoid of the ampulla of vater. Clinical characteristics and morphologic features. Cancer. 1994;73:1580–8.
2. Hartel M, Wente MN, Sido B, Friess H, Büchler MW. Carcinoid of the ampulla of Vater. J Gastroenterol Hepatol. 2005;20:676–81.
3. Waisberg J, Matos LLD, Waisberg DR, Santos HVBD, Fernezlian SM, Capelozzi VL. Carcinoid of the minor duodenal papilla associated with pancreas divisum: case report and review of the literature. Clinics. 2006;61:365–8.
4. Emory RE Jr, Emory TS, Goellner JR, Grant CS, Nagorney DM. Neuroendocrine ampullary tumors: spectrum of disease including the first report of a neuroendocrine carcinoma of non-small cell type. Surgery. 1994;115:762–6.
5. Carter JT, Grenert JP, Rubenstein L, Stewart L, Way LW. Neuroendocrine tumors of the ampulla of Vater: biological behavior and surgical management. Arch Surg. 2009;144:527–31.
6. Dumitrascu T, Dima S, Herlea V, Tomulescu V, Ionescu M, Popescu I. Neuroendocrine tumours of the ampulla of Vater: clinico-pathological features, surgical approach and assessment of prognosis. Langenbeck's Arch Surg. 2012; 397:933–43.
7. Nikfarjam M, McLean C, Muralidharan V, Christophi C. Neuroendocrine tumours of the ampulla of Vater. ANZ J Surg. 2002;72:531–3.
8. Bosman FT, Carneiro F, Hruban RH, Theise ND. WHO classification of tumours of the digestive system: World Health Organization, 2010.
9. Rindi G, Klöppel G, Alhman H, Caplin M, Couvelard A, de Herder WW, et al. TNM staging of foregut (neuro) endocrine tumors: a consensus proposal including a grading system. Virchows Arch. 2006;449:395–401.
10. Sobin LH, Gospodarowicz MK, Wittekind C. International Union Against Cancer. TNM Classification of Malignant Tumours. 7th ed. Oxford: Wiley-Blackwell; 2009.
11. Mayoral W, Salcedo J, Al-Kawas F. Ampullary carcinoid tumor presenting as acute pancreatitis in a patient with von Recklinghausen's disease: case report and review of the literature. Endoscopy. 2003;35:854–7.
12. Åkerström G. Management of carcinoid tumors of the stomach, duodenum, and pancreas. World J Surg. 1996;20:173–82.
13. Hwang S, Lee SG, Lee YJ, Han DJ, Kim SC, Kwon SH, et al. Radical surgical resection for carcinoid tumors of the ampulla. J Gastrointest Surg. 2008;12:713–7.
14. Yao JC, Hassan M, Phan A, Dagohoy C, Leary C, Mares JE, et al. One hundred years after "carcinoid": epidemiology of and prognostic factors for neuroendocrine tumors in 35,825 cases in the United States. J Clin Oncol. 2008;26:3063–72.
15. Randle RW, Ahmed S, Newman NA, Clark CJ. Clinical outcomes for neuroendocrine tumors of the duodenum and ampulla of Vater: a population-based study. J Gastrointest Surg. 2014;18:354–62.
16. Jayant M, Punia R, Kaushik R, Sharma R, Sachdev A, Nadkarni NK, et al. Neuroendocrine Tumors of the Ampulla of Vater: Presentation, Pathology and Prognosis. JOP. 2012;13:263–7.
17. Yano F, Hama Y, Abe K, Iwasaki Y, Hatsuse K, Kusano S. Carcinoid tumor of the ampulla of Vater: Magnetic resonance imaging findings. Clin Imaging. 2005;29:207–10.
18. Kim J, Lee WJ, Lee SH, Lee KB, Ryu JK, Kim YT, et al. Clinical features of 20 patients with curatively resected biliary neuroendocrine tumours. Dig Liver Dis. 2011;43:965–70.
19. Albores-Saavedra J, Hart A, Chablé-Montero F, Henson DE. Carcinoids and high-grade neuroendocrine carcinomas of the ampulla of vater: a comparative analysis of 139 cases from the surveillance, epidemiology, and end results program-a population based study. Arch Pathol Lab Med. 2010; 134:1692–6.

20. Cokmert S, Demir L, Akder Sari A, Kucukzeybek Y, Can A, Akyol M, et al. Synchronous Appearance of a High-Grade Neuroendocrine Carcinoma of the Ampulla Vater and Sigmoid Colon Adenocarcinoma. Case reports in oncological medicine. 2013:2013:4. Article ID 930359. http://dx.doi.org/10.1155/2013/930359.
21. Selvakumar E, Rajendran S, Balachandar TG, Kannan DG, Jeswanth S, Ravichandran P, et al. Neuroendocrine carcinoma of the ampulla of Vater: a clinicopathologic evaluation. Hepatobiliary Pancreat Dis Int. 2008;7:422–5.
22. Pyun DK, Han JM, Lee SS, Kim MH, Lee SS, Seo DW, et al. Case Reports: A Carcinoid Tumor of the Ampulla of Vater Treated by Endoscopic Snare Papillectomy. Korean J. Intern. Med. 2004;19:257–60.
23. Sakka N, Smith RA, Whelan P, Ghaneh P, Sutton R, Raraty M, et al. A preoperative prognostic score for resected pancreatic and periampullary neuroendocrine tumours. Pancreatology. 2009;9:670–6.
24. Rattner DW, CF-d C, Brugge WR, Warshaw AL. Defining the criteria for local resection of ampullary neoplasms. Arch Surg. 1996;131:366–71.
25. Salmi S, Ezzedine S, Vitton V, Ménard C, Gonzales JM, Desjeux A, et al. Can papillary carcinomas be treated by endoscopic ampullectomy? Surg Endosc. 2012;26:920–5.
26. Krishna SG, Lamps LW, Rego RF. Ampullary carcinoid: diagnostic challenges and update on management. Clin Gastroenterol Hepatol. 2010;8:e5–6.
27. Garcea G, Ladwa N, Neal C, Metcalfe MS, Dennison AR, Berry DP. Preoperative neutrophil-to-lymphocyte ratio (NLR) is associated with reduced disease-free survival following curative resection of pancreatic adenocarcinoma. World J Surg. 2011;35:868–72.

9

Protective effects of heme oxygenase-1 against severe acute pancreatitis via inhibition of tumor necrosis factor-α and augmentation of interleukin-10

Fei-hu Zhang[1], Yu-han Sun[2], Kai-liang Fan[1], Xiao-bin Dong[1], Ning Han[1], Hao Zhao[1] and Li Kong[1*]

Abstract

Background: Heme oxygenase-1 (HO-1) is an inducible defense gene which plays a significant role in inflammation. HO-1 protects cells and tissues through the mechanism of anti-oxidation, maintaining microcirculation and anti-inflammation. The aim of the current study is to investigate the role of HO-1 on systemic inflammatory response in severe acute pancreatitis (SAP).

Methods: Forty male Sprague-Dawley (SD) rats were randomly assigned into four groups: control group (n = 10); SAP group (n = 10), SAP model was induced by retrograde injection of 3% sodium taurocholate through pancreatic duct; HO-1 stimulation group (n = 10), SD rats were injected 75 μg/kg hemin intraperitoneally 30 min after induction of SAP; HO-1 inhibition group (n = 10), SD rats were injected 20 μg/kg Zinc porphyrin (Zn-PP) intraperitoneally 30 min after induction of SAP. After 24 h of SAP establishment, tissues were collected for HO-1, tumor necrosis factor-α (TNF-α) and interleukin-10 (IL-10) mRNA expression, and blood samples were collected for cytokines and biochemical measurements. Meanwhile, the histopathological changes of pancreas and liver tissues were observed.

Results: The expression of HO-1 mRNA and protein were significantly induced by SAP in rat pancreas and liver. Hemin treatment significantly decreased oxidative stress and TNF-α in plasma and tissues, while the IL-10 was significantly increased. Pancreas and liver injury induced by SAP was markedly attenuated by Hemin treatment. Moreover, inhibition of HO-1 expression by Zn-PP administration aggravated the injury caused by SAP.

Conclusions: Induction of HO-1 in early SAP may modulate systemic inflammatory response and prevent pancreas and nearby organs such as liver injury through inhibition of TNF-α and augmentation of IL-10.

Keywords: Heme oxygenase-1, Severe acute pancreatitis, Oxidative stress, Tumor necrosis factor-α, Interleukin-10

Background

Acute pancreatitis (AP), with a reported annual incidence of 13 ~ 45 cases per 100,000 people [1], and the mortality is up to 30% in severe cases [2], is one of the most common gastrointestinal disorders. It is widely accepted that inflammation plays a pivotal role in the pathogenesis of severe acute pancreatitis (SAP). The early acinar cell injury in SAP causes local inflammation, which subsequently activates the immune system inappropriately and eventually results in multiple organs dysfunction syndrome (MODS) [3]. Thus, the therapy strategy targeting to inhibit the pro-inflammatory cytokines and boost the anti-inflammatory cytokines attached much attention and might be an effective way for the treatment of SAP [4].

Several studies have demonstrated that heat shock proteins (HSPs) can inhibit both intrinsic and extrinsic pathways of apoptosis at multiple sites [5]. HSPs, which express in a variety of cells against stress and injury

* Correspondence: kongli_sdszyy@sina.com
[1]Department of Emergency Center, Affiliated Hospital of Shandong University of Traditional Chinese Medicine, Jingshi Road No.16369, Jinan, Shandong Province 250011, China

inciting stimulis, belong to a family of proteins which are highly conserved. Recent studies indicated that some HSPs, such as HSP-32/heme oxygenase-1 (HO-1), play important roles in the pathogenesis of SAP and some other several immune-mediated inflammatory diseases [6]. HO-1 (also referred to as HSP-32), an inducible isoform of heme oxygenase, catalyzes the degradation of heme into carbon monoxide (CO), iron and biliverdin [7]. Iron is sequestered by ferritin, and biliverdin is subsequently converted to bilirubin. Because of the anti-oxidization, anti-apoptotic, anti-proliferative, and anti-inflammatory effects of heme metabolites, HO-1 has been emerged as an important cytoprotective enzyme. Some studies showed that both transgenic overexpression and pharmacological activation of HO-1 alleviated and eventually eliminated the oxidative cell damage that occurs in some disease states [8]. Also, HO-1 plays an important role in mediating the pro-inflammatory effect of TNF-α and the anti-inflammatory effect of IL-10 [9, 10]. However, the role of HO-1 in the exocrine pancreas and its potential modulation role in pancreatic injury are still not fully elucidated [11].

In this study, we evaluated the effect of HO-1 on systemic inflammatory mediators: TNF-α and IL-10. Further research on the protective effects of HO-1 against SAP is necessary because it may be useful to improve organs function and survival rate via genetic or pharmacological strategies in SAP.

Methods

Animal ethics statement and experimental protocol

All animal experiments were conducted in accordance with the guidelines of the Shandong Committee on Animal Care of China which approved the study protocol. Male Sprague-Dawley (SD) rats weighting 220 g to 260 g were purchased from the Shandong Experimental Animal Center of Chinese Academy Science. All rats were housed in a temperature controlled (25 ± 1 °C) room under a 12-h light/12-h dark cycle with free access to drinking water and chow diet. Forty healthy male SD rats were randomly assigned into four groups: control group; SAP group; HO-1 stimulation group, Hemin (75 μg/kg; Sigma Chemical, St. Louis, MO) [12] was injected intraperitoneally 30 min after induction of SAP; and HO-1 inhibition group, Zn-PP (20 μg/kg; Sigma Chemical, St. Louis, MO) [9] was injected intraperitoneally 30 min after induction of SAP. Rats were anesthetized with sodium pentobarbital (40 mg/kg, intraperitoneally) and sacrificed 24 h after SAP establishment. Blood samples collected from the celiac artery were centrifuged and the serum were stored at −80 °C for the analysis of Amylase, Lipase, Alanine aminotransferase (ALT), Aspartate aminotransferase (AST), HO-1, TNF-α and IL-10 level. Pancreas and liver were immediately dissected from their attachments and divided for total RNA extraction. Portions of pancreas and liver were fixed in 40 g/L buffered formaldehyde for histological test.

Establishment of SAP model

Rats were anesthetized by intraperitoneal injection with sodium pentobarbital (40 mg/kg; Sigma Chemical, St. Louis, MO). Rats were then retrogradely injected 3% sodium taurocholate (0.1 mL/100 g; Sigma Chemical, St. Louis, MO) through pancreatic duct and the pressure was maintained for 5 min [3].

Measurement of HO-1, TNF-α and IL-10

The serum levels of HO-1, TNF-α and IL-10 were determined using enzyme-linked immunosorbent assay (ELISA) kits (EIAab, Shanghai, China) [3]. The mRNA levels of HO-1, TNF-α and IL-10 in tissues were determined using real-time PCR as described before and determined by the data from the real-time PCR instrument (ABI7900, Applied Biosystems, Foster City, CA) [3]. Briefly, total RNA was extracted from tissues with TRIzol reagent following the manufacturer's instructions and aliquots of 5 μg of total RNA were reverse-transcribed using the first-strand cDNA synthesis kit (Promega A3500, Madison, WI) [3]. The cDNA was then amplified by polymerase chain reaction using specific primers for HO-1, TNF-α and IL-10, and β-actin was used as internal control [3]. The primers used were in Table 1. PCR reactions were performed under the following conditions: denaturation at 95 °C for 15 s, annealing at 60 °C for 20 s and extension at 72 °C for 30 s [3].

Serum biochemical assays

The serum levels of Amylase, Lipase, ALT and AST were measured using automatic biochemical analyzer (UniCel DxC800, Beckman Coulter, CA) following the instructions.

Histopathological analysis

Paraffin-embedded pancreas and liver were cut into 5 μm thick sections, and stained with hematoxylin and eosin for light microscopic examination as described before [3]. Histological assessment was performed by an investigator blind to group assignment, and the pathological scores of pancreas and liver samples were determined by the standard of Schmidt et al. [13] and Sass et al. [14].

Table 1 PCR primer sequences (5′-3′)

Gene	Forward primer	Reverse primer
HO-1	ACCCCACCAAGTTCAAACAG	GAGCAGGAAGGCGGTCTTAG
TNF-α	CCCAATCTGTGTCCTTCTAACT	CACTACTTCAGCGTCTCGTGT
IL-10	GGCTCAGCACTGCTATGTTGCC	AGCATGTGGGTCTGGCTGACTG
β-actin	TGGTGGGTATGGGTCAGAAG	GACAATGCCGTGTTCAATGG

Statistical analysis

Data were analyzed using SPSS 16.0 software. All data in text and figures were expressed as mean ± SEM, and results were compared using the one-way analysis of variance followed by Tukey's test and unpaired Student's t test. A $p<0.05$ was considered to be statistically significant.

Results

Differential expression patterns of HO-1, TNF-α and IL-10 in serum, pancreas and liver

Compared with the control rats, the HO-1, TNF-α and IL-10 levels in serum and also the mRNA levels in pancreas and liver were significantly increased by SAP after 24 h of surgery ($p<0.05$) (Fig. 1a–i). While hemin administration significantly increased HO-1 and IL-10 levels both in serum and in pancreas and liver ($p<0.05$) (Fig. 1a–h). Though hemin administration increased TNF-α in serum and its mRNA expressions in pancreas and liver ($p<0.05$) (Fig. 1c–i), it significantly decreased TNF-α induced by SAP after 24 h of surgery ($p<0.05$) (Fig. 1c–i). In addition, Zn-PP treatment increased HO-1 and IL-10 both in serum and in pancreas and liver ($p<0.05$) (Fig. 1a–h). However, Zn-PP treatment significantly decreased HO-1 and IL-10 level in serum, pancreas and liver induced by SAP ($p<0.05$) (Fig. 1a–h). Moreover, Zn-PP

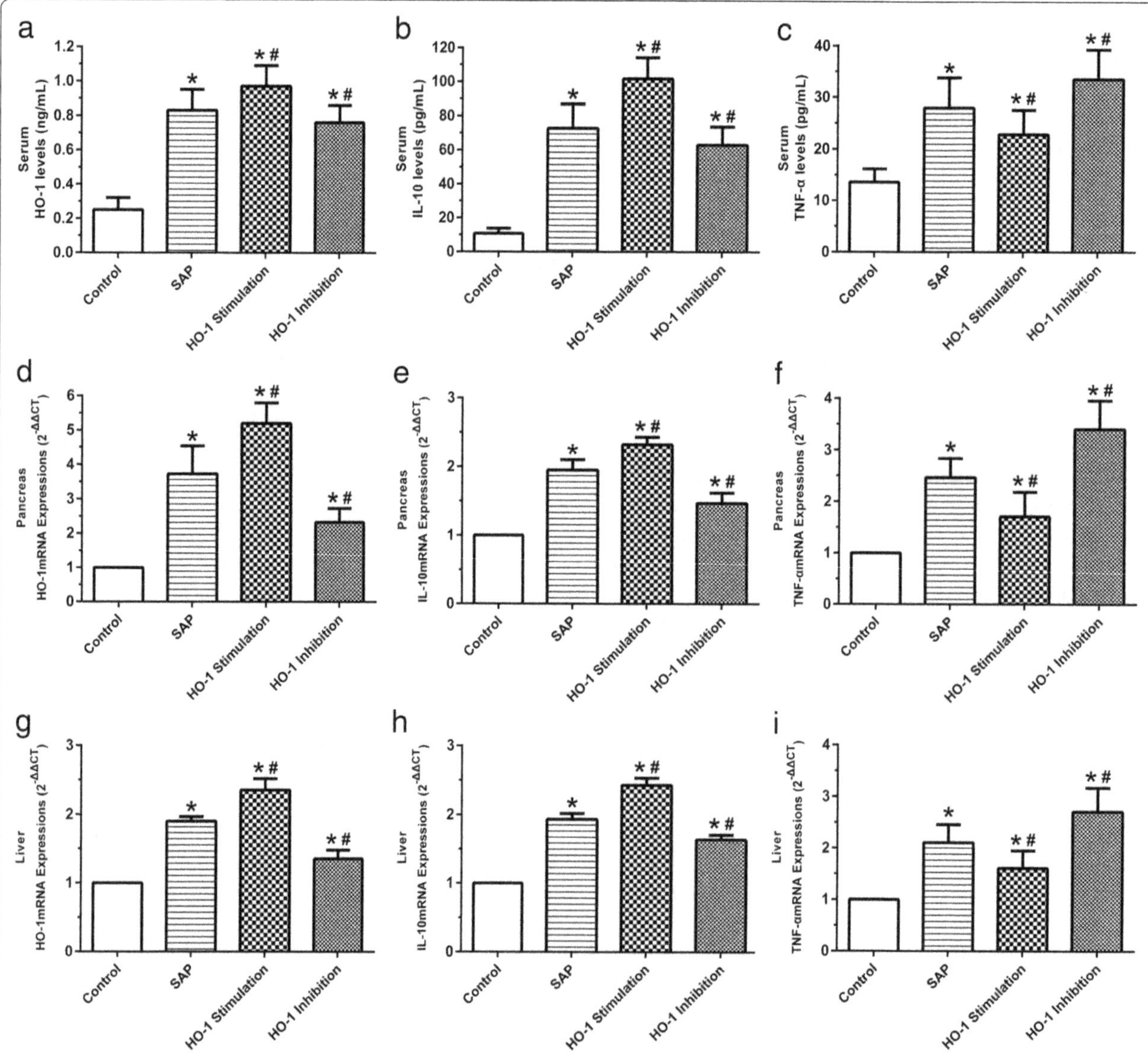

Fig. 1 Differential expression patterns of HO-1, IL-10 and TNF-α in serum, pancreas and liver after 24 h of SAP surgery. **a,** HO-1 levels in serum; **b,** IL-10 levels in serum; **c,** TNF-α levels in serum; **d,** HO-1mRNA expressions in pancreas; **e,** IL-10mRNA expressions in pancreas; **f,** TNF-αmRNA expressions in pancreas; **g,** HO-1mRNA expressions in liver; **h,** IL-10mRNA expressions in liver; **i,** TNF-αmRNA expressions in liver. Data are presented as mean ± SEM (n = 10). $^*p < 0.05$, compared with the control group; $^\#p < 0.05$, compared with the SAP group

administration increased TNF-α in the serum and the expressions of TNF-αmRNA in the pancreas and liver (p<0.05) (Fig. 1c–i).

Levels of biochemical parameters in serum

The levels of Amylase, Lipase, ALT and AST in the serum were significantly induced by SAP after 24 h of surgery (p<0.05) (Fig. 2a–d). Although hemin treatment increased the Amylase, Lipase, ALT and AST in the serum (p<0.05) (Fig. 2a–d), it significantly decreased these markers induced by SAP (p<0.05) (Fig. 2a–d). On the other hand, Zn-PP treatment significantly increased the level of Amylase, Lipase, ALT and AST in the serum (p<0.05) (Fig. 2a–d).

Histopathological evaluation and scores of pancreas and livers

The structure of pancreas of control rats showed morphologically normal, while the pancreas of SAP rats displayed partly hemorrhage, necrosis and infiltration of neutrophile granulocyte. Heme admistraton relieved pathological damage in pancreas caused by SAP, including the integrity of pancreatic duct and less infiltration of neutrophile granulocyte, while Zn-PP treatment caused more severe pathological pancreas damages including large scale pancreatic and vascular necrosis as well as mass infiltration of neutrophile granulocyte (Fig. 3a–d). The pathological scores were significantly reduced by stimulation of HO-1, whereas enhanced by inhibition of HO-1(p<0.05) (Fig. 3e).

The hepatic cells in control rats, showing morphologically normal, were observed in cord-like arrangement, and the structure of hepatic lobe was clear. While the cytoplasm became loosened, and the Kupffer cell proliferated in hepatic sinusoid in SAP rats. There were less Kupffer cells in sinusoid and the morphology of the hepatic cells was normal after heme admistration. In addition, the hepatocytes showed spotty necrosis with more loosened cytoplasm and lymphocyte infiltration after Zn-PP treatment (Fig. 3f–i). HO-1 stimulation significantly reduced the pathological scores induced by SAP, while HO-1 inhibition by Zn-PP significantly enhanced the pathological scores. (p<0.05) (Fig. 3j).

Discussion

Acute pancreatitis (AP), with severe complications and high mortality under severe condition which called SAP, is an inflammatory condition of the

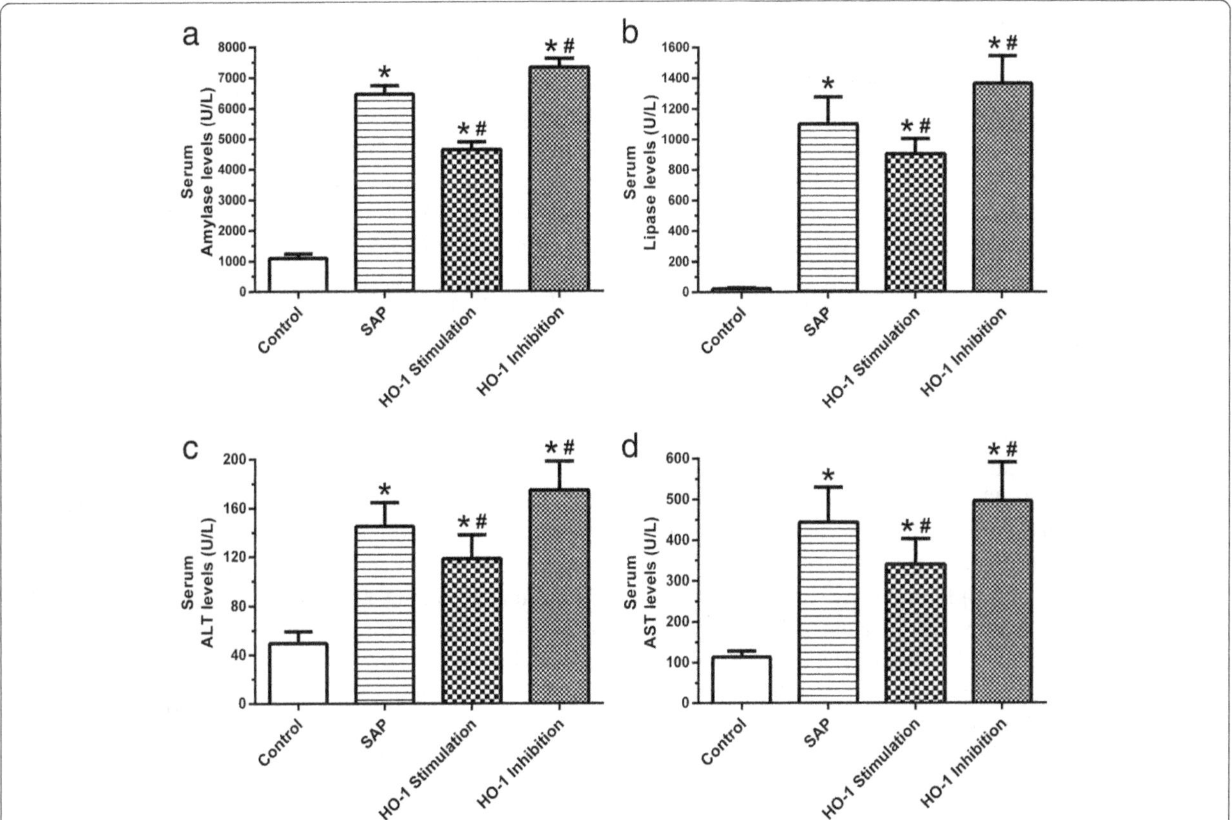

Fig. 2 Levels of Amylase, Lipase, ALT and AST in serum after 24 h of SAP surgery. **a,** Amylase levels in serum; **b,** Lipase levels in serum; **c,** ALT levels in serum; **d,** AST levels in serum. Data are presented as mean ± SEM (n = 10). $^{*}p$ < 0.05, compared with the control group; $^{\#}p$ < 0.05, compared with the SAP group

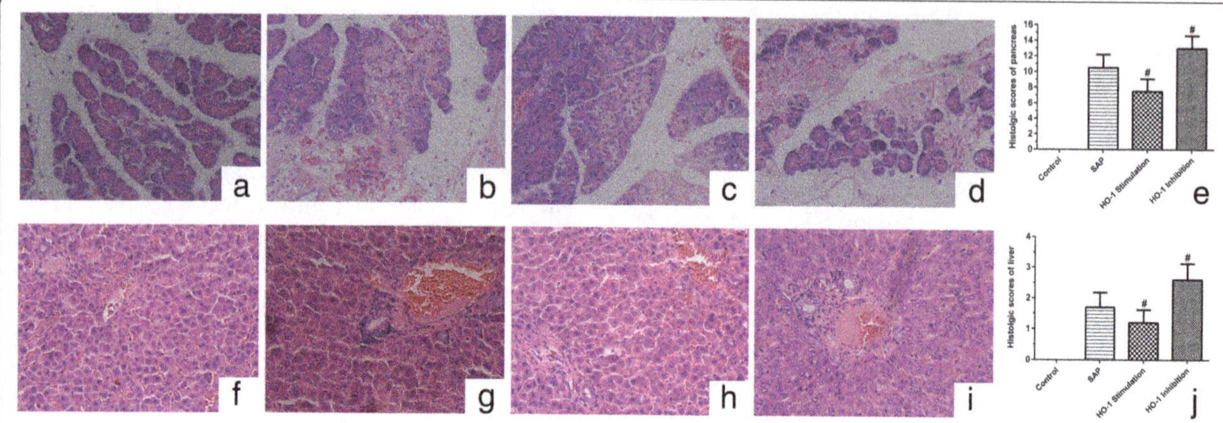

Fig. 3 Histopathological evaluation of pancreas and livers after 24 h of SAP surgery (HE × 400). **a**, pancreas of control group; **b**, pancreas of SAP group; **c**, pancreas of HO-1 stimulation group; **d**, pancreas of HO-1 inhibition group; **e**, pathological scores of pancreas; **f**, liver of control group; **g**, liver of SAP group; **h**, liver of HO-1 stimulation group; **i**, liver of HO-1 inhibition group; **j**, pathological scores of liver. Pathological scores are presented as mean ± SEM ($n = 10$). $^{\#}p < 0.05$, compared with the SAP group

pancreas. A manifestation of the inflammatory response is a hallmark of AP. In early SAP, the acinar cell injury causes the pancreatic cells secret inflammatory mediators like TNF-α and IL-10, which extend the inflammatory response and cause the organ injury. Our study showed that in the early stage of SAP, the HO-1 gene expression increased in the pancreas and liver. Also, induction of HO-1 by hemin treatment significantly increased plasma IL-10 and also decreased TNF-α, which modulated the inflammatory reaction, oxidative damage, and organs injury. These results demonstrated the beneficial effects of HO-1 in early SAP through mediating the systemic inflammatory response, indicating that HO-1 plays an important role in protecting pancreas and nearby organs from injury under SAP [3, 11, 15–17].

SAP is associated with the induction of several cytokines, including pro-inflammatory and anti-inflammatory mediators [18–20]. Some studies have demonstrated that TNF-α, which is secreted by activated macrophage and lymphocyte, plays an important role in the occurrence and development of SAP [21]. Induction of TNF-α subsequently induces the expression and secretion of IL-6, IL-8 as well as itself, causing the inflammatory cascade and the uncontrolled releasing of inflammatory mediators [18], which eventually cause the organs failure or even death. In contrast, IL-10, which is produced by macrophages, Th2 cells, hepatocytes and stellate cells, has the anti-inflammation effect in inflammatory diseases [22]. IL-10 inhibits the synthesis of pro-inflammatory cytokines, such as IL-2, IL-3 and TNF-α, and also prevents MODS caused by SAP [20, 23]. In our study, induction of HO-1 by Hemin in early SAP significantly decreased TNF-α in plasma and tissues, while the plasma and tissues IL-10 level was increased. In contrast, inhibition of HO-1 expression by Zn-PP treatment increased TNF-α and decreased IL-10 in plasma and tissues. So, it suggested that HO-1 plays a protective role in SAP through anti-inflammatory pathways. The heme metabolites catalyzed by HO-1 have anti-inflammatory effects through induction of IL-10 [10, 24]. It is still need to illuminate whether the protective effects of HO-1 in SAP is attributed to its metabolites, CO or the antioxidant bilirubin [25–28]. Dependent on the modulation of p38 mitogen-activated protein kinase (MAPK), CO showed anti-inflammation effect through inhibition of pro-inflammatory cytokines production [29, 30]. Our data demonstrated that the induction of HO-1 in early SAP can inhibit the inflammatory response through mediating the cytokines production and mitigate the damage to pancreas and nearby organs such as liver, indicating that HO-1 may function as therapeutic target for the treatment of SAP.

HO-1 is a stress-inducible enzyme which catalyzes the degradation of heme into CO, iron and biliverdin [7]. Under oxidative stress, such as inflammation and ischemia-reperfusion, HO-1 is induced and protects organs from damage, which in part by the anti-inflammatory effect of heme metabolites [31–35]. The expression of genes responsible for oxidative stress, especially HO-1 [16, 36, 37], are remarkably upregulated in the course of SAP, which suggests the existence of a compensatory mechanism against stress. Like most of the antioxidants, which protect organs from oxidative stress caused apoptosis and failure [38–40], hemin treatment induced HO-1 expression in early SAP and mitigated pancreas injury caused by oxidative stress and inflammation. In contrast, inhibition of HO-1 expression by Zn-PP aggravated the organs injury in SAP. These results indicated that induction of HO-1 in SAP may provide a new and effective therapeutic strategy for SAP.

Conclusions

In summary, our study demonstrated that HO-1 induction mitigated the pancreas injury through decreasing oxidative stress and TNF-α production, and also increasing IL-10 production in SAP. HO-1 overexpression also decreased the markers associated with pancreas and liver injury. Induction of HO-1 in early SAP, which reduced systemic inflammatory response and organs injury, may provide a new and effective therapeutic treatment for SAP.

Abbreviations

ALT: Alanine aminotransferase; AP: acute pancreatitis; AST: Aspartate aminotransferase; CO: carbon monoxide; ELISA: enzyme-linked immunosorbent assay; HO: Heme oxygenase; HSPs: heat shock proteins; IL: Interleukin; MAPK: mitogen-activated protein kinase; MODS: multiple organs dysfunction syndrome; SAP: severe acute pancreatitis; SD: Sprague-Dawley; TNF: Tumor necrosis factor; Zn-PP: Zinc porphyrin

Acknowledgements

Not applicable.

Funding

This study was supported by National Natural Science Foundation of China (No. 81503543) and Shandong Provincial Natural Science Foundation, China (No. ZR2015HL058).

Authors' contributions

FHZ and YHS drafted the manuscript. FHZ and LK conceived of the study, and participated in the design of the study. FHZ and KLF participated in the surgical procedure. XBD, NH and HZ carried out the histopathological analysis and serum biochemical assays. FHZ and XBD carried out the ELISA and real-time PCR. NH and HZ performed the statistical analysis. All authors have read and approved the final manuscript.

Consent for publication

Not applicable.

Competing interests

The authors declare that they have no competing interests.

Author details

[1]Department of Emergency Center, Affiliated Hospital of Shandong University of Traditional Chinese Medicine, Jingshi Road No.16369, Jinan, Shandong Province 250011, China. [2]Department of Traditional Chinese Medicine, Jinan Municipal Organs Hospital, Jianguoxiaojingsan Road No.35, Jinan, Shandong Province 250001, China.

References

1. Yadav D, Lowenfels AB. The epidemiology of pancreatitis and pancreatic cancer. Gastroenterology. 2013;144(6):1252–61.
2. Working Group IAP/APA Acute Pancreatitis Guidelines. IAP/APA evidence-based guideline for the management of acute pancreatitis. Pancreatology. 2013;13:e1–15.
3. Zhang F, Fei J, Zhao B, Chen E, Mao E. Protective effect of adenoviral transfer of heme oxygenase-1 gene on rats with severe acute pancreatitis. Am J Med Sci. 2014;348(3):224–31.
4. Anand N, Park JH, Wu BU. Modern management of acute pancreatitis. Gastroenterol Clin N Am. 2012;41(1):1–8.
5. Moretti AI, Rios EC, Soriano FG, de Souza HP, Abatepaulo F, Barbeiro DF, Velasco IT. Acute pancreatitis hypertonic saline increases heat shock proteins 70 and 90 and reduces neotrophil infiltration in lung injury. Pancreas. 2009;38(5):507–14.
6. Saluja A, Deduja V. Heat shock proteins in pancreatic diseaes. J Gastroenterol Hepatol. 2008;23:S42–5.
7. Nakamichil I, Habtezion A, Zhong B, Contag CH, Butcher EC, Omary MB. Hemin-activated macrophages home to the pancreas and protect from acute pancreatitis via heme oxygenase-1 induction. J Clin Invest. 2005;115: 3007–14.
8. Abraham NG, Asija A, Drummond G, Peterson S. Heme oxygenase-1 gene therapy : recent advances and therapeutic applications. Curr Gene Ther. 2007;7(2):89–108.
9. Tamion F, Richard V, Renet S, Thuillez C. Protective effects of heme-oxgenase expression against endotoxic shock: inhibition of tumor necrosis factor-alpha and augmentation of interleukin-10. J Trauma. 2006;61(5):1078–84.
10. Lee TS, Chau LY. Heme oxygenase-1 mediates the anti-inflammatory effect of interleukin-10 in mice. Nature Med. 2002;8:240–6.
11. Gulla A, Evans BJ, Navenot JM, Pundzius J, Barauskas G, Gulbinas A, Dambrauskas Z, Arafat H, Wang ZX. Heme oxygenase-1 gene promoter polymorphism is associateed with the development of necrotizing acute pancreatitis. Pancreas. 2014;43(8):1271–6.
12. Pellacani A, Wiesel P, Sharma A, Foster LC, Huggins GS, Yet SF, Perrella MA. Induction of heme oxygenase-1 during endotoxemia is downregulated by transforming growth factor-betal. Circ Res. 1998;83(4):396–403.
13. Schmidt J, Rattner DW, Lewandrowski K, Compton CC, Mandavilli U, Knoefel WT, Warshaw AL. A better model of acute pancreatitis for evaluating therapy. Ann Surg. 1992;215:44–56.
14. Sass G, Barikbin R, Tiegs G. The multiple functions of heme oxygenase-1 in the liver. Z Gastroenterol. 2012;50(1):34–40.
15. Zhu X, Fan WG, Li DP, Kung H, Lin MC. Heme oxygenase-1 system and gastronintestinal inflammation: a short review. World J Gastroenterol. 2011; 17(38):4283–8.
16. Saruc M, Yuceyar H, Turkel N, Ozutemiz O, Tuzcuoglu I, Ayhan S, Yuce G, Coker I, Huseyino A. The role of heme in hemolysis-induced acute pancreatitis. Med Sci Monit. 2007;13(3):BR67–72.
17. Castilho A, Aveleira CA, Leal EC, Simoes NF, Fernandes CR, Meirinhos RI, Baptista FI, Ambrosio AF. Heme oxygenase-1 protects retinal endothelial cells against high glucose- and oxidative/nitrosative stress-induced toxicity. PLoS One. 2012;7(8):e42428.
18. Malleo G, Mazzon E, Siriwardena AK, Cuzzocrea S. Role of tumor necrosis factor-alpha in avute pancreatitis: from biological basia to clinical evidence. Shock. 2007;28(2):130–40.
19. Bishehsari F, Sharma A, Stello K, Toth C, O'Connell MR, Evans AC, LaRusch J, Muddana V, Papachristou GI, Whitcomb DC. TNF-alpha gene (TNFA) variants increase risk for muti-origan dysfunction syndrome (MODS) in acute pancreatitis. Pancreatology. 2012;12(2):113–8.
20. Rongione AJ, Kusske AM, Kwan K, Ashley SW, Reber HA, McFadden DW. Interleukin 10 reduces the severity of acute pancreatitis in rats. Gastroenterology. 1997;112(3):960–7.
21. Grewal HP, Mohey el Din A, Gaber L, Kotb M, Gaber AO. Amelirorationof the physiologic and biochemical changes of acute pancreatitis using an anti-TNF-alpha polyclonal antibody. Am J Surg. 1994;167(1):214–8.
22. De Vries JE. Immunosuppressive and anti-inflammatory properties of interleukin 10. Ann Med. 1995;27(5):537–41.

23. Chen ZQ, Tang YQ, Zhang Y, Jiang ZH, Mao EQ, Zou WG, Lei RQ, Han TQ, Zhang SD. Adenoviral transfer of human interleukin-10 gene in lethal pancreatitis. World J Gastroenterol. 2004;10(20):3021–5.
24. Morse D, Choi AM. Heme-oxygenase-1: the "emerging molecule" has arrived. Am J Respir Cell Mol Biol. 2002;283:L476–84.
25. Tosaki A, Das DK. The role of heme oxygenase signaling in various disorders. Mol Cell Biochem. 2002;232:149–57.
26. Petrache I, Otterbein LE, Alam J, Wiegand GW, Choi AM. Heme oxygenase-1 inhibits TNF-alpha-induced apoptosis in cultured fibroblasts. Am J Physiol Lung Cell Mol Physiol. 2000;278:L312–9.
27. Ryter SW, Tyrrell RM. The heme synthesis and degradation pathways: role in oxidant sensitivity. Heme oxygenase has both pro- and antioxidant properties. Free Radic Biol Med. 2000;28:289–309.
28. Morse D, Choi AM. Heme oxygenase-1: from bench to bedside. Am J Respir Crit Care Med. 2005;172(6):660–70.
29. Otterbein LE, Bach FH, Alam J, Soares M, Tao Lu H, Wysk M, Davis RJ, Flavell RA, Choi AM. Carbon monoxide has anti-inflammatory effects involving the mitogen-activated protein kinase pathway. Nat Med. 2000;6:4222–428.
30. Morse D, Pischke SE, Zhou Z, Davis RJ, Flavell RA, Loop T, Otterbein SL, Otterbein LE, Choi AM. Suppression of inflammatory cytokine production by carbon monoxide involves the JNK pathway and AP-1. J Biol Chem. 2003; 278:36993–8.
31. Liao YF, Zhu W, Li DP, Zhu X. Heme oxygenase-1 and ischemia/reperfusion injury: a short review. World J Gastroenterol. 2013;19(23):3555–61.
32. Liu B, Qian JM. Cytoprotective role of heme oxygenase-1 in liver ischemia reperfusion injury. Int J Clin Exp Med. 2015;8(11):19867–73.
33. Scharn CR, Collins AC, Nair VR, Stamm CE, Marciano DK, Graviss EA, Shiloh MU. Heme oxygenase-1 regulates inflammation and mycobacterial survival in human macrophages during mycobacterium tuberculosis infection. J Immunol. 2016;196(11):4641–9.
34. Ciesla M, Marona P, Kozakowska M, Jez M, Seczynska M, Loboda A, Bukowska-Strakova K, Szade A, Walawender M, Kusior M, et al. Heme oxygenase-1 controls an HDAC4-miR-206 pathway of oxidative stress in rhabdomyosarcoma. Cancer Res. 2016;76(19):5707–18.
35. Wang L, Zhao B, Chen Y, Ma L, Chen EZ, Mao EQ. Biliary tract external drainage increases the expression levels of heme oxygenase-1 in rat livers. Eur J Med Res. 2015;22(20):61.
36. Weis S, Jesinghaus M, Kovacs P, Schleinitz D, Schober R, Ruffert C, Herms M, Wittenburg H, Stumvoll M, Bluher M, et al. Genetic analyses of heme oxygenase 1 (HMOX1) in different forms of pancreatitis. PLoS One. 2012;7(5): e37981.
37. Habtezion A, Kwan R, Yang AL, Morgan ME, Akhtar E, Wanaski SP, Collins SD, Butcher EC, Kamal A, Omary MB. Heme oxygenase-1 is induced in peripheral blood mononuclear cells of patients with acute pancreatitis: a potential therapeutic target. Am J Physiol Gastrointest Liver Physiol. 2011; 300(1):G12–20.
38. Singh U, Devaraj S, Jialal I. Vitamin E, oxidative stress, and inflammation. Annu Rev Nutr. 2005;25:151–74.
39. Lorente JA, Marshall JC. Neutralization of tumor necrosis factor in preclinical models of sepsis. Shock. 2005;1:107–19.
40. Malleo G, Mazzon E, Siriwardena AK, Cuzzocrea S. TNF-alpha as a therapeutic target in acute pancreatitis-lessons from experimental models. Sci World J. 2007;7:431–48.

10

Endocrine and exocrine pancreatic insufficiency after acute pancreatitis

Jianfeng Tu[1,2†], Jingzhu Zhang[1†], Lu Ke[1], Yue Yang[3], Qi Yang[1], Guotao Lu[1], Baiqiang Li[1], Zhihui Tong[1*], Weiqin Li[1*] and Jieshou Li[1]

Abstract

Background: Patients could develop endocrine and exocrine pancreatic insufficiency after acute pancreatitis (AP), but the morbidity, risk factors and outcome remain unclear. The aim of the present study was to evaluate the incidence of endocrine and exocrine pancreatic insufficiency after AP and the risk factors of endocrine pancreatic insufficiency through a long-term follow-up investigation.

Methods: Follow-up assessment of the endocrine and exocrine function was conducted for the discharged patients with AP episodes. Oral Glucose Tolerance Test (OGTT) and faecal elastase-1(FE-1) test were used as primary parameters. Fasting blood-glucose (FBG), fasting insulin (FINS), glycosylated hemoglobin HBA1c, 2-h postprandial blood glucose (2hPG), Homa beta cell function index (HOMA-β), homeostasis model assessment of insulin resistance (HOMA-IR) and FE-1 were collected. Abdominal contrast-enhanced computed tomography (CECT) was performed to investigate the pancreatic morphology and the other related data during hospitalization was also collected.

Results: One hundred thirteen patients were included in this study and 34 of whom (30.1%) developed diabetes mellitus (DM), 33 (29.2%) suffered impaired glucose tolerance (IGT). Moreover, 33 patients (29.2%) developed mild to moderate exocrine pancreatic insufficiency with 100μg/g<FE-1<200μg/g and 7 patients (6.2%) were diagnosed with severe exocrine pancreatic insufficiency with FE-1<100μg/g. The morbidity of DM and IGT in patients with pancreatic necrosis was significant higher than that in the non-pancreatic necrosis group ($X^2 = 13.442, P = 0.001$). The multiple logistic regression analysis showed that extent of pancreatic necrosis<30% ($P = 0.012$, OR = 0.061) were the protective factors of endocrine pancreatic insufficiency. HOMA-IR ($P = 0.002$, OR = 6.626), Wall-off necrosis (WON) ($P = 0.013$, OR = 184.772) were the risk factors.

Conclusion: The integrated morbidity of DM and IGT after AP was 59.25%, which was higher than exocrine pancreatic insufficiency. 6.2% and 29.2% of patients developed severe and mild to moderate exocrine pancreatic insufficiency, respectively. The extent of pancreatic necrosis>50%, WON and insulin resistance were the independent risk factors of new onset diabetes after AP.

Keywords: Endocrine pancreatic insufficiency, Exocrine pancreatic insufficiency, Acute pancreatitis, Follow-up study, Insulin resistance, Pancreatic necrosis

* Correspondence: njzyantol@hotmail.com; njzy_pancrea@163.com
†Equal contributors
[1]Research Institute of General Surgery, Jinling Hospital, Medical School of Nanjing University, 305 East Zhongshan Road, Nanjing 210002, China
Full list of author information is available at the end of the article

Background

Patients could develop endocrine and exocrine pancreatic insufficiency after AP, but the morbidity, risk factors, treatment and outcome remain unclear. The most controversial part is about the risk factors of endocrine pancreatic insufficiency. Das et al. [1] reported that prediabetes and diabetes were common after AP with about 40% prevalence. Reccurent attacks, hyperglycaemia, obesity, age above 45 years, family history of DM were the risk factors,but severity of AP showed minimal effect on it. Hsiu-Nien Shen et al. found that the overall risk of DM increased by two-fold after the first-attack of AP and the risk of diabetes for mild AP patients were similar to those for all AP [2]. However,other studies suggested that the severity of AP was a risk factor of the DM after AP [3, 4]. But it was the insufficient of these studies with small size and short follow-up time. In the present study,we conduct a long-term follow-up investigation to assess the incidence of endocrine and exocrine pancreatic insufficiency after AP attacks and the risk factors of endocrine pancreatic insufficiency.

Methods

Patients

From January to April 2016, this study was undertaken in the sever acute pancreatitis(SAP) care center of Nanjing University, which is one of the largest SAP centers in China. One hundred twenty four discharged patients in our outpatients database were randomly invited to the hospital to participate in the follow-up study by phone or mail. The written informed consent was obtained from each subject. The study was approved by the ethics committee of the Jinling Hospital, Medical School of Nanjing University.

The exclusion criteria were as follows: I. Patients who suffered recurrent AP; II. Patients with chronic pancreatitis; III. Patients with diagnosed DM before AP episodes; IV. Patients suffered from chronic diarrhea before AP; V. Patients with intestinal tuberculosis or Crohn's disease; VI. Patients with family history of DM; VII. Patients with incomplete medical record. VIII. Patients who died during hospitalization or after discharge from hospital.

Assessment methods and data collection:

Simplified OGTT [5] and FE-1 test were applied to assess the endocrine and exocrine pancreatic function. The value of FBG, FINS, HBA1C, 2hPG, HOMA-β, HOMA-IR and FE-1 from the two tests were collected as evaluation indexes. Abdominal CECT was performed for pancreatic morphology. The stool samples were collected and stored in −20 °C for FE-1 test. The symptoms such as abdomen pain, diarrhea, diet, exercise, medication were inquired and recorded. The other information of each patient during their hospitalization such as onset time, admission time, discharge time, diagnosis time for DM or IGT, family history of DM, smoking and alcoholism history, Etiology, the classification of AP, APACHE II score [6], Balthazar score [7], systemic complications such as Acute Kidney Injury (AKI), Acute Respiratory Distress Syndrome (ARDS), etc., local complications (pancreatic infection, pancreatic necrosis, etc.); location and extent of pancreatic necrosis from CT scan image, treatment such as percutaneous catheter drainage (PCD), Operative Necrosectomy, etc. were also collected.

Evaluation index

Endocrine pancreatic function index included DM symptoms (polydipsia, polyphagia, urorrhagia, loss of weight, etc.), FBG, FINS, Fasting c-peptide, HBA1C, 2hPG. The HOMA-β which represents the function of β-cell and HOMA-IR which represents the condition of insulin resistance were respectively calculated by the formula of [HOMA-β = 20 × FINS/(FPG-3.5)] [8] and [HOMA-IR = FPG × FINS/22.5] [9]. Exocrine pancreatic function index included the symptoms of exocrine pancreatic insufficiency (abdominal pain, abdominal distension, diarrhea, fat diarrhea, etc.), value of FE-1 and blood albumin.

Definition

Diabetes

Diabetes was defined using the 1999 World Health Organization criteria. It was diagnosed by Typical diabetes symptoms with any of the following items:

A. FPG ≥ 7.0 mmol/L.
B. Random blood glucose ≥ 11.1 mmol/L.
C. FPG<7.0 mmol/L and 2hPG>11.1 mmol/L after a 75-g OGTT.

Diabetes was also diagnosed by any of the following items if without classical diabetes symptom:

A. FPG>7.0 mmol/L for 2 times.
B. 2hPG ≥ 11.1 mmol/L for 2 times.

Igt

IGT was diagnosed by FPG<7.0 mmol/L and 7.8 mmol/L<2hPG<11.1 mmol/L after a 75-g OGTT.

Exocrine pancreatic insufficiency

FE-1 test (BIOSERV Diagnostics GmbH, Rostock, Germany) was used to assess the exocrine pancreatic function. Reference concentration for FE-1 in stool was as follows:

- Normal exocrine pancreatic function: above 200μg/g stool,
- mild to moderate exocrine pancreatic function: 100 to 200μg/g stool,
- severe exocrine pancreatic function: less than 100μg/g stool [10, 11].

Statistical analysis:

Statistical analysis was performed using SPSS 22.0 for Windows (SPSS Inc., Chicago, Ill). Non-parametric tests were used to analyze the data. When comparing more than 3 groups, the Kruskal-Wallis test was used. Comparison between 2 groups was made with Mann-Whitney U test. The X^2 test was used to compare categorical variables. Fisher test was used when expected frequencies were less than 5. Multiple logistic regression analysis was used to analysis the risk factors of endocrine pancreatic insufficiency. Odds ratios (ORs) are expressed with 95% confidence intervals (CIs).A P value of<0.05 was considered significant.

Results

General information

Finally, 113 patients were included and 11 patients were excluded due to meeting the exclusion criteria, change of address or declining to participating in the study. Among the 11 cases, 7 patients (5.6% in all patients) died during hospitalization or after discharge from hospital due to different reasons(4 for septic shock, 2 for major bleeding and 1 died out of hospital for unknown reason). Of the 113 eligible patients, there were 75 male and 38 female with a mean age of 47.2 ± 1.3 years (median, 46 years). The shortest interval from the AP onset to follow-up assessment was 1 month and the longest was 260 months with a mean value of 42.93 ± 4.03 months (median, 30 months). 83.2% patients were first episode. For the severity, 10 patients (8.8%) were classified as Mild AP (MAP), 12 patients (10.6%) as Moderate Severe AP (MSAP) and the remaining 91 patients (80.6%) were all diagnosed as Severe AP(SAP). The detail data was listed in the Tables 1 and 2.

Morbidity of endocrine and exocrine pancreatic insufficiency

Thirty four of 113 patients (30.1%) was diagnosed with DM, 33 patients (29.2%) with IGT and 46 patients (40.7%) with normal endocrine function as shown in Fig. 1. The incidence of abdominal pain, abdominal distension and diarrhea (including fat diarrhea) was respectively 5.3%, 10.6% and 15.04%. Body Mass Index (BMI) of 4.4% study subjects was lower than 18. Seventy three patients (64.6%), 33 patients (29.2%) and 7 patients (6.2%) were defined as normal, mild to moderate and severe exocrine pancreatic function, respectively as shown in Fig. 2.

Comparison of endocrine and exocrine pancreatic function between the patients with different follow-up time interval

According to the time interval from the AP onset to follow-up assessment, the patients were divided into 3 groups, respectively as "group<3 months", "group 3 months-5 years" and "group>5 years". The morbidity of endocrine pancreatic insufficiency and the value of FE-1 among the 3 groups showed no significant difference ($X^2 = 4.751, P = 0.235$ and $X^2 = 3.262$, $P = 0.515$, respectively). The difference regarding the value of HBA1C among the 3 groups was also no significant ($X^2 = 0.731$, $P = 0.484$). The detail data was listed in the Table 3.

Endocrine and exocrine pancreatic function of patients with different location and extent of pancreatic necrosis

According to the ECET images, the patients were divided into group pancreatic necrosis and group non-pancreatic necrosis. The morbidity of DM and IGT in patients with pancreatic necrosis was significant higher than group non-pancreatic necrosis ($X^2 = 13.442, P = 0.001$). The value of FE-1 between the 2 groups showed no significant difference ($X^2 = 0.242, P = 0.886$)as listed in Table 4. The cases were also divided into group necrosis area<30%,group 50%>necrosis area>30% and group necrosis area>50% on the basis of different extent of pancreatic necrosis. The morbidity of DM and IGT and the value of FE-1 between the 3 groups showed no significant difference. But the value of HBA1C ($X^2 = 7.525$, $P = 0.001$) and HOMA-β ($X^2 = 13.088$, $P = 0.000$) among the 3 groups were significantly different as shown in Table 5. According to the CECT images, group pancreatic necrosis was divided into 4 sub-groups again, such as group head of pancreas, group body of pancreas, group tail of pancreas and group whole pancreas. The value of HOMA-β ($X^2 = 5.173$, $P = 0.002$) and the morbidity of DM and IGT ($X^2 = 12.79$, $P = 0.046$) in group tail of pancreas and group whole pancreas was significant different with the other 2 groups. But it showed no significant difference in the value of FE-1 between 4 sub-groups ($X^2 = 3.267$, $P = 0.775$) as listed in Table 6.

Table 1 General characteristics of the patients with AP (1)

Variable	$\overline{X}$	S.E.	Median	Minimum	Maximum	Percentile25	Percentile75
Age(year)	47.2	1.3	46.0	13.0	80.0	38.5	54.0
Time Interval(month)	42.93	4.03	30	1.0	260.0	10.0	66.0
APACHE II	9.24	0.64	7.0	0	32	4.0	13.0
Balthazar Score	6.83	0.25	8.0	1.0	10.0	5.0	9.5
Recurrence Rate	1.51	0.19	1.0	1.0	20.0	1.0	1.0

Time Interval, the time from AP onset to follow-up visit; APACHE II, Acute Physiology and Chronic Health Evaluation II

Table 2 General characteristics of the patients with AP (2)

Variable	N	%
Sex		
Male	75	66.4
Female	38	33.6
Classification		
MAP	10	8.8
MSAP	12	10.6
SAP	91	80.6
Etiology		
Biliary	65	57.5
HTG	39	34.5
Alcoholic	3	2.7
Others	6	5.3
ARDS		
Mild	23	20.4
Moderate	20	17.7
Severe	15	13.3
No	55	48.7
AKI		
AKI-I	13	11.5
AKI-II	12	10.6
AKI-III	23	20.4
No	65	57.5
Pancreatic Necrosis		
Yes	89	78.8
No	24	21.2
WON		
Yes	7	6.2
No	106	93.8
Pancreatic Infection		
Yes	73	64.6
No	40	35.4
Part of Pancreatic Necrosis		
Head of pancreas	11	12.36
Body of pancreas	12	13.48
Tail of pancreas	51	57.3
Whole pancreas	15	16.85
Area of Pancreatic Necrosis		
<1/3	31	34.83
1/3–50%	26	35.96
>50%	89	29.21
PCD		
Yes	81	71.7
No	32	28.3
ON		

Table 2 General characteristics of the patients with AP (2) *(Continued)*

Variable	N	%
Yes	32	28.3
No	81	71.7
Morphology of Pancreas		
Absence or atrophy of the Head of Pancreas	17	15.0
Absence or atrophy of the Body and/or tail of Pancreas	40	35.4
Absence or atrophy of the whole pancreas	11	9.7
Normal area of pancreas	45	39.8

HTG hypertriglyceridemia, *WON* wall-off necrosis, *PCD* percutaneous catheter drainage, *ON* operative necrosectomy; Morphology of Pancreas, outline of pancreas by CT scan at follow-up time

Endocrine and exocrine pancreatic function of patients with pancreatic infection and different AP classification. The morbidity of DM and IGT in patients with pancreatic infection was significant higher than those without (X^2 = 9.139,P = 0.01). But the difference of the value of FE-1 between the 2 groups was not significant (X^2 = 0.29, P = 0.865) as shown in Table 7. According to the Atlanta criteria, 113 patients were divided into group MAP (n = 10, 8.9%), group MSAP (n = 12, 10.6%) and group SAP (n = 91, 80.5%). Both the morbidity of DM and IGT (X^2 = 8.439, P = 0.069) and the value of FE-1 (X^2 = 1.272, P = 0.906) between 3 groups was no significant difference as listed in Table 8.

Risk factors analyzed by multiple logistic regression analysis

These factors such as sex, age, part and area of pancreatic necrosis, pancreatic infection et al. were included into the logistic regression analysis according the above mentioned results and clinical characteristics. The results showed that male (P = 0.01, OR = 0.083), 18–44 years age (P = 0.018, OR = 0.018), PCD (P = 0.001,OR = 0.006),

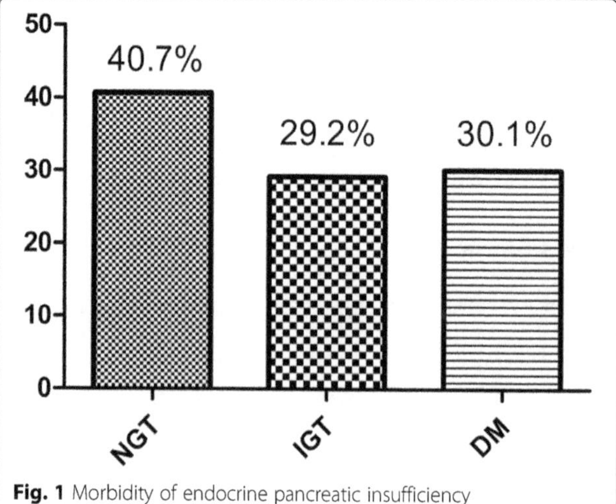

Fig. 1 Morbidity of endocrine pancreatic insufficiency

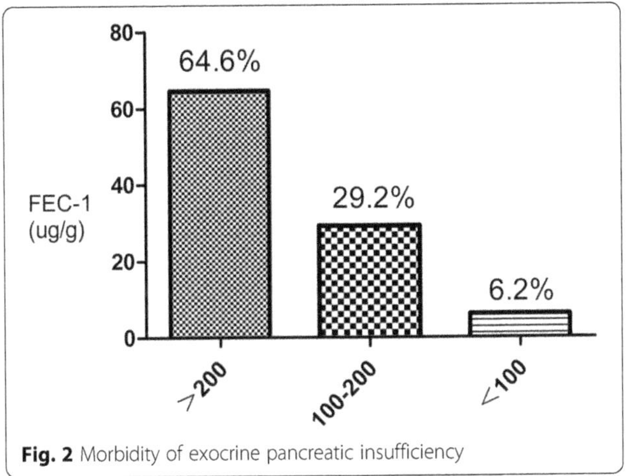

Fig. 2 Morbidity of exocrine pancreatic insufficiency

Table 4 Comparison of endocrine and exocrine pancreatic function between group pancreatic necrosis and group non-pancreatic necrosis

	Pancreatic Necrosis (*n* = 89,78.8%)	Non- Pancreatic Necrosis (*n* = 24, 21.2%)	F/X^2 Value	*P* Value
Endocrine function			13.442	0.001
NGT	34.8%	62.5%		
IGT	27%	37.5%		
DM	38.2%	0		
FE-1			0.242	0.886
>200	64.1%	66.6%		
100–200	29.2%	29.2%		
<100	6.7%	4.2%		

necrosis of the head of the pancreas ($P = 0.007$, OR = 0.009), extent of pancreatic necrosis<30% ($P = 0.012$, OR = 0.061) was the protective factors of endocrine pancreatic insufficiency. HOMA-IR ($P = 0.002$, OR = 6.626) and WON ($P = 0.013$, OR = 184.772) were the risk factors as shown in detail in Table 9.

Discussion

A few patients will develop endocrine and exocrine pancreatic insufficiency after recovering from AP episodes, which catch more and more attention than before in recent years as more patients survive from severe AP. In traditional opinion, disturbance of carbohydrate metabolism should resulted from acute stress, pancreatic microcirculation disorder and excessive secretion of catecholamine after AP, which leading to transient rising in blood glucose. After the improvement of disease, the blood glucose will return to normal soon [12–14]. But part of the patients could not fully recover from the hyperglycemia in the end and some patients' blood glucose could rise again after a short time recovery. Some patients even develop DM and need treatment with antidiabetic or insulin in their rest of lives [15, 16]. In our study, DM and IGT occurred in 34 and 33 of the study patients respectively. Symersky assessed the endocrine pancreatic function of patients who recovered from AP and found out 32% MAP patients and 42% SAP patients still suffered from disturbance of carbohydrate metabolism. He also suggested that patients who received pancreas surgery had higher risk of glucose metabolism disorder [13]. However, the risk factors of endocrine pancreatic insufficiency were controversial and need further verification.

The diagnosis of the new-onset diabetes after AP was not unified and usually confused by type2 diabetes mellitus. But the World Health Organization and American Diabetes Association has defined it as "pancreatogenic diabetes" and classified it as a form type 3c diabetes mellitus (T3c DM) with a prevalence of 5–10% among

Table 3 Comparison of endocrine and exocrine pancreatic function between the different time interval groups

	<3 m (*N* = 9, 7.9%)	3 m-5y (*N* = 75, 66.4%)	>5y (*N* = 29,25.7%)	X^2/F Value	*P* Value
Endocrine function				4.751	0.235*
DM	22.2%	25.3%	44.8%		
IGT	44.4%	29.3%	24.1%		
NGT	33.3%	45.3%	31.1%		
HOMA-β(%) (X ± S.E.)	78.81 ± 15.23	80.31 ± 6.13	66.82 ± 8.92	0.731	0.484
FE-1				3.262	0.515*
>200	66.7%	66.7%	58.6%		
100–200	33.3%	25.3%	37.9%		
<100	0	8%	3.4%		

IGT impaired glucose tolerance, *NGT* normal glucose tolerance, *FE-1* faecal elastase-1; * Fish Exact Test

Table 5 Comparison of endocrine and exocrine pancreatic function between the different area of pancreatic necrosis groups

	<30%	30%–50%	>50%	X^2/F Value	*P* Value
Endocrine function				8.957	0.062
NGT	45.2%	34.4%	23.1%		
IGT	35.5%	25.0%	19.2%		
DM	19.4%	40.6%	57.7%		
HBA1C%(HPLC) (X ± S.E.)	5.54 ± 0.32	5.69 ± 0.11	6.57 ± 0.27	7.525	0.001
HOMA-β(%) (X ± S.E.)	101.65 ± 10.12	60.65 ± 6.91	43.54 ± 6.60	13.088	0.000
FE-1				4.435	0.35
>200	67.7%	71.9%	50.0%		
100–200	22.6%	25.0%	42.3%		
<100	9.7%	3.1%	7.7%		

Table 6 Comparison of endocrine and exocrine pancreatic function between the different part of pancreatic necrosis groups

	Head of Pancreas	Body of Pancreas	Tail of Pancreas	Whole Pancreas	F/X^2 Value	*P* Value
Endocrine function					12.79	0.046
NGT	63.6%	50.0%	29.4%	20.0%		
IGT	18.2%	41.7%	23.5%	33.3%		
DM	18.2%	8.3%	47.1%	46.7%		
HOMA-β(%)(X ± S.E.)	100.16 ± 15.42	104.44 ± 19.42	61.34 ± 6.11	49.39 ± 9.11	5.173	0.002
FE-1					3.267	0.775
>200	54.5%	75.0%	60.8%	73.3%		
100–200	36.4%	25.0%	31.4%	20.0%		
<100	9.1%	0	7.8%	6.7%		

all diabetic subjects in western population [17–20]. About 80% of T3cDM patients were diagnosed as a complication of chronic pancreatitis. Acute pancreatitis, pancreatic cancer, pancreatectomy et al. are the other common causes of T3cDM [21, 22]. Thus studies about pathomechanism of T3cDM mostly focused on chronic pancreatitis. Persistent chronic inflammation of the pancreatic tissue in patients with chronic pancreatitis could lead to pancreatic fibrosis and islet damage both of which result in islet β-cell insufficiency, hepatic insulin resistance and finally occurrence of DM [23, 24].

Compare to endocrine pancreatic insufficiency, exocrine pancreatic insufficiency is more difficult to diagnose. Usually the symptoms such as abdominal pain, abdominal extension and fat diarrhea combined with radiological examination and stool test are used for precise diagnosis [25, 26]. In our study, 5.3%, 10.6% and 15.04% of patients respectively suffered from abdominal pain, abdominal extension and diarrhea (including fat diarrhea) after discharge. The BMI of 4.4% of patients was lower than 18. Thus it can be seen that the symptom of exocrine pancreatic insufficiency is neither usual nor specific which is of less value for diagnosis. In contrast, FE-1 was much better with relatively high stability and specificity and was verified to be a good indirect index of exocrine pancreatic insufficiency by a few studies [27, 28]. We found 6.2% of patients could be diagnosed with severe exocrine pancreatic insufficiency (<100μg/g)and 29.2% of patients only showed mild to moderate (100-200μg/g) insufficiency. There are some scholars doubt it's specificity and sensitivity. Leeds found that FE-1<100μg/g was highly specific for exocrine pancreatic insufficiency, however 100-200μg/g could only offer limited specificity and sensitivity [29]. On the other hand, we couldn't know the patients' baseline value of FE-1 before AP and the stool sample preparation is complicated. So the diagnosis of exocrine pancreatic insufficiency by FE-1 should be strengthened by other diagnostic tools such as MRI of pancreatic duct [30].

In our study, the morbidity of DM and IGT showed no significant difference between the different time interval groups. But we also found that as time goes on, the value of HBA_1C gradually increased in the study patients. This phenomenon suggests that endocrine pancreatic function could weaken over time. But we could not confirm if it resulted from the disease or the natural course. Therefore, more long-term studies with

Table 7 Comparison of endocrine and exocrine pancreatic function between the group pancreatic infection and group non-pancreatic infection

	Pancreatic Infection (*n* = 73, 64.6%)	Non-Pancreatic Infection (*n* = 40,35.4%)	F/X^2 Value	*P* Value
Endocrine function			9.139	0.01
NGT	35.6%	50%		
IGT	24.7%	37.5%		
DM	39.7%	12.5%		
FE-1			0.29	0.865
>200	63.0%	67.5%		
100–200	30.1%	27.5%		
<100	6.8%	5.0%		

Table 8 Comparison of endocrine and exocrine pancreatic function between the different AP classification

	(N = 10, 8.9%)	MSAP (*N* = 12, 10.6%)	SAP (*N* = 91, 80.5%)	X^2/F Value	*P* Value
DM Morbidity				8.439	0.069
NGT	70%	58.33%	35.16%		
IGT	30%	25%	29.67%		
DM	0	16.67%	35.16%		
FEC-1				1.272	0.906
>200	80%	66.67%	62.64%		
100–200	20%	33.33%	29.67%		
<100	0	0	7.69%		

Table 9 Risk factors of endocrine pancreatic insufficiency by multiple logistic regression analysis

	Wald	P	Exp(B)	95% C.I. lower	95% C.I. upper
Sex(male)	6.616	0.01	0.083	0.012	0.553
Age	13.532	0.001			
age(18-44y)	5.583	0.018	0.018	0.001	0.506
age(45-64y)	0.012	0.913	1.153	0.091	14.646
HOMA-IR	9.666	0.002	6.626	2.011	21.825
PCD(yes)	10.636	0.001	0.006	0.000	0.134
WON(yes)	6.195	0.013	184.772	3.032	11,258.328
Part of pancreatic necrosis	11.779	0.008			
Head of pancreas	7.290	0.007	0.009	0.000	0.27
Body of pancreas	3.698	0.054	0.045	0.002	1.061
Tail of pancreas	0.066	0.798	0.746	0.080	6.994
Pancreatic infection(yes)	2.843	0.328	1.237	0.067	11.215
Area of pancreatic necrosis	7.154	0.028			
<30%	6.276	0.012	0.024	0.001	0.446
30%–50%	5.819	0.016	0.061	0.006	0.592
AKI(No)	3.741	0.291			
AKI-1	0.038	0.845	0.428	0.037	4.889
AKI-2	0.066	0.797	6.887	1.206	3.331
AKI-3	3.419	0.064	2.851	0.028	1.359

larger sample size is needed to verify the role of time interval from onset of AP to follow-up time.

It is reported in previous studies that the disease severity of AP had no relationship with new-onset diabetes [1, 2]. We also found that the morbidity of endocrine and exocrine pancreatic insufficiency among group MAP, group MSAP and group SAP was not significantly different. But pancreatic necrosis, which is an important marker for disease severity, was found as an independent risk factor in multiple logistic regression analysis. We also found the difference of the disease severity indexes and complications between group NGT, group IGT and group DM as detailed in Additional file 1: Tables S1-S2 of the additional file. Compare to the DM after pancreatectomy, large scale pancreatic necrosis may has similar pathogenesis to secondary diabetes which could also lead to great decline in the number of β-cell and insulin secretion [31–33]. Garip reported that the patients with SAP, pancreatectomy and pancreatic necrosis especially those with large extent of necrosis had higher risk of endocrine pancreatic insufficiency than patients with MAP [14]. The significant difference of pancreatic necrosis between the three groups was revealed as listed in Table A3 of the additional file. Above all, we may could not simply deny the effect of disease severity on the endocrine pancreatic insufficiency. Pancreatic necrosis may play an important role in the new-onset diabetes.

We also observe that female, age>45 years, pancreatic necrosis, extent of pancreatic necrosis>50%, WON, insulin resistance are the independent risk factors of endocrine pancreatic insufficiency, while PCD is the protective factor. For the age, it is recognized that prevalence of DM increase exponentially after 45 years of age [33, 34]. But Hsiu-Nien Shen et al. found that the highest age-specific HR of DM was observed in men aged<45 years (HR = 7.46) [2]. So according to the current research outcome, we couldn't affirm the effect of gender and age and it needs more studies to verify.

Conclusions

The integrated morbidity of DM and IGT after AP was 59.25%, which was much higher than that of exocrine pancreatic insufficiency. Only 6.2% and 29.2% of patients respectively developed severe exocrine pancreatic insufficiency and mild to moderate exocrine pancreatic insufficiency in the present study. Pancreatic necrosis, extent of pancreatic necrosis>50%, WON and insulin resistance were the independent risk factors of new onset diabetes after AP. For the diagnosis of exocrine pancreatic insufficiency, the FE-1 test is easy, but still not an ideal evaluation index for exocrine pancreatic function.

Additional file

Additional file 1: Tables S1-S3. Comparision on the disease severity, complication and pancreatic necrosis between NGT, IGT and DM groups. The APACHE II score and Balthazar score in group DM was significant higher than that in group IGT and group NGT (X^2 = 5.257, P = 0.007; X^2 = 13.03, P = 0.000). The value of the HOMA-IR in group DM and group IGT was significant higher than group NGT (X^2 = 4.025, P = 0.021). Morbidity of AKI in group DM was higher than in group IGT and group NGT (F = 20.885, P = 0.001), but the complication of ARDS in 3 groups showed no significant difference(X^2 = 4.453, P = 0.627). Compare to group IGT and group NGT, the morbidity of pancreatic necrosis in group DM was significant higher and 100% patients in group DM got pancreatic necrosis (X^2 = 13.442, P = 0.001). For pancreatic necrosis, the proportion of the tail of pancreas and whole pancreas during hospitalization in group DM was higher than other two groups (X^2 = 11.788, P = 0.063, likely attributed to type II error). The area of pancreatic necrosis>50% and the area<1/3 in group DM was higher and lower than in group IGT and group NGT respectively (X^2 = 8.957, P = 0.062, likely attributed to type II error). The atrophy or absence of the body and tail of pancreas in group DM at follow-up time was significant more than the other two groups (X^2 = 43.92, P = 0.000). The morbidity of pancreatic infection in group DM was also showed much higher than group IGT and group NGT (X^2 = 9.139, P = 0.01).

Abbreviations

2hPG: 2-h postprandial blood glucose; AKI: Acute kidney injury; AP: Acute pancreatitis; ARDS: Acute respiratory distress syndrome; BMI: Body mass index; CECT: Contrast-enhanced computed tomography; DM: Diabetes mellitus; FBG: Fasting blood-glucose; FE-1: Faecal elastase-1; FINS: Fasting insulin; HOMA-IR: Homeostasis model assessment of insulin resistance; HOMA-β: Homa beta cell function index; IGT: Impaired glucose tolerance; MAP: Mild AP; MSAP: Moderate Severe AP; OGTT: Oral Glucose Tolerance Test; PCD: Percutaneous catheter drainage; SAP: Sever acute pancreatitis; WON: Wall-off necrosis

Acknowledgements

The authors are indebted to all doctors for the follow-up assessment and data collection during the study from the severe acute pancreatitis care center of Jinling Hospital, Medical School of Nanjing University. The authors would also like to thank professor Hanqing He from the Center for Disease Control, Zhejiang Province, China for his help with the statistical analysis.

Funding

The article processing charge was funded by the Natural Science Foundation of China (No.81570584, 81,670,588). The collection, analysis and interpretation of data was funded by the Science and Technology Foundation of Zhejiang Province, China (No. 2013C37022). Natural Science Foundation of Zhejiang Province, China (LY18H150005).

Authors' contributions

JFT and JZZ: Study concept and design; JFT: Drafting of the manuscript; QY and GTL: Statistical analysis; YY and BQL: Acquisition of data, analysis and interpretation of data; WQL: Critical revision of the manuscript for important intellectual content; LK and ZHT: Administrative, technical, or material support; WQL and JSL: Study supervision. All authors have read and approved the final version of this manuscript, including the authorship.

Consent for publication

Not applicable.

Competing interests

The authors declare that they have no competing interests.

Author details

[1]Research Institute of General Surgery, Jinling Hospital, Medical School of Nanjing University, 305 East Zhongshan Road, Nanjing 210002, China. [2]Zhejiang Provincial People's Hospital, People's Hospital of Hangzhou Medical College, Shangtang road 158#, Hangzhou 310014, China. [3]Hangzhou Medical College, Binwen road 481#, Hangzhou 310053, China.

References

1. Das SL, Singh PP, Phillips AR, et al. Newly diagnosed diabetes mellitus after acute pancreatitis: a systematic review and meta-analysis[J]. Gut. 2013;0:1–14.
2. Shen H-N, Yang C-C, Chang Y-H, et al. Risk of diabetes mellitus after first-attack acute pancreatitis: a National Population-Based Study[J]. Am J Gastroenterol. 2015;110:1698–706.
3. Vipperla K, Papachristou GI, Slivka A, et al. Risk of new-onset diabetes is determined by severity of acute pancreatitis [J]. Pancreas. 2016;45:e14–5.
4. Uomo G, Gallucci F, Madrid E, et al. Pancreatic functional impairment following acute necrotizing pancreatitis: long-term outcome of a non-surgically treated series. Dig Liver Dis. 2010;42:149–52.
5. Rämö JT, Kaye SM, Jukarainen S, et al. Liver Fat and Insulin Sensitivity Define Metabolite Profiles During a Glucose Tolerance Test in Young Adult Twins. J Clin Endocrinol Metab. 2016;3:jc20153512.
6. Saito N, Kawasaki A, Kim A, et al. APACHE II SCORE AND AT III ACTIVITY ON ADMISSION RELATES TO MORTALITY IN ICU PATIENTS. Crit Care Med. 2016; 44(12 Suppl 1):354.
7. Raghuwanshi S, Gupta R, Vyas MM, et al. CT Evaluation of Acute Pancreatitis and its Prognostic Correlation with CT Severity Index. J Clin Diagn Res. 2016; 10(6):TC06–11.
8. Ha CH, Swearingin B, Jeon YK. Relationship of visfatin level to pancreatic endocrine hormone level, HOMA-IR index, and HOMA β-cell index in overweight women who performed hydraulic resistance exercise. J Phys Ther Sci. 2015;27(9):2965–9.
9. Peplies J, Börnhorst C, Günther K, et al. Longitudinal associations of lifestyle factors and weight status with insulin resistance (HOMA-IR) in preadolescent children: the large prospective cohort study IDEFICS. Int J Behav Nutr Phys Act. 2016;13(1):97.
10. DominiciR FC. Fecal elastase-1 as a test for pancreatic function: a review. Clin Chem Lab Med. 2002;40:325–32.
11. Martinez J, Lvaeda R, Trigo C, et al. Fecal elastase-1 determination in the diagnosis of chronic pancreatitis. Gastroenterol Hepatol. 2002;25:377–82.
12. Kaya E, Dervisoglu A, Polat C. Evaluation of diagnostic findings and scoring systems in outcome prediction in acute pancreatitis[J]. World J Gastroenterol. 2007;13(22):3090–4.
13. Symersky T, van Hoom B, Masclee AA. The outcome of a long-term follow-up of pancreatic function after recovery from acute pancreatitis[J]. JOP. 2006;7(5):447–53.
14. Garip G, Sarand E, Kaya E. Effects of disease severity and necrosis on pancreatic dysfunction after acute pancreatitis[J]. World J Gastroenterol. 2013;19(44):8065–70.
15. Mentula P, Kylnp ML, Kemppainen E, et al. Obesity correlates with early hyperglycemia inpatients with acute pancreatitis who developed organ failure[J]. Pancreas. 2008;36(1):e21–5.
16. Czakó L, Hegyi P, Rakonczay Z Jr, et al. Interactions between the endocrine and exocrine pancreas and their clinical relevance[J]. Pancreatology. 2009; 9(4):351–9.
17. Hardt PD, Brendel MD, Kloer HU. Et al.is pancreatic diabetes (type 3c diabetes) under diagnosed and misdiagnosed?[J]. Diabetes Care. 2008; 31(Suppl 2):S165–9.
18. Expert Committee on the Diagnosis and Classification of Diabetes mellitus. Report of the expert committee on the diagnosis and classification of diabetes mellitus. Diabetes Care. 2003;26:5–20.
19. Ewald N, Kaufmann C, Raspe A, et al. Prevalence of diabetes mellitus secondary to pancreatic diseases (type 3c). Diabetes Metab Res Rev. 2012; 28:338–42.
20. American Diabetes Association. Diagnosis and classification of diabetes mellitus. Diabetes Care. 2011;34:62–9.
21. Cui Y, Andersen DK. Pancreatogenic diabetes: special considerations for management[J]. Pancreatology. 2011;11(3):279–94.
22. Rickels MR, Bellin M, Toledo FG, et al. Detection, evaluation and treatment

of diabetes mellitus in chronic pancreatitis: recommendations from pancreas fest 2012[J]. Pancreatology. 2013;13(4):336–42.

23. Stram M, Liu S, Singhi AD. Chronic pancreatitis[J]. Surg Pathol Clin. 2016;9(4):643–59.
24. Brock A, Aldag I, Edskes S, et al. Novel ciliate lipases for enzyme replacement during exocrine pancreatic insufficiency[J]. Eur J Gastroenterol Hepatol. 2016;28(11):1305–12.
25. Sabater L, Ausania F, Bakker OJ, et al. Evidence-based guidelines for the Management of Exocrine Pancreatic Insufficiency after Pancreatic Surgery[J]. Ann Surg. 2016;264(6):949–58.
26. Löser C, Möllgaard A, Fölsch UR. Faecal elastase 1:a novel,highly sensitive,and specific tubeless pancreatic function test[J]. Gut. 1996; 39(4):580–6.
27. Nousia-Arvanitakis S. Fecal elastase-1 concentration: an indirect test of exocrine pancreatic function and a marker of an enteropathy regardless of cause [J]. J Pediatr Gastroenterol Nutr. 2003;36(3):314–5.
28. Leeds JS, Opporg K, Sanders DS. The role of fecal elastase-1 in detecting exocrine pancreatic disease[J]. Nat Rev Gastroenterol Hepatol. 2011;8(7):405–15.
29. Madzak A, Engjom T, Wathle GK, et al. Secretin-stimulated MRI assessment of exocrine pancreatic function in patients with cystic fibrosis and healthy controls[J]. Abdom Radiol (NY). 2016. [Epub ahead of print].
30. Ewald N, Bretzel RG. Diabetes mellitus secondary to pancreatic diseases (type 3c) — are we neglecting an important disease?[J]. Eur J Intern Med. 2013;24(3):203–6.
31. Dugnani E, Gandolfi A, Balzano G, et al. Diabetes associated with pancreatic ductal adenocarcinoma is just diabetes: results of a prospective observational study in surgical patients[J]. Pancreatology. 2016;16(5):844–52.
32. Riveline JP, Boudou P, Blondeau B, et al. Glucagon-secretion inhibition using somatostatin: an old hormone for the treatment of diabetes-associated pancreatectomy[J]. Diabetes Metab. 2017;43(3):269–71.
33. Narayan K, Boyle JP, Thompson TJ, et al. Lifetime risk for diabetes mellitus in the United States. JAMA. 2003;290:1884–90.
34. Halter JB. Diabetes mellitus in an aging population: the challenge ahead. J Gerontol A Biol Sci Med Sci. 2012;67:1297–9.

11

A small pancreatic hamartoma with an obstruction of the main pancreatic duct and avid FDG uptake mimicking a malignant pancreatic tumor

Hiroaki Nagano[1*], Masayuki Nakajo[1], Yoshihiko Fukukura[5], Yoriko Kajiya[1], Atsushi Tani[1], Sadao Tanaka[2], Mari Toyota[3], Toru Niihara[3], Masaki Kitazono[4], Toyokuni Suenaga[4] and Takashi Yoshiura[5]

Abstract

Background: Pancreatic hamartomas are extremely rare and may be misdiagnosed as malignant tumors. We report herein a case of a small, solid-type pancreatic hamartoma.

Case presentation: A 72-year-old female was incidentally detected pancreatic lesion by ultrasonography. Computed tomography and magnetic resonance imaging revealed a 2.0-cm solid lesion. The main pancreatic duct (MPD) was obstructed by the lesion in the head of the pancreas, and the upstream MPD was dilated. ^{18}F-fluorodeoxyglucose (FDG) accumulated avidly in the lesion and increased in FDG intensity from the early to the delayed images. The histopathological studies confirmed the diagnosis of pancreatic hamartoma. Immunohistochemically, the cell membrane of the accessory glands and ducts showed homogeneous expression of glucose transporter type I and hexokinase II.

Conclusion: Pancreatic hamartomas causing dilatation of the MPD are extremely rare, and this appears to be the first case of a hamartoma to take up FDG avidly. It was a rare occurrence and should be noted that pancreatic hamartomas can cause an obstruction of the MPD and show avid FDG uptake, thereby mimicking malignant pancreatic tumors.

Keywords: Hamartoma, Pancreas, CT, MRI, FDG, PET/CT

Background

Hamartomas are benign, tumor-like nodules composed of an overgrowth of mature cells and tissues that normally occur in the affected tissue, but often with one predominant element. Pancreatic hamartomas are composed of three disarranged cellular components in varying proportions: acinar, islet, and ductal cells [1]. These hamartomas are extremely rare and may be misdiagnosed as malignant tumors. Herein, we report a case of pancreatic hamartoma resembling a malignant pancreatic tumor.

* Correspondence: hi-naga@m3.kufm.kagoshima-u.ac.jp
[1]Departments of Radiology, Nanpuh Hospital, 14-3 Nagata, Kagoshima 892-8512, Japan
Full list of author information is available at the end of the article

Case presentation

A 72-year-old asymptomatic woman was referred to our hospital for examination of a pancreatic lesion detected on abdominal ultrasonography during a health screening. Her past medical history and physical examination were unremarkable. On laboratory testing, the serum levels of amylase, bilirubin, carcinoembryonic antigen, and carbohydrate antigen 19-9 were within normal limits.

Abdominal ultrasonography revealed a heterogeneous, hypoechoic mass in the pancreatic head. Dynamic computed tomography (CT) demonstrated a non-deforming mass in the pancreatic head measuring 2.0 cm in maximum diameter and a dilated upstream of the main pancreatic duct (MPD) (Fig. 1a and b). The lesion

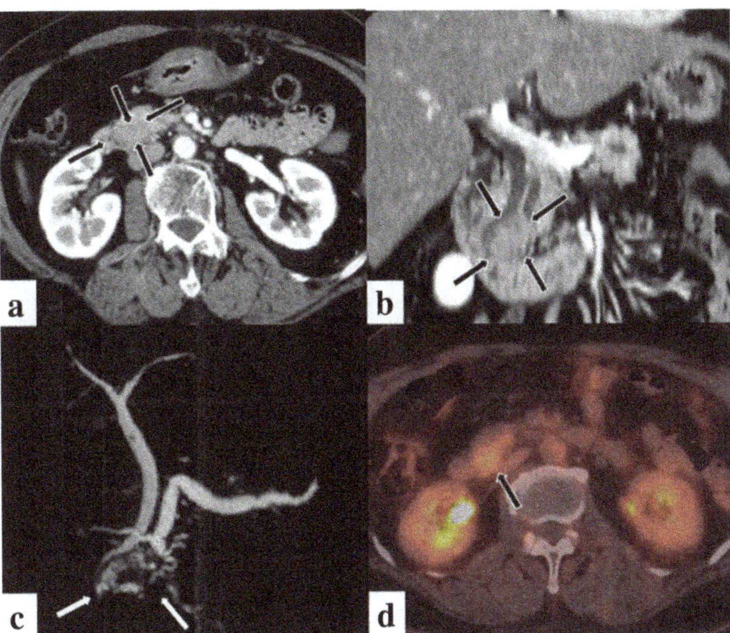

Fig. 1 Contrast-enhanced CT axial (**a**) and coronal (**b**) images demonstrates a 2.0 cm, non-deforming mildly hypoattenuating mass in the pancreatic head (arrows) associated with obstruction of the pancreatic duct. MRCP (**c**): Confirms the dilatation of the pancreatic duct (8 mm in diameter) in the body of the pancreas. Note the associated dilatation of the Santorini duct (small arrows). FDG-PET/CT (**d**): The pancreatic lesion (arrow) shows avid ^{18}F-fluorodeoxyglucose (FDG) uptake on the early image. The lesion increases in visual intensity on the delayed image on FDG-PET/CT

showed isoattenuation on unenhanced CT, mild hypoattenuation during the pancreatic parenchymal phase, and isoattenuation during the portal venous and delayed phases relative to the surrounding pancreatic parenchyma. On magnetic resonance imaging (MRI), the lesion showed heterogeneous low-signal intensity on T1-weighted imaging and mild high-signal intensity on T2-weighted imaging compared to the surrounding pancreatic parenchyma. On diffusion-weighted imaging, the lesion showed mild high-signal intensity with an apparent diffusion coefficient value of 1.4×10^{-3} mm^2/s. On MR cholangiopancreatography (MRCP) (Fig. 1c), the lesion obstructed the MPD in the head of the pancreas, and the upstream pancreatic duct was smoothly dilated (8 mm in diameter). Endoscopic retrograde cholangiopancreatography (ERCP) showed a stricture of the MPD with a dilated upstream. Endoscopic ultrasound (EUS) showed a 24 mm mural hyperechoic mass in the MPD. On positron emission tomography/CT (PET/CT), the pancreatic lesion showed avid ^{18}F-fluorodeoxyglucose (FDG) uptake with a maximum standardized uptake value (SUVmax) of 3.6 at the early imaging (1 h after intravenous FDG injection) (Fig. 1d), which increased to 5.0 at the delayed imaging (2 h after intravenous FDG injection).

The patient then underwent a subtotal pyloric-preserving pancreaticoduodenectomy. Macroscopically, a well-demarcated, homogeneous, white-to-yellow-colored solid lesion measuring 2.0 cm was noted in the pancreas head. Microscopically, the solid lesion was composed of accessory glands and ducts, lined by cuboidal to flattened epithelium without atypia (Fig. 2a). The accessory glands and ducts were embedded in a fibrotic stroma, and the islets of Langerhans were not evident within the lesion. Lymphocyte and follicle formation infiltrated diffusely around the MPD. Immunohistochemically, the ductal cells were positive for epithelial markers, but negative for synaptophysin and chromogranin A. The cell membrane of the accessory glands and ducts showed homogeneous expression of glucose transporter type I (GLUT-1) (Fig. 2b) and hexokinase II (HK-II). The expressions were especially strong along the basilar membrane of the accessory glands. The pathological diagnosis was solid-type pancreatic hamartoma. After surgical resection, the patient received follow-up CT examinations every three to 6 months and there has been no recurrence for 36 months.

Discussion

Pancreatic hamartomas are extremely rare, and their radiologic features have not been fully evaluated. To the best of our knowledge, there have been only 30 previous reports of pancreatic hamartomas in the literature, and there are very few reports regarding their imaging appearance [1–20]. Age at presentation ranged from 34 weeks to 78 years (mean, 48.6 years). Both sexes were

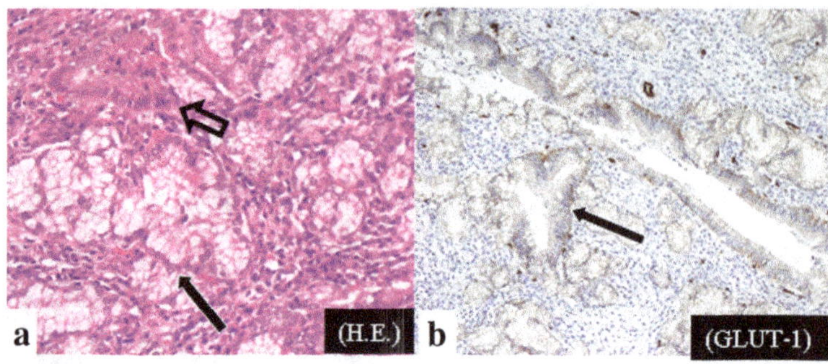

Fig. 2 Macroscopic and immunohistochemical findings. **a**: The lesion is composed of accessory glands (closed arrows) and ducts lined by cuboidal to flattened epithelium, without atypia (open arrows). **b**: On immunohistochemistry, the cell membrane of the accessory glands and ducts show homogeneous expression of glucose transporter type I. The expressions are especially strong along the basilar membrane of the accessory glands (closed arrows)

equally affected, with a male-to-female ratio of 1:0.82. Most patients were either asymptomatic or they exhibited symptoms related to local mass effect, including abdominal pain, weight loss, and a palpable mass; and only one patient had jaundice, caused by obstruction of the common bile duct [17]. Pancreatic hamartomas were reported to arise from all parts of the pancreas, although the pancreatic head was the most common site (64.5%, 20/31). Their size ranged from 1.0–14.0 cm (mean, 4.5 cm).

Morphologically, there are two types of pancreatic hamartoma: solid, and solid and cystic [2, 3]. Nine of the previously reported cases of pancreatic hamartoma seemed to fit the criteria of solid type; however, only three reports included the radiological appearance [1, 16, 17]. One showed that the MPD was compressed by the hamartoma located in the pancreatic body, and the upstream was dilated [16]. The remaining two cases had no stricture or dilatation of the MPD [1, 17]. On enhanced CT, one case showed a hyperattenuating hamartoma during the portal venous phase [17], and the other two cases demonstrated delayed enhancement on contrast-enhanced CT or MRI [1, 16]. In the present case, a pancreatic hamartoma measuring 2.0 cm in diameter was located in the head of the pancreas and caused an obstruction of the MPD, with a dilated upstream on CT, MRCP, and ERCP. Contrast-enhanced CT demonstrated an ill-defined lesion with mild hypoattenuation during the pancreatic parenchymal phase and isoattenuation during the portal venous and delayed phases.

Pancreatic ductal adenocarcinomas may present as a non-deforming iso- or hypoattenuation mass during the pancreatic parenchymal to portal venous phase on enhanced CT [21], and have an obstruction of the MPD with upstream ductal dilatation on CT or MRI [21, 22]. Pancreatic neuroendocrine tumors usually show hypervascular patterns during the arterial to the portal venous phase. However, high-grade pancreatic neuroendocrine tumors tend to show hypovascular patterns and an interruption of the MPD with upstream ductal dilatation [23–25]. Therefore, in the present case, it was difficult to differentiate pancreatic hamartoma from ductal adenocarcinoma, neuroendocrine tumor, or pancreatic metastases.

On FDG-PET, no avid FDG uptake was noted in the three previously reported cases of pancreatic hamartoma [9, 14, 15]. Ours appears to be the first case of a pancreatic hamartoma to show avid FDG uptake, which may be related to the GLUT-1 and HK-II expression of the accessory glands and ducts. Yoshioka et al. [26] reported that an FDG SUVmax of 2.5 would be justified as a cut-off value to differentiate between malignant and benign pancreatic tumors. Kawada et al. [27] reported that the FDG SUVmax increased from the early to the delayed images in 89% (39/44) of the small malignant pancreatic tumors (< 25 mm). In the present case, the FDG SUVmax was 3.6 at the early phase and increased to 5.0 at the delayed phase, in concordance with malignant pancreatic tumors. In our case, therefore, it was difficult to differentiate from malignant tumors based on US, CT, MRI, and FDG-PET/CT findings. Pancreatic hamartoma is benign entity, and does not require surgical treatment. EUS-Fine-Needle-Aspiration might have been effective for definitive diagnosis if we had performed it.

Conclusion

Pancreatic hamartomas causing dilatation of the MPD were extremely rare, and showed no avid FDG uptake in the previously reported cases. We described a rare case of a small, solid-type pancreatic hamartoma that showed an obstruction of the main pancreatic duct and avid FDG uptake. Radiologists should be aware that pancreatic hamartomas may be associated with these findings.

Abbreviations

CT: Computed tomography; ERCP: Endoscopic retrograde cholangiopancreatography; EUS: Endoscopic ultrasound; FDG: ^{18}F-fluorodeoxyglucose; GLUT-1: Glucose transporter type I; HE: Hematoxylin-eosin staining; HK-II: Hexokinase II; MPD: Main pancreatic duct; MRCP: MR cholangiopancreatography; MRI: Magnetic resonance imaging; PET/CT: Positron emission tomography/CT; SUVmax: Maximum standardized uptake value

Acknowledgements
Not applicable.

Funding
The authors have no funding to report.

Authors' contributions
All authors participated in clinical examinations, diagnosis, surgical operation and follow up for of this patient. MN, YF, YK, AT and TY took part in the design of this study and helped to draft the manuscript. All authors read and approved the final manuscript.

Consent for publication
Written informed consent was obtained from the patient for publication of this case report and any accompanying images. A copy of the written consent is available for review by the Editor of this journal.

Competing interests
The authors declare that they have no competing interests.

Author details
[1]Departments of Radiology, Nanpuh Hospital, 14-3 Nagata, Kagoshima 892-8512, Japan. [2]Departments of Pathology, Nanpuh Hospital, 14-3 Nagata, Kagoshima 892-8512, Japan. [3]Departments of Gastroenterology, Nanpuh Hospital, 14-3 Nagata, Kagoshima 892-8512, Japan. [4]Departments of Surgery, Nanpuh Hospital, 14-3 Nagata, Kagoshima 892-8512, Japan. [5]Department of Radiology, Kagoshima University Graduate School of Medical and Dental Sciences, 8-35-1 Sakuragaoka, Kagoshima-shi, Kagoshima 890-8544, Japan.

References

1. Nagata S, Yamaguchi K, Inoue T, Yamaguchi H, Ito T, Gibo J, et al. Solid pancreatic hamartoma. Pathol Int. 2007;57:276–80.
2. Pauser U, Kosmahl M, Kruslin B, Kilmstra DS, Klöppel G. Pancreatic solid and cystic hamartoma in adults: characterization of a new tumorous lesion. Am J Surg Pathol. 2005;29:797–800.
3. Pauser U, da Silva MT, Placke J, Kilmstra DS, Klöppel G. Cellular hamartoma resembling gastrointestinal stromal tumor: a solid tumor of the pancreas expressing c-kit (CD117). Med Pathol. 2005;18:1211–6.
4. Anthony PP, Faber RG, Russell RC. Pseudotumours of the pancreas. Br Med J. 1977;1:814.
5. Burt TB, Condon VR, Matlak ME. Fetal pancreatic hamartoma. Pediatr Radiol. 1983;13:287–9.
6. Flaherty MJ, Benjamin DR. Multicystic pancreatic hamartoma: a distinctive lesion with immunohistochemical and ultrastructural study. Hum Pathol. 1992;23:1309–12.
7. Izbicki JR, Knoefel WT, Müller-Höcker J, Mandelkow HK. Pancreatic hamartoma: a benign tumor of the pancreas. Am J Gastroenterol. 1994;89:1261–2.
8. Wu SS, Vargas HI, French SW. Pancreatic hamartoma with Langerhans cell histiocytosis in a draining lymph node. Histopathology. 1998;33:485–7.
9. McFaul CD, Vitone LJ, Campbell F, Azadeh B, Hughes ML, Garvey CJ, et al. Pancreatic hamartoma. Pancreatology. 2004;4:533–8.
10. Thrall M, Jessurun J, Edwaard B, Stelow N, Adsay V, Selwyn M, et al. Multicystic adenomatoid hamartoma of the pancreas: a hitherto undescribed pancreatic tumor occurring in a 3-year-old boy. Pediatr Dev Pathol. 2008;11:314–20.
11. Sampelean D, Adam M, Muntean V, Hanescu B, Domsa I. Pancreatic hamartoma and SAPHO syndrome: a case report. J Gastrointestin Liver Dis. 2009;18:483–6.
12. Sueyoshia R, Okazakia T, Lane GJ, Arakawa A, Yao T, Yamataka A. Multicystic adenomatoid pancreatic hamartoma in a child: case report and literature review. Int J Surg Case Rep. 2013;4:98–100.
13. Kim H, Cho CK, Hur YH, Koh YS, Kim JC, Kim HJ, et al. Pancreatic hamartoma diagnosed after surgical resection. J Korean Surg Soc. 2012;83:330–4.
14. Kersting S, Janot MS, Munding J, Suelberg D, Tannapfel A, Chromik AM, et al. Rare solid tumors of the pancreas as differential diagnosis of pancreatic adenocarcinoma. JOP. 2012;13:268–77.
15. Kawakami F, Shimizu M, Yamaguchi H, Hara S, Matsumoto I, Ku Y, et al. Multiple solid pancreatic hamartomas: a case report and review of the literature. World J Gastrointest Oncol. 2012;4:202–6.
16. Addeo P, Tudor G, Oussoultzoglou E, Averous G, Bachellier P. Pancreatic hamartoma. Surg. 2014;156:1284–5.
17. Inoue H, Tameda M, Yamada R, Tano S, Kasturahara M, Hamada Y, et al. Pancreatic hamartoma: a rare cause of obstructive jaundice. Endoscopy. 2014;46:E157–8.
18. Yamaguchi H, Aishima S, Oda Y, Mizukami H, Tajiri T, Yamada S, et al. Distinctive histopathologic findings of pancreatic hamartomas suggesting their "hamartomatous" nature: a study of 9 cases. Am J Surg Pathol. 2013;37:1006–13.
19. Durczynski A, Wiszniewski M, Olejniczak W, Polkowski M, Sporny S, Strzekzyk J. Asymptomatic solid pancreatic hamartoma. Arch Med Sci. 2011;7(6):1082–4.
20. Matsushita D, Kurahara H, Mataki Y, Maemura K, Michiyo H, Satoshi I, et al. Pancreatic hamartoma: a case report and literature review. BMC Gastroenterol. 2016;16:3.
21. Kim JH, Park SH, Yu ES, Kim MH, Kim J, Byun JH, et al. Visually isoattenuating pancreatic adenocarcinoma at dynamic-enhanced CT: frequency, clinical and pathologic characteristics, and diagnosis at imaging examinations. Radiology. 2010;257:87–96.
22. Fukukura Y, Takumi K, Kamimura K, Shindo T, Kumagae Y, Tateyama A, et al. Pancreatic Adenocarcinoma: variability of diffusion-weighted MR imaging findings. Radiology. 2012;263(3):732–40.
23. Luo Y, Dong Z, Chen J, Chan T, Lin Y, Chen M, et al. Pancreatic neuroendocrine tumours: correlation between MSCT features and pathological classification. Eur Radiol. 2014;24:2945–52.
24. Kim DW, Kim HJ, Kim KW, Byun JH, Song KB, Kim JH, et al. Neuroendocrine neoplasms of the pancreas at dynamic enhanced CT: comparison between grade 3 neuroendocrine carcinoma and grade 1/2 neuroendocrine tumour. Eur Radiol. 2015;25:1375–83.
25. Kim JH, Eun HW, Kim YJ, Han JK, Choi BI. Staging accuracy of MR for pancreatic neuroendocrine tumor and imaging findings according to the tumor grade. Abdom Imaging. 2013;38:1106–14.
26. Yoshioka M, Uchinami H, Watanabe G, Sato T, Shibata S, Kume M, et al. F-18 fluorodeoxyglucose positron emission tomography for differential diagnosis of pancreatic tumors. Spring. 2015;31(4):154.
27. Kawada N, Uehara H, Hosoki T, Takami M, Shiroeda H, Arisawa T, et al. Usefulness of dual-phase 18F-FDG PET/CT for diagnosing small pancreatic tumors. Pancreas. 2015;44:655–9.

12

Palliative chemotherapy for pancreatic adenocarcinoma: a retrospective cohort analysis of efficacy and toxicity of the FOLFIRINOX regimen focusing on the older patient

Anne Katrin Berger[1*†], Georg Martin Haag[1†], Martin Ehmann[2], Anne Byl[3], Dirk Jäger[1] and Christoph Springfeld[1]

Abstract

Background: Pancreatic cancer occurs more frequently in older patients, but these are underrepresented in the phase III clinical studies that established the current treatment standards. This leads to uncertainty regarding the treatment of older patients with potentially toxic but active regimens like FOLFIRINOX.

Methods: We conducted a retrospective analysis of patients treated according to the FOLFIRINOX protocol at our institution between 2010 and 2014 with a focus on older patients.

Results: Overall survival in our cohort was 10.2 months. Only 43% of patients did not need dose adaptations, but dose reductions did not lead to an inferior survival. We did not find evidence that patients aged 65 years and older deemed fit enough for palliative treatment had more toxicities or a worse outcome than younger patients.

Conclusion: We conclude that treatment with the FOLFIRINOX protocol in patients with pancreatic cancer should not be withhold from patients solely based on their chronological age but rather be based on the patient's performance status and comorbidities.

Keywords: Pancreatic cancer, Elderly patients, Folfirinox, Toxicity

Background

Cancer occurs more frequently in elderly people, and the current demographic changes with an aging population in Western countries will therefore result in a rising incidence of cancer and an increasing amount of older cancer patients [1–3]. For the US, it has been estimated that by 2030, approximately 70% of all cancers will be diagnosed in adults older than 65 years [4]. In contrast to this development, older patients remain underrepresented in the clinical cancer studies that establish standard treatment regimens [5]. There is widespread critique concerning this issue, but to date, trial results have to be extrapolated to the older population, although this approach remains questionable [6]. Fear of increased toxicities and uncertainty concerning both clinical treatment benefit and the patient's physical resources may cause limitation of tumor-specific therapies in older patients. Ensuring an adequate antitumor treatment while avoiding toxicity is a challenging task for geriatric oncology in daily routine.

For pancreatic adenocarcinoma, the fourth common cause of cancer-related death in the US [7], approximately two-thirds of cases are diagnosed in patients over 65 years [8]. The overall 5-year survival rate is about 6% and remains the poorest of all major malignancies [9, 10]. Because the majority of tumors is irresectable or recurs after surgery, systemic palliative treatment is needed for almost every patient [11]. Despite its limited activity, single-agent gemcitabine was the standard palliative first-

* Correspondence: anne.berger@med.uni-heidelberg.de
†Equal contributors
[1]Department of Medical Oncology, National Center for Tumor Diseases (NCT), Heidelberg University Hospital, Im Neuenheimer Feld 460, 69120 Heidelberg, Germany
Full list of author information is available at the end of the article

line treatment for patients with advanced disease for more than a decade [12], until therapy options improved in 2011. In the landmark PRODIGE 4 trial, the FOLFIRINOX protocol had an impressive response rate of 31.6%, and it significantly improved median overall survival (OS) from 6.8 months in the gemcitabine monotherapy arm to 11.1 months [13]. More recently, this protocol has also been used successfully in patients with irresectable, locally advanced disease to achieve resectability and therefore offering a chance for cure [14]. The impressive results of the FOLFIRINOX protocol are accompanied by significantly increased grade 3 and 4 toxicities, mainly myelosuppression, diarrhea and peripheral neuropathy. Concerns regarding safety in the palliative setting have been raised immediately [15]. Likewise, the study population was criticized as heavily selected (young age, excellent performance status, mostly "non-head" tumors), not representing the average "real-life" patient. Subsequent retrospective clinical analyses confirmed the substantial toxicity profile, and modifications of the regimen are commonly recommended [16–18]. In 2013, therapeutic options further increased with publication of the MPACT trial. In this study, the addition of nab-paclitaxel to gemcitabine therapy increased the median overall survival from 6.6 to 8.7 months [19].

Thus, oncologists might be reluctant to apply FOLFIRINOX to older patients. Given the undoubted advantages in response rate and survival, older cancer patients might be at risk for therapeutic disparity and undertreatment. We conducted a retrospective analysis of patients with advanced pancreatic cancer under palliative first-line treatment with FOLFIRINOX at the National Center for Tumor Diseases, Heidelberg, to assess efficacy and toxicity in academic practice, especially focusing on older patients.

Methods

Patients

Requirements for inclusion were (1) histologically proven diagnosis of ductal pancreatic adenocarcinoma, (2) irresectable (metastasized or locally advanced) disease and (3) palliative first-line treatment with FOLFIRINOX at the NCT Heidelberg, Germany between January 2010 and June 2014. The observation period for each patient started with initiation of first-line treatment (i.e. first systemic chemotherapy after primary diagnosis of metastatic or inoperable disease or, in resected patients, after diagnosis of recurrence). The follow-up period for this analysis ended on July, 15th 2015. Survival data were available for all patients. The patients were identified with permission of two own institutional databases (the *NCT clinical cancer registry, a* prospectively maintained database and the registry of the pharmacy department of the University hospital Heidelberg, respectively).

Treatment

Full dose FOLFIRINOX consisted of oxaliplatin 85 mg/m^2, irinotecan 180 mg/m^2, leucovorin 400 mg/m^2, fluorouracil 400 mg/m^2 bolus and 2400 mg/m^2 over 46 h, q2w, as originally described [13]. Dose modifications were at the discretion of the treating physician.

Assessment

Clinical data were documented via an electronic medical record system. Information included Eastern Cooperative Oncology Group performance status (ECOG PS) [20], presence and site of metastases at diagnosis, date of previous surgery and adjuvant chemotherapy, start and stop date of FOLFIRINOX treatment, type and severity of toxicities and consecutive dose reductions, response to first-line therapy, date of progression, and date of death. Toxic effects were registered according to the National Cancer Institute's common terminology criteria for adverse events (CTCAE). Tumor response was routinely evaluated according to the response evaluation criteria in solid tumors (RECIST, [21]).

Statistical analysis

Man Whitney U-Test and Fisher's exact test were used for comparing independent samples of quantitative and binary data, respectively. Progression-free survival (PFS) was defined as time from start of palliative first-line treatment to documented tumor progression or death. Overall survival (OS) was defined as the time from start of palliative first-line treatment to death. Time-to event data were analyzed using standard methods, including Kaplan-Meier product-limit estimates. All analyses of prognostic factors were of an exploratory nature. Statistical analysis was performed using the SPSS statistical software, Version 22.

Results

Patients' demographics

We identified 88 patients meeting the inclusion criteria. Median duration of observation was 10.4 months. The median age at diagnosis of advanced disease was 56 years (range 32–78), 15 patients (17%) were 65 years or older, and 8 patients (9%) were ≥70 years. 80 patients (91%) had died at the time of analysis. 50 patients (57%) had pancreatic head tumors, and 79 patients (90%) had metastatic disease. 22 patients (25%) had undergone prior tumor resection, and 13 (15%) had initially received adjuvant chemotherapy. 85 patients (97%) started therapy with an ECOG of 0 or 1. The main characteristics concerning both tumor disease and patient demographics did not differ significantly between younger (< 65 years) and older (≥ 65 years) patients. The patient characteristics are summarized in Table 1.

Table 1 Patient characteristics

Patient characteristics	all	<65 years	≥ 65 years
Number of Patients	88	73	15
Median age (range), years	56 (32–78)		
	n (%)		
Gender			
Female	31 (35.2)	29 (39.7)	2 (13.3)
Male	57 (64.8)	44 (60.3)	13 (86.7)
ECOG PS			
0	49 (55.7)	43 (58.9)	6 (40.0)
1	36 (40.9)	27 (37.0)	9 (60.0)
2	3 (3.4)	3 (4.1)	0
Metastatic disease	79 (89.8)	64 (87.7)	15 (100.0)
Locally advanced tumor	9 (10.2)	9 (12.3)	0
Primary palliative treatment	66 (75.0)	55 (75.3)	11 (73.3)
Previous resection	22 (25.0)	18 (24.7)	4 (26.7)
Prior (neo-) adjuvant CTX	13 (14.8)	11 (15.1)	2 (13.3)
Site of Tumor			
Pancreatic head	50 (56.8)	42 (57.5)	8 (53.3)
Pancreatic corpus	22 (25.0)	20 (27.4)	2 (13.3)
Pancreatic tail	16 (18.2)	11 (15.1)	5 (33.3)

Table 2 Grade 3 or 4 toxicity according to the CTCAE (version 4)

	all, n (%)	<65 years	≥ 65 years
Any grade ≥ 3 toxicity	46 (52.3)	41 (56.2)	5 (33.3)
Hematological toxicity grade ≥ 3			
Neutropenia	2 (2.3)	2 (2.7)	0
Febrile neutropenia	1 (1.1)	1 (1.4)	0
Thrombopenia/Anemia	3 (3.4)	3 (4.1)	0
Fatigue	6 (6.8)	4 (5.5)	2 (13.3)
Nausea/Vomiting	3 (3.4)	1 (1.4)	2 (13.3)
Diarrhea	6 (6.8)	5 (6.8)	1 (6.7)
Cholangitis	6 (6.8)	5 (6.8)	1 (6.7)
Thrombosis/Pulmonary embolism	18 (20.5)	17 (23.3)	1 (6.7)
Treatment modifications due to tocixity	50 (56.8)	43 (58.9)	7 (46.7)
Permanent treatment stop due to toxicity	7 (8.0)	4 (5.5)	3 (20.0)

FOLFIRINOX and toxicities

Median duration of first-line therapy with FOLFIRINOX was 150 days (range 14–787). Thirty-eight patients (43%) received therapy per protocol without any modifications during the course of treatment. Forty-six patients (52%) developed side effects that were classified as CTCAE grade 3 or higher: Hematologic side effects were found in 11 patients (13%), and 8 (9%) developed severe peripheral neuropathy. Six patients (7%) suffered from severe diarrhea, fatigue or cholangitis, respectively. Seven patients (8%) stopped therapy due to toxicity. There was no therapy-related death. Modifications of the FOLFIRINOX protocol were necessary in 50 patients. Median time to the first reduction was 74 days (range 0–287) after initiation of therapy. 12 patients (13.6%) had dosage modifications of only oxaliplatin of which 7 totally stopped and 5 continued therapy with 80% dosage. In 7 patients (8.0%), solely irinotecan, and in 5 patients (5.7%) the 5-fluorouracil bolus was dropped. 12 patients (13.6%) had a fixed reduction of all 3 cytotoxic drugs of 75–80% of the per-protocol dosage. 12 patients (13.6%) had dose reduction of varying degrees of two (4 patients) or three components (8 patients).

A summary of CTCAE Grade 3 and 4 toxicities is given in Table 2.

Progression and survival

Median PFS of our cohort was 6.4 months [95% CI 5.7;7.2]. It differed significantly between the ECOG groups: it was 6.9 months [95% CI 6.2;7.6] for patients with an ECOG PS 0, 5.4 months [95% CI 3.8;6.9] for ECOG PS 1 and 2.3 months [95% CI 1.0;3.6] for ECOG PS 2 (overall comparison $p = 0.019$) (Fig. 1). Patients needing dose reductions had a longer median PFS than those in the per-protocol group (7.4 months [95% CI 5.6;9.2] vs. 3.8 months [95% CI 0.9;6.8]; $p = 0.003$), however duration of therapy was significantly longer in this group: 180 days vs. 59 days ($p < 0.001$). Patients with therapy discontinuation due to toxicity had a significantly shorter PFS (2.5 months [95% CI 1.3;3.8] vs. 6.7 months [95% CI 6.0;7.4] $p = 0.01$). There were no apparent PFS associations for metastasized compared to locally advanced tumors or for different tumor localizations.

Median OS in our patients was 10.2 months [95% CI 7.1;13.3], and also differed significantly between the ECOG groups with 11.8 months [95% CI 11.0;12.6] for ECOG PS 0, 7.9 months [95% CI 6.4;9.3] for ECOG PS 1 and 3.6 months [95% CI 2.4;4.8] for ECOG PS 2 (overall comparison $p = 0.003$) (Fig. 2). While dose modifications did not significantly influence OS ($p = 0.078$), patients with permanent therapy discontinuation due to toxicity lived significantly shorter (2.8 months [95% CI 2.3;3.3] vs. 11.5 months [95% CI 9.6;13.4], $p < 0.001$). OS did not significantly differ between the groups of patients with metastasized compared to locally advanced tumors or for different tumor localizations.

Comparison of different age groups

When we compared older patients (≥ 65 years) and younger patients, we did not find significant differences

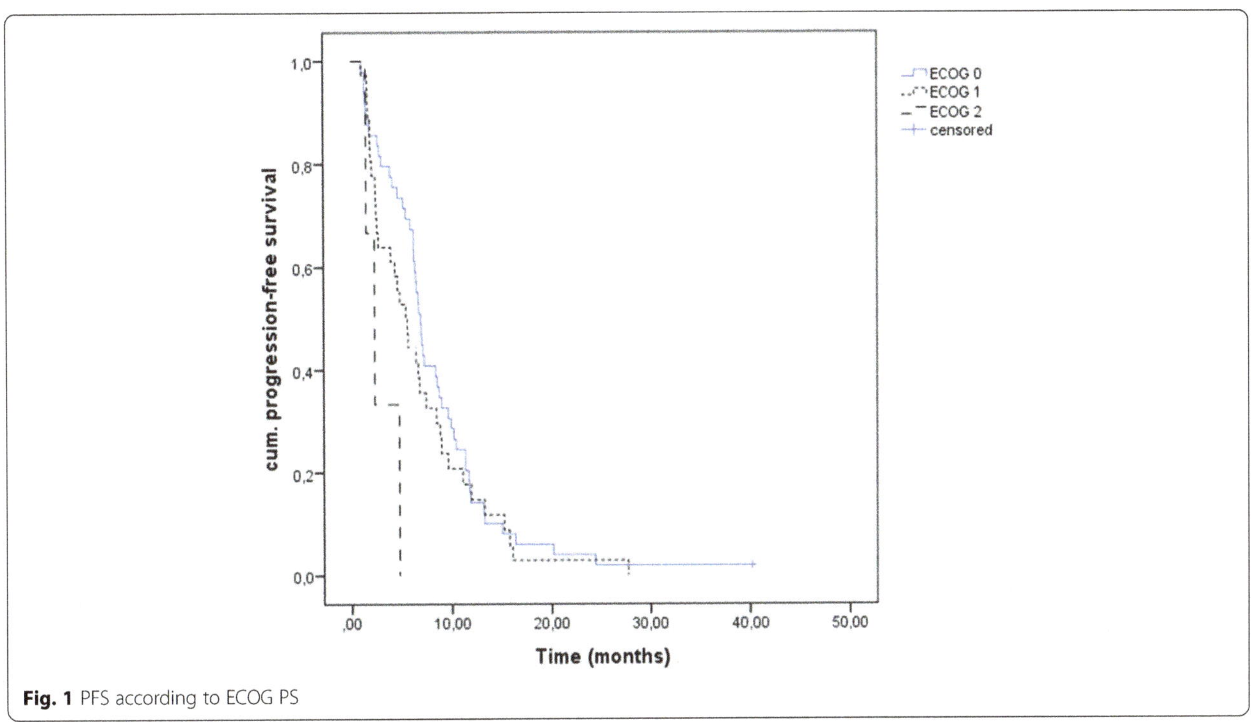

Fig. 1 PFS according to ECOG PS

in frequency of therapy interruptions, dosage modifications, or appearance of any toxicity CTCAE grade 3 or higher (Table 2). An age ≥ 65 years was not associated with significantly different PFS or OS. Median OS of patients ≥65 years was 7.9 months [95% CI 5.8;10.0] compared to 11.2 months [95%CI 8.9;13.6] for patients aged younger than 65 years, but this difference was not significant ($p = 0.83$).

Discussion

In the U.S., the median age at diagnosis of pancreatic cancer is 71 years (data for 2006–2010, seer.cancer.gov).

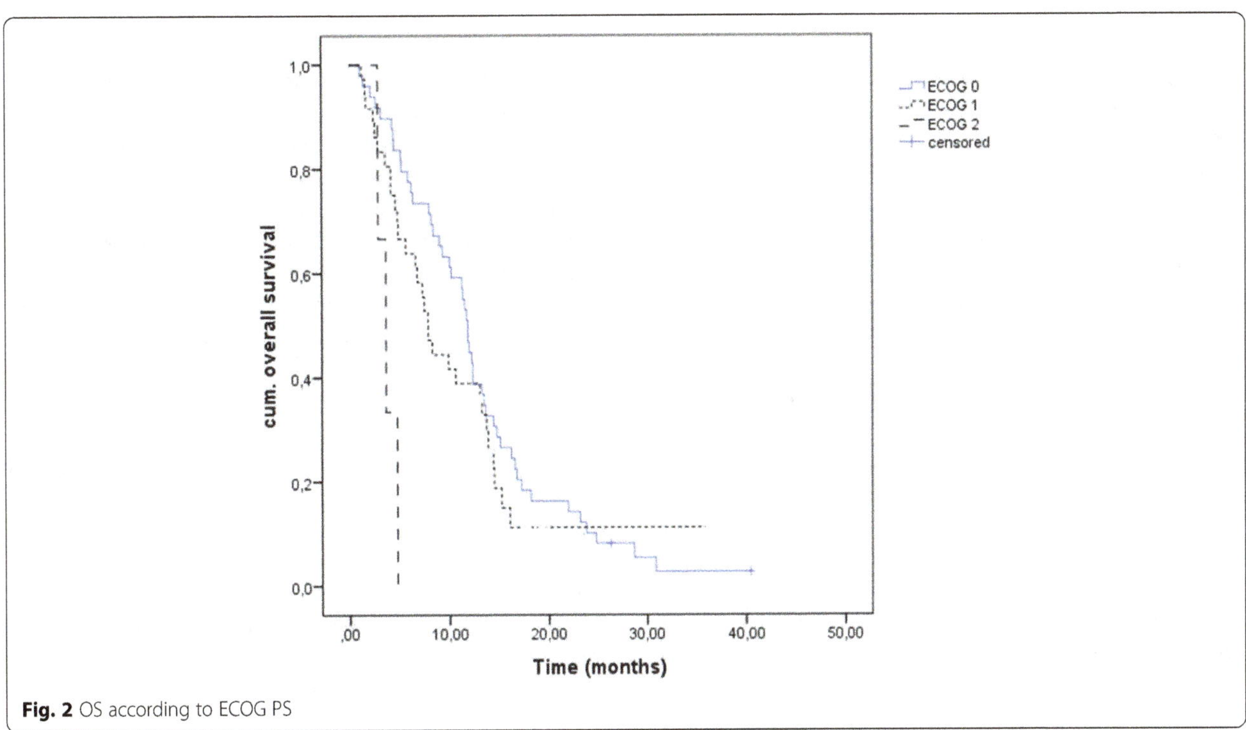

Fig. 2 OS according to ECOG PS

Two-thirds of patients are 65 years and older, and 41% are even 75 years or older. However, the FOLFIRINOX trial excluded patients older than 75 years (median age 61), and the vast majority of patients was even younger than 66 years (71%, 244 out of 342). Similarly, other clinical trials establishing the standard treatments for advanced pancreatic cancer had median ages between 62 and 64 years [12, 22, 23]. Although the MPACT trial introducing nab-paclitaxel + gemcitabine did not have an age limit, median age was also 63 years (range 27–88), with 42% of patients older than 65 years and 10% of patients older than 75 years [24].

In our heterogeneous academic outpatient collective, the survival times for first-line FOLFIRINOX treatment were in good accordance with the PRODIGE 4 trial collective and other retrospective analyses [17, 18]. 57% of our patients needed dose reductions, confirming the regimen's substantial toxicity profile. Several authors have recommended using modified FOLFIRINOX regimens with reduced doses of chemotherapy to decrease the frequency of side effects. In our cohort, survival times for patients with dose reductions were not inferior to those receiving full-dose FOLFIRINOX, supporting the thesis that dose reductions might be possible without reducing efficacy [25]. The superior PFS of our patients with protocol adjustments is probably associated with the fact that dose reductions occurred more frequently in patients with a longer treatment period, reflecting the cumulative toxicity with prolonged chemotherapy. It might be a reasonable approach to start with full-dose FOLFIRINOX but to carefully monitor side effects and quickly adapt the doses if necessary. In patients that are deemed borderline fit for FOLFIRINOX, it might be wise to immediately start with a reduced dose to avoid toxicity-induced treatment discontinuation since this seems to be associated with a worse outcome. In terms of toxicities, no data for the different age groups were reported by the PRODIGE 4 trial authors. We did not find evidence that the subgroup of patients ≥65 years that was initially deemed fit enough for FOLFIRINOX treatment had an increased incidence of toxicities. In the PRODIGE 4 trial, the subgroup analysis showed no hint for a worse survival for patients between 65 and 74 years [13] and also in our analysis, the difference in OS for the age groups did not reach statistical significance. However, the small sample size of our old patients should be noted.

For gemcitabine-based palliative regimes, we have previously found that older patients with advanced pancreatic cancer with an ECOG PS of 0 or 1 do not have an inferior outcome or more toxicities than younger patients [26]. These findings are consistent with studies in other solid malignancies [27–29]. Thus, for advanced pancreatic cancer, the feasibility and efficacy of modern palliative chemotherapy regimens seems to be independent of chronological age. Our analysis highlights the prognostic impact of the initial ECOG PS, which allows a rapid evaluation of the patients′ resources with respect to tumor-specific treatment. In the pivotal PRODIGE 4 trial, only patients with an ECOG PS of 0 or 1 were included, and the MPACT trial included less than 10% of patients with an Karnofsky-score of less than 80%. Contrasting clinical trials with very strict inclusion criteria, "real-life" analyses include patients with more comorbidities and/or a reduced general condition. However, differences in the rated ECOG score between different physicians as well as different medical disciplines have been observed [30]. There is no doubt that older patients will have on average a worse ECOG PS and more comorbidities than younger patients, but the decision to withhold FOLFIRINOX from old patients based only on chronological age would not be reasonable and reflects a form of "ageism". Whether a more intensive comprehensive geriatric assessment will translate into a superior rating regarding the tolerability of oncological treatment remains unknown. Some authors suggest that gemcitabine + nab-paclitaxel might be the preferred option in older patients given the lower incidence of several adverse events such as diarrhea in comparison to FOLFIRINOX. However, although independent phase III trials should only be directly compared very cautiously, the median overall survival rates clearly favor the FOLFIRINOX protocol (median OS 11.1 months for FOLFIRINOX vs. 8.7 months for gemcitabine/nab-paclitaxel) and this active combination should therefore be considered as a valuable treatment option for old patients in good PS.

The main limitation of our study is the small number of older patients and the retrospective, non-randomized nature of the analysis. It seems unlikely that a new randomized study on FOLFIRINOX in older patients will formally prove the benefit compared to gemcitabine monotherapy or gemcitabine/nab-paclitaxel in this patient group, but our study could serve as an encouragement to offer FOLFIRINOX also to older patients with good performance status. Finally, larger retrospective analyses, e.g. from cancer registers, might put our conclusions on a more solid fundament.

Conclusion

Our single-center experience confirms the FOLFIRINOX protocol being associated with a high rate of substantial side effects requiring dose reductions in more than half of the patients. We find some evidence, that dose reductions are possible without reducing clinical efficacy. Additionally, FOLFIRINOX seems to be a safe and efficient regimen for selected old patients with a good ECOG PS. It should not be withhold from patients solely based on the chronological age, avoiding any form of "ageism".

Abbreviations

CTCAE: Common terminology criteria for adverse events; ECOG PS: Eastern Cooperative Oncology Group performance status; NCT: National Center for Tumor Diseases; OS: Overall survival; PFS: Progression-free survival; RECIST: Response evaluation criteria in solid tumors

Acknowledgements

Not applicable

Author contributions

AKB participated in study concepts and design, data acquisition, data analysis and interpretation, manuscript preparation and editing. GMH participated in quality control of data and algorithms, data analysis and interpretation, statistical analysis and manuscript preparation. AB and ME participated in data acquisition and manuscript preparation. DJ and CS participated in data analysis and interpretation and manuscript preparation and review. All authors read and approved the final manuscript.

Consent for publication

Not applicable

Competing interests

The authors state that there are no competing interests.

Author details

[1]Department of Medical Oncology, National Center for Tumor Diseases (NCT), Heidelberg University Hospital, Im Neuenheimer Feld 460, 69120 Heidelberg, Germany. [2]Pharmacy Department, Heidelberg University Hospital, Heidelberg, Germany. [3]NCT Clinical Cancer Registry, German Cancer Research Center, Heidelberg, Germany.

References

1. Yancik R. Cancer burden in the aged: an epidemiologic and demographic overview. Cancer. 1997;80(7):1273–83.
2. Yancik R. Population aging and cancer: a cross-national concern. Cancer J. 2005;11(6):437–41.
3. Weir HK, Thompson TD, Soman A, Moller B, Leadbetter S. The past, present, and future of cancer incidence in the United States: 1975 through 2020. Cancer. 2015;121(11):1827–37. doi: 10.1002/cncr.29258.
4. Smith BD, Smith GL, Hurria A, Hortobagyi GN, Buchholz TA. Future of cancer incidence in the United States: burdens upon an aging, changing nation. J Clin Oncol. 2009;27(17):2758–65. doi: 10.1200/JCO.2008.20.8983.
5. Kumar A, Soares HP, Balducci L, Djulbegovic B, National Cancer I. Treatment tolerance and efficacy in geriatric oncology: a systematic review of phase III randomized trials conducted by five National Cancer Institute-sponsored cooperative groups. J Clin Oncol. 2007;25(10):1272–6. doi: 10.1200/JCO.2006.09.2759.
6. Pallis AG, Fortpied C, Wedding U, Van Nes MC, Penninckx B, Ring A, Lacombe D, Monfardini S, Scalliet P, Wildiers H. EORTC elderly task force position paper: approach to the older cancer patient. Eur J Cancer. 2010; 46(9):1502–13. doi: 10.1016/j.ejca.2010.02.022.
7. Siegel R, Naishadham D, Jemal A. Cancer statistics, 2013. CA Cancer J Clin. 2013;63(1):11–30. doi: 10.3322/caac.21166.
8. Niederhuber JE, Brennan MF, Menck HR. The National Cancer Data Base report on pancreatic cancer. Cancer. 1995;76(9):1671–7.
9. Hidalgo M. Pancreatic cancer. N Engl J Med. 2010;362(17):1605–17. doi: 10.1056/NEJMra0901557.
10. Vincent A, Herman J, Schulick R, Hruban RH, Goggins M. Pancreatic cancer. Lancet. 2011;378(9791):607–20. doi: 10.1016/S0140-6736(10)62307-0.
11. Werner J, Combs SE, Springfeld C, Hartwig W, Hackert T, Buchler MW. Advanced-stage pancreatic cancer: therapy options. Nat Rev Clin Oncol. 2013;10(6):323–33. doi: 10.1038/nrclinonc.2013.66.
12. Burris HA 3rd, Moore MJ, Andersen J, Green MR, Rothenberg ML, Modiano MR, Cripps MC, Portenoy RK, Storniolo AM, Tarassoff P, Nelson R, Dorr FA, Stephens CD, Von Hoff DD. Improvements in survival and clinical benefit with gemcitabine as first-line therapy for patients with advanced pancreas cancer: a randomized trial. J Clin Oncol. 1997;15(6):2403–13.
13. Conroy T, Desseigne F, Ychou M, Bouche O, Guimbaud R, Becouarn Y, Adenis A, Raoul JL, Gourgou-Bourgade S, de la Fouchardiere C, Bennouna J, Bachet JB, Khemissa-Akouz F, Pere-Verge D, Delbaldo C, Assenat E, Chauffert B, Michel P, Montoto-Grillot C, Ducreux M, Groupe Tumeurs Digestives of U, Intergroup P. FOLFIRINOX versus gemcitabine for metastatic pancreatic cancer. N Engl J Med. 2011;364(19):1817–25. doi: 10.1056/NEJMoa1011923.
14. Blazer M, Wu C, Goldberg RM, Phillips G, Schmidt C, Muscarella P, Wuthrick E, Williams TM, Reardon J, Ellison EC, Bloomston M, Bekaii-Saab T. Neoadjuvant modified (m) FOLFIRINOX for locally advanced unresectable (LAPC) and borderline resectable (BRPC) adenocarcinoma of the pancreas. Ann Surg Oncol. 2015;22(4):1153–9. doi: 10.1245/s10434-014-4225-1.
15. Ko AH. FOLFIRINOX: a small step or a great leap forward? J Clin Oncol. 2011; 29(28):3727–9. doi: 10.1200/JCO.2011.37.3464.
16. Peddi PF, Lubner S, McWilliams R, Tan BR, Picus J, Sorscher SM, Suresh R, Lockhart AC, Wang J, Menias C, Gao F, Linehan D, Wang-Gillam A. Multi-institutional experience with FOLFIRINOX in pancreatic adenocarcinoma. JOP. 2012;13(5):497–501. doi: 10.6092/1590-8577/913.
17. Gunturu KS, Yao X, Cong X, Thumar JR, Hochster HS, Stein SM, Lacy J. FOLFIRINOX for locally advanced and metastatic pancreatic cancer: single institution retrospective review of efficacy and toxicity. Med Oncol. 2013; 30(1):361. doi: 10.1007/s12032-012-0361-2.
18. Mahaseth H, Brutcher E, Kauh J, Hawk N, Kim S, Chen Z, Kooby DA, Maithel SK, Landry J, El-Rayes BF. Modified FOLFIRINOX regimen with improved safety and maintained efficacy in pancreatic adenocarcinoma. Pancreas. 2013;42(8):1311–5. doi: 10.1097/MPA.0b013e31829e2006.
19. Goldstein D, El-Maraghi RH, Hammel P, Heinemann V, Kunzmann V, Sastre J, Scheithauer W, Siena S, Tabernero J, Teixeira L, Tortora G, Van Laethem JL, Young R, Penenberg DN, Lu B, Romano A, Von Hoff DD (2015) nab-Paclitaxel plus gemcitabine for metastatic pancreatic cancer: long-term survival from a phase III trial. J Natl Cancer Inst 107 (2). doi:10.1093/jnci/dju413
20. Oken MM, Creech RH, Tormey DC, Horton J, Davis TE, McFadden ET, Carbone PP. Toxicity and response criteria of the eastern cooperative oncology group. Am J Clin Oncol. 1982;5(6):649–55.
21. Eisenhauer EA, Therasse P, Bogaerts J, Schwartz LH, Sargent D, Ford R, Dancey J, Arbuck S, Gwyther S, Mooney M, Rubinstein L, Shankar L, Dodd L, Kaplan R, Lacombe D, Verweij J. New response evaluation criteria in solid tumours: revised RECIST guideline (version 1.1). Eur J Cancer. 2009;45(2): 228–47. doi: 10.1016/j.ejca.2008.10.026.
22. Moore MJ, Goldstein D, Hamm J, Figer A, Hecht JR, Gallinger S, Au HJ, Murawa P, Walde D, Wolff RA, Campos D, Lim R, Ding K, Clark G, Voskoglou-Nomikos T, Ptasynski M, Parulekar W, National Cancer Institute of Canada Clinical Trials G (2007) Erlotinib plus gemcitabine compared with gemcitabine alone in patients with advanced pancreatic cancer: a phase III trial of the National Cancer Institute of Canada clinical trials group. J Clin Oncol 25 (15):1960-1966. doi: 10.1200/JCO.2006.07.9525.
23. Cunningham D, Chau I, Stocken DD, Valle JW, Smith D, Steward W, Harper PG, Dunn J, Tudur-Smith C, West J, Falk S, Crellin A, Adab F, Thompson J, Leonard P, Ostrowski J, Eatock M, Scheithauer W, Herrmann R, Neoptolemos JP. Phase III randomized comparison of gemcitabine versus gemcitabine plus capecitabine in patients with advanced pancreatic cancer. J Clin Oncol. 2009;27(33):5513–8. doi: 10.1200/JCO.2009.24.2446.
24. Von Hoff DD, Ervin T, Arena FP, Chiorean EG, Infante J, Moore M, Seay T, Tjulandin SA, Ma WW, Saleh MN, Harris M, Reni M, Dowden S, Laheru D, Bahary N, Ramanathan RK, Tabernero J, Hidalgo M, Goldstein D, Van Cutsem E, Wei X, Iglesias J, Renschler MF. Increased survival in pancreatic cancer with nab-paclitaxel plus gemcitabine. N Engl J Med. 2013;369(18):1691–703. doi: 10.1056/NEJMoa1304369.
25. James ES, Cong X, Yao X, Hahn C, Kaley K, Li J, Kortmansky JS, Fischbach NA, Cha C, Salem RR, Stein S, Hochster HS, Lacy J. Final analysis of a phase II

study of Yale-modified FOLFIRINOX (mFOLFIRINOX) in metastatic pancreatic cancer (MPC). J Clin Oncol (Meeting Abstracts). 2015;33(3_suppl):395.

26. Berger AK, Abel U, Komander C, Harig S, Jager D, Springfeld C. Chemotherapy for advanced pancreatic adenocarcinoma in elderly patients (>/=70 years of age): a retrospective cohort study at the National Center for tumor diseases Heidelberg. Pancreatology. 2014;14(3):211–5. doi: 10.1016/j.pan.2014.03.004.
27. Hutson TE, Bukowski RM, Rini BI, Gore ME, Larkin JMG, Figlin RA, Barrios CH, Escudier B, Lin X, Fly KD, Martell B, Matczak E, Motzer RJ. A pooled analysis of the efficacy and safety of sunitinib in elderly patients (pts) with metastatic renal cell carcinoma (mRCC). J Clin Oncol (Meeting Abstracts). 2011;29(15):4604.
28. Folprecht G, Seymour MT, Saltz L, Douillard JY, Hecker H, Stephens RJ, Maughan TS, Van Cutsem E, Rougier P, Mitry E, Schubert U, Kohne CH. Irinotecan/fluorouracil combination in first-line therapy of older and younger patients with metastatic colorectal cancer: combined analysis of 2,691 patients in randomized controlled trials. J Clin Oncol. 2008;26(9):1443–51. doi: 10.1200/JCO.2007.14.0509.
29. Berger AK, Zschaebitz S, Komander C, Jager D, Haag GM. Palliative chemotherapy for gastroesophageal cancer in old and very old patients: a retrospective cohort study at the National Center for tumor diseases, Heidelberg. World J Gastroenterol. 2015;21(16):4911–8. doi: 10.3748/wjg.v21.i16.4911.
30. Kim YJ, Hui D, Zhang Y, Park JC, Chisholm G, Williams J, Bruera E. Differences in performance status assessment among palliative care specialists, nurses, and medical oncologists. J Pain Symptom Manag. 2015; 49(6):1050–1058 e1052. doi: 10.1016/j.jpainsymman.2014.10.015.

13

Neutrophil to lymphocyte ratio and platelet to lymphocyte ratio can predict the severity of gallstone pancreatitis

Seung Kook Cho, Saehyun Jung, Kyong Joo Lee* and Jae Woo Kim*

Abstract

Background: Neutrophil to lymphocyte ratio (NLR) and platelet to lymphocyte ratio (PLR) predict severity in various diseases. In this study, we evaluated the value of NLR and PLR as prognostic factors in acute pancreatitis (AP).

Methods: Patients with AP were prospectively enrolled from March 2014 to September 2016 at Yonsei University Wonju College of Medicine. NLR and PLR were obtained at admission and were compared with other known prognostic scoring systems.

Results: A total of 243 patients were enrolled with an etiology of gallstone ($n = 134$) or alcohol ($n = 109$). NLR (17.7 ± 18.3 vs. 8.8 ± 8.4, $P < 0.001$) and PLR (344.1 ± 282.6 vs. 177.8 ± 150.1, $P < 0.001$) were significantly higher in the gallstone AP group than in the alcoholic AP group. For gallstone AP, NLR and PLR were significantly higher in severe AP, whereas high NLR and PLR were not related to severe AP in alcoholic AP. For the gallstone AP group, NLR and PLR demonstrated a predictive value significantly superior to C-reactive protein (CRP), whereas NLR, PLR, and CRP were not significant predictors for alcoholic AP.

Conclusion: Our study demonstrated that NLR and PLR can predict the severity of AP, but only in gallstone AP.

Keywords: Acute pancreatitis, Gallstone, Neutrophil to lymphocyte ratio, Platelet to lymphocyte ratio, Severity

Background

Acute pancreatitis (AP) is an inflammatory process in which local pancreatic injury leads to systemic inflammation through activation of cytokine cascades [1]. The clinical extent of AP varies widely from no symptoms to systemic inflammatory response syndrome (SIRS), persistent organ failure (POF), and death [2]. The clinical presentation of AP is both unreliable and nonspecific and exhibits a sensitivity less than 40% for the prediction of adverse outcomes [3]. Also, the underlying pathophysiology behind the progression of local pancreatic injury to SIRS is not fully understood [4]. Due to the diverse presentations of AP and its unknown pathophysiology, multiple severity scoring systems have been designed to help clinicians in triaging AP patients and predicting their prognosis. The Ranson score, the Acute Physiologic Assessment and Chronic Health Evaluation II (APACHE II) score, the Bedside Index for Severity in Acute Pancreatitis (BISAP) score, and the Glasgow-Imrie criteria are currently in wide use. However, these systems are time-consuming and difficult to apply to patients outside of intensive care settings because they use many variables [5]. Also, they are unsuitable for the evaluation of patients at the time of admission or shortly thereafter. Simplified serum markers such as C-reactive protein (CRP), procalcitonin, interleukin-6, and interleukin-8 have been applied to predict the prognosis or severity of AP, but they are expensive, not readily available, and cannot adequately predict the prognosis or severity of AP [6].

Recently, many research groups have studied the value of hematological components, such as the neutrophil to lymphocyte ratio (NLR) and the platelet to lymphocyte ratio (PLR), in predicting disease severity and outcomes across a variety of diseases, including inflammation, cardiovascular disease, and neoplastic states [2]. The superiority of NLR over total white blood cell (WBC) count, which is used in the Ranson, APACHE-II, and

* Correspondence: smild123@yonsei.ac.kr; jawkim96@yonsei.ac.kr
Department of Internal Medicine, Yonsei University Wonju College of Medicine, 20 Ilsan-ro, Wonju-si 26426, Republic of Korea

Glasgow-Imrie scoring systems, has been demonstrated in a variety of medical conditions [7]. Furthermore, a few studies have shown that PLR is superior to NLR as a prognostic factor in certain disease conditions [8–10]. Increased NLR and PLR ratios have been associated with inflammatory conditions, and poor outcomes in severe AP are explained by uncontrolled SIRS and its progression to multi-organ dysfunction syndrome [6].

Although a few studies have considered NLR and its prognostic value in AP, no studies have yet examined the prognostic value of PLR in AP. In the present study, we evaluated NLR and PLR values as independent prognostic factors for adverse outcomes in AP and sought to improve previous scoring systems by incorporating NLR and PLR.

Methods

Patients

Patients with AP were prospectively enrolled in Yonsei University Wonju College of Medicine from March 2014 to September 2016. The International Review Board for Human Research of Yonsei University Wonju College of Medicine approved this study (CR315005–002). We only included patients who visited our hospital for a primary visit: patients referred from other clinics were excluded. Written informed consent was obtained from all patients. The diagnosis of AP requires 2 of the following 3 criteria [1]: typical abdominal pain; serum amylase or lipase elevation ≥ 3 times the upper limit of normal; and characteristic findings of AP on contrast-enhanced computed tomography, magnetic resonance imaging, or abdominal ultrasonography. During the study period, a total of 274 patients were diagnosed with AP (Fig. 1). Etiologies other than gallstone and alcohol were excluded. All patients were followed until discharge from the hospital or hospital mortality.

Data collection

Blood samples for hematological and biochemical data were obtained within 1 h of admission. NLR and PLR were defined as the quotient of absolute neutrophil count to absolute lymphocyte count and that of absolute platelet count to absolute lymphocyte count, respectively. Ranson score, computed tomography scoring index (CTSI), and BISAP score were also calculated upon admission.

Definition of persistent organ failure

Organ failure was diagnosed as a score ≥ 2 in one or more of the three organ systems described in the modified Marshall score: respiratory failure if the ratio of PaO_2/FiO_2 was < 300 mmHg; renal failure if serum creatinine was ≥ 1.9 mg/dL; and cardiovascular failure if systolic blood pressure was < 90 mmHg despite fluid replacement. POF was defined as organ failure lasting more than 48 h. That definition is in accordance with the revised Atlanta classification [1].

Statistical analysis

Continuous variables are presented as mean and standard deviation. Categorical variables are presented as frequency and percentage. Continuous variables in 2 groups were compared using Student's *t*-test, and categorical variables were compared using the chi-square test. In addition, comparisons of area under the curve (AUC) were used to assess the predictive ability for POF. *P* values less than 0.05 were considered statistically significant, and all statistical analyses were performed using SPSS software, version 18.0 (SPSS Inc., Chicago, IL).

Results

Patient characteristics

A total of 243 patients were enrolled (Table 1). The etiologies of acute pancreatitis were gallstone ($n = 134$) and alcohol ($n = 109$). Mean age was higher in the gallstone AP group, whereas the male-to-female ratio and proportion of smokers were lower. We found no significant difference in body mass index or proportion of patients with diabetes mellitus in the two groups. Hypertension and liver cirrhosis were more frequent in patients with alcoholic AP than in

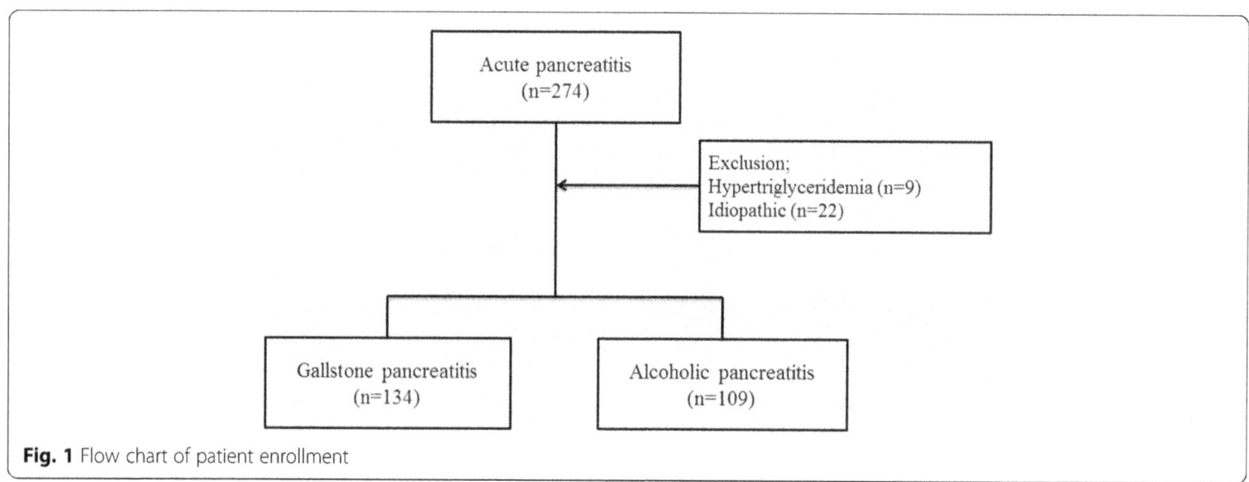

Fig. 1 Flow chart of patient enrollment

Table 1 Baseline Characteristics

Characteristics	Overall (*N* = 243)	Gallstone (*N* = 134)	Alcohol (*N* = 109)	*P* value
Age (year)	59.3 ± 17.9	66.3 ± 17.2	50.8 ± 14.8	< 0.001
Sex (male)	166 (68.3%)	72 (53.7%)	94 (86.2%)	< 0.001
Smoking	114 (46.9%)	37 (27.6%)	77 (70.6%)	< 0.001
BMI (kg/m2)	23.8 ± 3.9	24 ± 3.4	23.7 ± 4.4	0.591
Diabetes mellitus	62 (25.5%)	35 (26.1%)	27 (24.8%)	0.810
Hypertension	85 (35%)	56 (41.8%)	29 (26.6%)	0.014
Liver cirrhosis	21 (8.6%)	7 (5.2%)	14 (12.8%)	0.036
Atlanta classification				< 0.001
Mild	161 (66.3%)	107 (79.9%)	54 (49.5%)	
Moderately severe	57 (23.5%)	21 (15.7%)	36 (33%)	
Severe	25 (10.3%)	6 (4.5%)	19 (17.4%)	
Scoring systems				
Ranson	2.4 ± 1.7	2.4 ± 1.5	2.4 ± 1.8	0.998
CTSI	1.9 ± 1.7	1.2 ± 1.3	2.6 ± 1.8	< 0.001
BISAP	1.3 ± 1.1	1.2 ± 1.1	1.4 ± 1.3	0.236
Laboratory data				
WBC (/mm^3)	11,936 ± 5569	12,023 ± 5172	11,828 ± 6043	0.787
Neutrophil (/mm^3)	10.2 ± 7.1	10.8 ± 8.1	9.4 ± 5.4	0.126
Lymphocyte (/mm^3)	1.2 ± 1.0	1.1 ± 1.0	1.5 ± 0.9	< 0.001
Platelet (/mm^3)	210,000 ± 88,000	220,000 ± 74,000	198,000 ± 102,000	0.001
NLR	13.8 ± 15.3	17.7 ± 18.3	8.8 ± 8.4	< 0.001
PLR	269.5 ± 246.6	344.1 ± 282.6	177.8 ± 150.1	< 0.001
CRP (mg/dL)	4.9 ± 6.9	4.4 ± 5.7	5.5 ± 8.1	0.192
Hospital stay (day)	7.2 ± 6.5	6.9 ± 5.9	7.7 ± 7.2	0.292
ICU admission, n	52 (21.4%)	15 (11.2%)	37 (33.9%)	< 0.001
Mortality, n	15 (6.2%)	3 (2.2%)	12 (11%)	0.005

BMI indicates body mass index, *CTSI* computed tomography severity index, *BISAP* Bedside Index for Severity in Acute Pancreatitis, *WBC* white blood count, *NLR* neutrophil to lymphocyte ratio, *PLR* platelet to lymphocyte ratio, *CRP* C-reactive protein, *ICU* intensive care unit

those with gallstone AP. According to the Atlanta classification, more patients with moderately severe and severe pancreatitis were classified into the alcoholic AP group. Mean Ranson and BISAP scores on admission did not differ between gallstone and alcoholic AP, but mean CTSI was significantly higher in the gallstone AP group. The mean duration of hospital stay did not differ between the two groups. However, the number of admissions to the intensive care unit (ICU) and mortality were significantly higher in the alcoholic AP group.

WBC, neutrophil, lymphocyte, NLR, PLR, and CRP levels on admission

Although the total WBC and neutrophil counts were similar between the two AP groups, the gallstone AP group showed significantly lower lymphocyte count and higher platelet count (Table 1). NLR (17.7 ± 18.3 vs. 8.8 ± 8.4, $P <$ 0.001) and PLR (344.1 ± 282.6 vs. 177.8 ± 150.1, $P < 0.001$) were significantly higher in the gallstone AP group than in the alcoholic AP group. CRP did not differ significantly between the groups (4.4 ± 5.7 vs. 5.5 ± 8.1 mg/dL, $P = 0.192$).

We performed subgroup analysis according to AP etiology (Tables 2 and 3). For gallstone AP, NLR was significantly higher in severe pancreatitis, as defined by the revised Atlanta classification (32.4 ± 30.9 vs. 17.1 ± 17.4, $P = 0.045$), Ranson score ≥ 3 (24.8 ± 19.6 vs. 12.1 ± 15.1, $P < 0.001$), and BISAP score ≥ 3 (28.6 ± 20.7 vs. 16.3 ± 17.6, $P = 0.012$) (Table 2). A similar pattern was found for PLR in gallstone AP. In the alcoholic AP group, higher NLR was significantly correlated only with Ranson score ≥ 3 (11.9 ± 109 vs. 6.5 ± 4.7, $P < 0.001$) (Table 3).

Predictive value of NLR and PLR in comparison to CRP in both groups

We calculated the AUCs of NLR, PLR, and CRP for predicting POF in all patients (Fig. 2a). For all AP patients, NLR, PLR, and CRP failed to predict POF with statistical significance. The AUC was recalculated for the etiology

Table 2 Neutrophil to Lymphocyte Ratio and Platelet to Lymphocyte Ratio in Gallstone Pancreatitis

Parameters	NLR	*P* value	PLR	*P* value
Atlanta classification		0.045		0.008
Mild/moderate	17.1 ± 17.4		330.2 ± 263.7	
Severe	32.4 ± 30.9		641 ± 498.6	
Ranson		< 0.001		< 0.001
< 3	12.1 ± 15.1		258.5 ± 219.3	
≥ 3	24.8 ± 19.6		449.7 ± 316.3	
CTSI		0.083		0.095
< 3	16.3 ± 17.9		323.1 ± 273.7	
≥ 3	23.1 ± 19.1		423.6 ± 306.5	
BISAP		0.012		0.020
< 3	16.3 ± 17.6		323.2 ± 267.6	
≥ 3	28.6 ± 20.7		498.1 ± 347.9	

CTSI computed tomography severity index, *BISAP* Bedside Index for Severity in Acute Pancreatitis, *NLR* neutrophil to lymphocyte ratio, *PLR* platelet to lymphocyte ratio

subgroups. For the gallstone AP group, NLR and PLR demonstrated a predictive value significantly superior to that of CRP (NLR-AUC 0.663, 95% CI 0.56–0.77; PLR-AUC 0.638, 95% CI 0.53–0.75; CRP-AUC 0.475, 95% CI 0.35–0.60, Fig. 2b), whereas NLR, PLR, and CRP were not significant for alcoholic AP (NLR-AUC 0.618, 95% CI 0.51–0.72; PLR-AUC 0.446, 95% CI 0.34–0.55; CRP-AUC 0.598, 95% CI 0.49–0.71, Fig. 2c). The best NLR and PLR cutoffs for predicting POF in gallstone AP patients were 7.8 and 229.1, respectively, with sensitivity and specificity of 88.9% and 41.1% for NLR and 70.4% and 52.3% for PLR.

Table 3 Neutrophil to lymphocyte ratio and platelet to lymphocyte ratio in alcoholic pancreatitis

Parameters	NLR	*P* value	PLR	*P* value
Atlanta classification		0.606		0.218
Mild/moderate	8.7 ± 8.3		186 ± 150.5	
Severe	9.8 ± 8.8		139.1 ± 145.4	
Ranson		0.001		0.511
< 3	6.5 ± 4.7		169.5 ± 115.4	
≥ 3	11.9 ± 10.9		188.7 ± 187.1	
CTSI		0.107		0.805
< 3	7.5 ± 7.8		181.4 ± 147.4	
≥ 3	10.1 ± 8.7		174.3 ± 153.9	
BISAP		0.417		0.876
< 3	8.5 ± 7.2		179 ± 130.7	
≥ 3	10.1 ± 11.6		173.5 ± 208.2	

CTSI computed tomography severity index, *BISAP* Bedside Index for Severity in Acute Pancreatitis, *NLR* neutrophil to lymphocyte ratio, *PLR* platelet to lymphocyte ratio

Discussion

In the present study, we investigated the value of NLR and PLR as predictive markers of AP severity. We found that NLR and PLR were well correlated with other scoring systems in patients with gallstone AP. In addition, NLR and PLR showed significant predictive ability for POF in patients with gallstone AP. However, in patients with alcoholic AP, NLR and PLR were not correlated with other scoring systems.

NLR was first introduced as an easily measurable parameter assessing systemic inflammation and stress in critically ill patients [11]. Later, PLR was also found to be an inflammatory marker, and the role of platelets as a critical link between inflammation and microvascular dysfunction has since been investigated [12–14]. The prognostic value of these two parameters has been confirmed in a variety of clinical conditions, and PLR was shown to be superior to NLR in certain cancers [8–10]. AP is an inflammatory condition characterized by activation of both innate and adaptive immune responses. Activation and modulation of neutrophils and platelets play a core role in establishing host defenses in settings of systemic inflammation; however, excessive inflammatory response causes massive cell transmigration to the pancreas and subsequent release of aggressive defense molecules, resulting in destruction of the pancreas and organ failure [15–18].

A few studies have investigated the relationship between NLR and outcome in patients with AP. Azab et al. [7] first applied the concept of NLR to patients with AP in 2011. They found that NLR was a better predictor of ICU admission or prolonged hospitalization in AP than was total WBC count and suggested a cutoff value of < 4.7 as a predictor of a poor outcome [7]. However, in-hospital mortality was extremely low in that study, and the investigators failed to assess records of organ failure. Suppiah et al. [6] revealed an association between NLR measured in the first 48 h and the risk of AP developing into a more severe form. However, that study was limited by a small sample size (*n* = 146), and the AP cases included were mostly mild, with no local/systemic complications or organ failure. Recently, Gulen et al. [19] investigated the association between NLR and early mortality and argued that NLR is not a significant independent prognostic factor. Zhang et al. [2] demonstrated that elevated NLR is associated with POF, ICU stay longer than > 7 days, and increased in-hospital mortality in a Chinese population.

However, despite the demonstrated superiority of PLR over NLR in predicting the outcome of inflammation in several clinical conditions, no previous study has investigated the predictive value of PLR at the time of admission on outcomes in patients with AP. Furthermore, although they are grouped together as pancreatitis, gallstone AP and alcoholic AP each has a distinct pathophysiology, and no study has compared NLR or PLR between them.

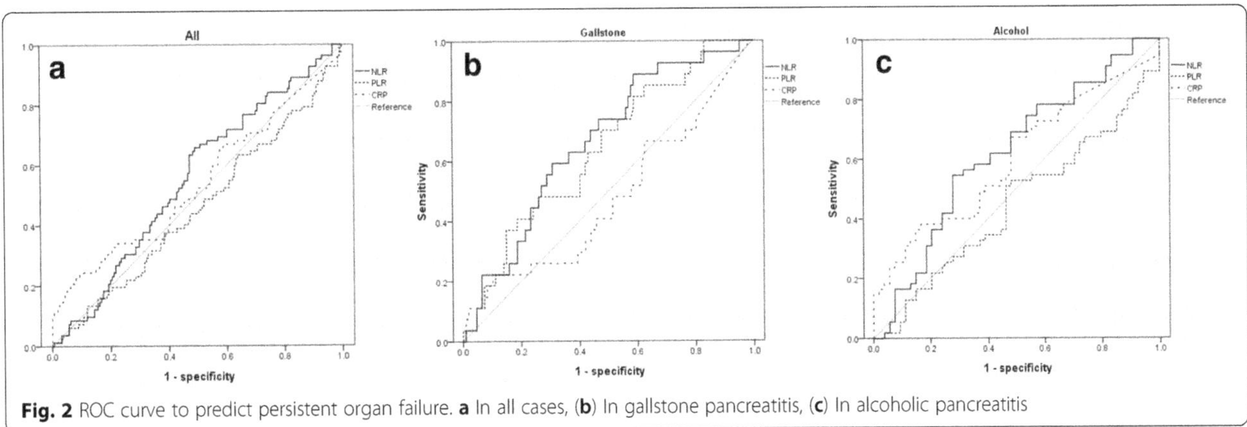

Fig. 2 ROC curve to predict persistent organ failure. **a** In all cases, (**b**) In gallstone pancreatitis, (**c**) In alcoholic pancreatitis

Therefore, we investigated the value of PLR in predicting AP outcomes and compared differences between NLR and PLR patterns in two distinct forms of AP. We excluded pancreatitis caused by factors other than gallstone or alcohol. When all AP cases were combined, NLR and PLR were not significant independent predictive factors of POF. However, after subgrouping AP by etiology, both NLR and PLR were independent predictive factors of POF in gallstone AP. In alcoholic AP, NLR was a significant predictor, but PLR was not. This can be explained by the different mechanism of alcohol AP. Alcoholic AP is usually associated with chronic liver disease. In our results, the number of liver cirrhosis patients was larger and the platelet count was lower in alcoholic AP compared to gallstone AP. Thrombocytopenia is related to chronic liver disease due to impaired platelet production and decreased hepatic synthesis of thrombopoietin [20]. Therefore, PLR can vary according to liver function as well as systemic inflammation. Interestingly, CRP, a marker traditionally used to assess the severity of inflammation [21–23], failed to predict POF in gallstone AP and alcoholic AP. This suggests the superiority of NLR and PLR to CRP in predicting the course of gallstone AP.

Although the exact mechanism of alcoholic AP has not been elucidated, our findings imply a fundamental difference in pathophysiology between the two subgroups. Although elevated NLR and PLR can be used as predictive biomarkers in AP, interpretation should follow confirmation of the etiology. Furthermore, our findings challenge the rationale of applying a uniform prognostic scoring system to all AP. Replacing WBC count with NLR or PLR in traditional prognostic scoring systems could improve their performance [10].

Also, pancreatic cancer can induce impairment of the patient's immune system through systemic inflammation [24]. In this aspect, NLR and PLR can reflect the status of the immune system in patients with pancreatic cancer. Several studies have reported that NLR and PLR were correlated with poor overall survival in patients with pancreatic cancer [25, 26]. A recent study demonstrated that NLR was a predictive marker for the presence of invasive carcinoma in patients with intraductal papillary mucinous neoplasm [27]. Therefore, NLR and PLR have a role as biomarkers in pancreatic malignancy.

This study has several limitations. First, the number of patients enrolled in this study was small, and this study was performed in a tertiary care center, which could have resulted in disproportional inclusion of patients with severe disease status and tendency to progress to POF. Such selection bias might have overestimated the predictive value of elevated NLR or PLR. Second, we did not compare NLR or PLR with other biochemical markers, such as procalcitonin and IL-6. Third, we did not describe changes in NLR or PLR during treatment, which could estimate the prognosis of AP. Despite these limitations, this study also has strengths. This is the first prospective study investigating the predictive value of PLR in AP and the difference between NLR and PLR in two subgroups of AP. Also, all laboratory values were obtained within 1 h of initial presentation, minimizing changes in WBC and platelet counts caused by hydration and medication.

Conclusions

In conclusion, both NLR and PLR were significant independent predictive factors of POF in gallstone AP, and they were better predictors of POF than was CRP, a traditionally used inflammatory marker and independent prognostic factor. Future studies including a larger number of patients across both subgroups of AP should be performed to further compare differences between NLR and PLR in the two etiologies.

Abbreviations

AP: Acute pancreatitis; APACHE II: Acute Physiologic Assessment and Chronic Health Evaluation II; AUC: Area under the curve; BISAP: Bedside Index for Severity in Acute Pancreatitis; CRP: C-reactive protein; CTSI: Computed tomography scoring index; NLR: Neutrophil to lymphocyte ratio; PLR: Platelet to lymphocyte ratio; POF: Persistent organ failure; SIRS: Systemic inflammatory response syndrome; WBC: Total white blood cell

Acknowledgments
We thank to Geun Sook Lee for coordinating this study.

Funding
This work was supported by the National Research Foundation of Korea (NRF) grant funded by the Korea government (MSIP). (No. NRF-2016R1C1B1007909).

Authors' contributions
SKC, KJL, and JWK designed the study. SKC and SHJ collected the data. KJL and JWK analyzed and interpreted the results. SKC and KJL drafted and revised the manuscript. All authors approved the final manuscript.

Consent for publication
Not applicable

Competing interests
The authors declare that they have no competing interests.

References

1. Banks PA, Bollen TL, Dervenis C, Gooszen HG, Johnson CD, Sarr MG, Tsiotos GG, Vege SS, Acute Pancreatitis Classification Working G. Classification of acute pancreatitis–2012: revision of the Atlanta classification and definitions by international consensus. Gut. 2013;62(1):102–11.
2. Zhang Y, Wu W, Dong L, Yang C, Fan P, Wu H. Neutrophil to lymphocyte ratio predicts persistent organ failure and in-hospital mortality in an Asian Chinese population of acute pancreatitis. Medicine. 2016;95(37):e4746.
3. Steinberg WM. Predictors of severity of acute pancreatitis. Gastroenterol Clin N Am. 1990;19(4):849–61.
4. Oiva J, Mustonen H, Kylanpaa ML, Kyhala L, Kuuliala K, Siitonen S, Kemppainen E, Puolakkainen P, Repo H. Acute pancreatitis with organ dysfunction associates with abnormal blood lymphocyte signaling: controlled laboratory study. Crit Care. 2010;14(6):R207.
5. Pavlidis TE, Pavlidis ET, Sakantamis AK. Advances in prognostic factors in acute pancreatitis: a mini-review. Hepatobiliary Pancreat Dis Int. 2010; 9(5):482–6.
6. Suppiah A, Malde D, Arab T, Hamed M, Allgar V, Smith AM, Morris-Stiff G. The prognostic value of the neutrophil-lymphocyte ratio (NLR) in acute pancreatitis: identification of an optimal NLR. J Gastrointest Surg. 2013;17(4): 675–81.
7. Azab B, Jaglall N, Atallah JP, Lamet A, Raja-Surya V, Farah B, Lesser M, Widmann WD. Neutrophil-lymphocyte ratio as a predictor of adverse outcomes of acute pancreatitis. Pancreatology. 2011;11(4):445–52.
8. Feng JF, Huang Y, Chen QX. Preoperative platelet lymphocyte ratio (PLR) is superior to neutrophil lymphocyte ratio (NLR) as a predictive factor in patients with esophageal squamous cell carcinoma. World J Surg Oncol. 2014;12:58.
9. Acharya S, Rai P, Hallikeri K, Anehosur V, Kale J. Preoperative platelet lymphocyte ratio is superior to neutrophil lymphocyte ratio to be used as predictive marker for lymph node metastasis in oral squamous cell carcinoma. J Investig Clin Dent. 2016;8(3):e12219.
10. Que Y, Qiu H, Li Y, Chen Y, Xiao W, Zhou Z, Zhang X. Preoperative platelet-lymphocyte ratio is superior to neutrophil-lymphocyte ratio as a prognostic factor for soft-tissue sarcoma. BMC Cancer. 2015;15:648.
11. Zahorec R. Ratio of neutrophil to lymphocyte counts–rapid and simple parameter of systemic inflammation and stress in critically ill. Bratislavske lekarske listy. 2001;102(1):5–14.
12. Stokes KY, Granger DN. Platelets: a critical link between inflammation and microvascular dysfunction. J Physiol. 2012;590(5):1023–34.
13. Thomas MR, Storey RF. The role of platelets in inflammation. Thromb Haemost. 2015;114(3):449–58.
14. Klinger MH, Jelkmann W. Role of blood platelets in infection and inflammation. J Interferon Cytokine Res. 2002;22(9):913–22.
15. Bermejo-Martin JF, Tamayo E, Ruiz G, Andaluz-Ojeda D, Herran-Monge R, Muriel-Bombin A, Fe Munoz M, Heredia-Rodriguez M, Citores R, Gomez-Herreras J, et al. Circulating neutrophil counts and mortality in septic shock. Crit Care. 2014;18(1):407.
16. Soehnlein O, Lindbom L. Phagocyte partnership during the onset and resolution of inflammation. Nat Rev Immunol. 2010;10(6):427–39.
17. Nauseef WM, Borregaard N. Neutrophils at work. Nat Immunol. 2014;15(7): 602–11.
18. Maitre B, Magnenat S, Heim V, Ravanat C, Evans RJ, de la Salle H, Gachet C, Hechler B. The P2X1 receptor is required for neutrophil extravasation during lipopolysaccharide-induced lethal endotoxemia in mice. J Immunol. 2015; 194(2):739–49.
19. Gulen B, Sonmez E, Yaylaci S, Serinken M, Eken C, Dur A, Turkdogan FT, Sogut O. Effect of harmless acute pancreatitis score, red cell distribution width and neutrophil/lymphocyte ratio on the mortality of patients with nontraumatic acute pancreatitis at the emergency department. World J Emerg Med. 2015;6(1):29–33.
20. Afdhal N, McHutchison J, Brown R, Jacobson I, Manns M, Poordad F, Weksler B, Esteban R. Thrombocytopenia associated with chronic liver disease. J Hepatol. 2008;48(6):1000–7.
21. Mayer AD, McMahon MJ, Bowen M, Cooper EH. C reactive protein: an aid to assessment and monitoring of acute pancreatitis. J Clin Pathol. 1984;37(2):207–11.
22. Del Prete M, Castiglia D, Meli M, Perri S, Nicita A, Dalla Torre A, Moraldi A. Prognostic value of C reactive protein in acute pancreatitis. Chir Ital. 2001; 53(1):33–8.
23. Digalakis MK, Katsoulis IE, Biliri K, Themeli-Digalaki K. Serum profiles of C-reactive protein, interleukin-8, and tumor necrosis factor-alpha in patients with acute pancreatitis. HPB Surg. 2009;2009:878490.
24. Sideras K, Braat H, Kwekkeboom J, van Eijck CH, Peppelenbosch MP, Sleijfer S, Bruno M. Role of the immune system in pancreatic cancer progression and immune modulating treatment strategies. Cancer Treat Rev. 2014;40(4):513–22.
25. Luo G, Guo M, Liu Z, Xiao Z, Jin K, Long J, Liu L, Liu C, Xu J, Ni Q, et al. Blood neutrophil-lymphocyte ratio predicts survival in patients with advanced pancreatic cancer treated with chemotherapy. Ann Surg Oncol. 2015;22(2):670–6.
26. Martin HL, Ohara K, Kiberu A, Van Hagen T, Davidson A, Khattak MA. Prognostic value of systemic inflammation-based markers in advanced pancreatic cancer. Intern Med J. 2014;44(7):676–82.
27. Gemenetzis G, Bagante F, Griffin JF, Rezaee N, Javed AA, Manos LL, Lennon AM, Wood LD, Hruban RH, Zheng L, et al. Neutrophil-to-lymphocyte ratio is a predictive marker for invasive malignancy in Intraductal papillary Mucinous Neoplasms of the pancreas. Ann Surg. 2017;266(2):339–45.

14

Significantly different clinical features between hypertriglyceridemia and biliary acute pancreatitis: a retrospective study of 730 patients from a tertiary center

Xiaoyao Li†, Lu Ke†, Jie Dong, Bo Ye, Lei Meng, Wenjian Mao, Qi Yang*, Weiqin Li* and Jieshou Li

Abstract

Background: Unlike western world, gallstones and hypertriglyceridemia (HTG) are among the first two etiologies of acute pancreatitis (AP) in China. But yet, detailed differences in clinical features and outcomes between hypertriglyceridemia and biliary acute pancreatitis have not been well described.

Methods: This retrospective study enrolled 730 acute pancreatitis patients from July 1, 2013 to October 1, 2016 in Jinling Hospital. The causes of the study patients were defined according to specific diagnostic criteria. The clinical features and outcomes of patients with hypertriglyceridemia acute pancreatitis (HTG-AP) and biliary acute pancreatitis (BAP) were compared in terms of general information, disease severity, laboratory data, system complications, local complications, and clinical outcome.

Results: In the enrolled 730 AP patients, 305 (41.8%) were HTG-AP, and 425 (58.2%) were BAP. Compared to BAP, the HTG-AP patients were found to be younger, with higher body mass Index (BMI), and much higher proportion of diabetes, fatty liver and high fat diet. Besides that, HTG-AP patients had significantly higher C-reactive protein (CRP) ($p<0.01$) and creatinine ($p = 0.031$), together with more acute respiratory distress syndrome (ARDS) ($p = 0.039$), acute kidney injury (AKI) ($p<0.001$), deep venous thrombosis ($p = 0.008$) and multiple organ dysfunction syndrome (MODS) ($p = 0.032$) in systematic complications. As for local complications, HTG-AP patients had significantly less infected pancreatitis necrosis ($p = 0.005$). However, there was no difference in mortality, hospital duration and costs between the groups.

Conclusion: HTG-AP patients were younger, more male, having high fat diet and with higher BMI compared to BAP patients. The prevalence of AKI/ARDS/DVT/MODS in HTG-AP patients was higher than BAP patients, while BAP patients had a greater possibility in development of infected pancreatitis necrosis (IPN). According to the multivariate analysis, only the complication of AKI was independently related with the etiology of HTG, however, BMI contributes to AKI, ARDS and DVT.

Keywords: Biliary acute pancreatitis, Hypertriglyceridemia acute pancreatitis, Acute kidney injury(AKI), Body Mass Index(BMI), Infected pancreatic necrosis

* Correspondence: yangqi_nj@163.com; njzy_pancrea@163.com
†Xiaoyao Li and Lu Ke contributed equally to this work.
Surgical Intensive Care Unit (SICU), Department of General Surgery, Jinling Hospital, Medical School of Nanjing University, Nanjing, China

Background

Acute pancreatitis (AP) is an acute inflammatory disease which is characterized by local pancreatic inflammation and consequently systemic inflammatory response. The imaging of AP manifests as pancreatic edema or necrosis involving the pancreas as well as peripancreatic tissues and even distant organs [1, 2]. In the western countries, the most common etiology of AP was gallstones, followed by alcohol abuse and hypertriglyceridemia [3, 4]. While the incidence of hypertriglyceridemia acute pancreatitis (HTG-AP) was much higher in China and has been increasing year by year according to the recent studies [5–10].

Previous studies well reported the clinical features of AP with different etiologies, rather than the detailed differences between HTG-AP and BAP. In this retrospective study from July 2013 to October 2016, we compared the clinical features, complications and outcomes between hypertriglyceridemia and biliary acute pancreatitis patients, as the two leading etiologies of acute pancreatitis in China.

Methods

Patient selection

This study retrospectively screened 999 AP cases admitted to the Surgical Intensive Care Unit (SICU), Department of General Surgery from July,1 2013 to October,1 2016, Jinling Hospital, Medical School of Nanjing University.

Patients who met the following criteria were excluded: (1) re-admission to the SICU; (2) traumatic, neoplastic, parathyroidal or other idiopathic pancreatitis; (3) younger than 18 years old. Eventually, 730 AP patients were enrolled in this study. The diagnosis and classification of the severity of AP were defined according to the 2012 revision of the Atlanta Classification.

Data collection

The data analyzed in this study included general information as sex, age, body mass index (BMI), diabetes, fatty liver, high fat diet, transfer from other hospitals and clinical features as pancreatitis severity, incidence of systemic and local complications, mortality. Levels of hemoglobin, hematocrit, platelet, C-reactive protein (CRP), IL-6, creatinine, alanine aminotransferase (ALT) and other laboratory results were included in the comparison. All the laboratory results were obtained from the Central Laboratory of Jinling Hospital according to the standard protocols. Meanwhile, acute physiology and chronic health evaluation II (APACHE II) score was manually calculated for each single patient.

According to the 2012 revised of the Atlanta Classification the etiology of AP and the definition of complications, including portal vein thrombosis, intra-abdominal hypertension and hemorrhage, deep vein thrombosis (DVT) and gastrointestinal fistula, were judged by two independent physicians [1]. Different severity of AP as mild, moderate and severe, was assessed based on the presence of local or systemic complications and transient/persistent organ failure [2].

Definition

The diagnosis of AP requires at least two of the following three features: (1) abdominal pain consistent with the disease (2) serum lipase activity (or amylase activity) at least three times greater than the upper limit of normal; and (3) characteristic findings from abdominal imaging [1].

The etiology of AP was analyzed by the following criteria. Biliary acute pancreatitis required the confirmation of gallstones or biliary sludge by any kind radiological imaging, including endoscopic ultrasonography(EUS), computed tomography (CT) and magnetic resonance cholangiopancreatography (MRCP), or elevated serum levels of ALT (> 60 U/L) and a BMI < 30 kg/m^2 indicates an episode of acute pancreatitis with a biliary origin [3]. Hypertriglyceridemia acute pancreatitis was confirmed by triglyceride levels > 1000 mg/dL or triglyceride levels between 500 mg/dL to 1000 mg/dL together with emulsion plasma and without any other obvious causes [1, 4].

The diagnosis of local complications was performed according to the 2012 revision of the Atlanta Classification. Infected pancreatitis necrosis (IPN) could be diagnosed by the presence of extra luminal gas in the pancreatic and/or peripancreatic tissues on CECT or by a positive bacterial culture of the necrosis from the fine-needle aspiration or drainage [1]. As this study being retrospectively, one clinical feature as "high fat diet" could not be defined exactly according to the standard definition. So here, we inquired the patients or their relatives to describe the normal typical 1-day diet. By calculating the constituent ratio, we defined the "high fat diet" as fat accounts over 30–35%.

This study was performed according to the principles of the Declaration of Helsinki (modified 2000) and was approved by the institutional review board of Jinling Hospital.

Statistical analysis

We used SPSS 18.0 statistical software package (IBM Analytics, Armonk, NY) for statistical analyses. As the following tables show, datas were presented as median plus interquartile range (IQR) for continuous variables and absolute numbers and percentages for categorical variables. The x^2 test was used for analyzing categorical variables and Student-test or Mann–Whitney test was used for analyzing continuous variables. Statistical significance was considered as a P value of < 0.05 (2-tailed).

Results

Baseline characteristics and clinical features

Nine hundred and ninety-nine patients were initially screened and eventually 730 patients were enrolled. The guidelines and procedures were shown in Fig. 1. Firstly, 141 patients were excluded, who were re-admitted to ICU not because of AP but other complications, such as intestinal fistula, from the recovery ward. Secondly, the patients were divided into different groups by the etiology according to the revised Atlanta criteria, which were done by two independent physicians [1]. Traumatic acute pancreatitis patients ($n = 9$), parathyroidal acute pancreatitis patients ($n = 1$), idiopathic acute pancreatitis patients ($n = 76$), alcoholic acute pancreatitis patients ($n = 37$) were also exclude. After that, we got 426 biliary acute pancreatitis (BAP) patients and 309 hypertriglyceridemia acute pancreatitis (HTG-AP) patients. Thirdly, we excluded five patients with age < 18, as 1 BAP patient and 4 HTG-AP patients. Ultimately, two groups were enrolled in this study, namely, biliary acute pancreatitis (BAP) ($n = 425$) and hypertriglyceridemia acute pancreatitis (HTG-AP) ($n = 305$) group.

The baseline characteristics of BAP and HTG-AP were displayed in Table 1. Compared to BAP patients, the HTG-AP patients were younger (40 vs 51, $p < 0.01$), with higher BMI (27 vs 22.7, $p < 0.01$), and more males (214/91 vs 242/183, $p < 0.01$), and higher incidence of diabetes (32.1% vs 12.9%, $p < 0.01$) and fatty liver (43.9% vs 15.1%, $p < 0.01$) and higher fat diet rate (42.6% vs14.6%, $p < 0.01$). Meanwhile, HTG-AP patients had significantly higher APACHEII score ($p < 0.01$) than BAP. Besides that, some similarities were also found between two groups, such as hypertension history, and duration from AP onset to transfer to our center.

All the patients initially received standard medical treatment according to the recent international guidelines [5]. Following a standard protocol (Additional file 1: Figure S1), fluid resuscitation was performed for each patient. The protocol includes the timing to initiation of hydration, rate of hydration and the appropriate solution. Moreover, 91 HTG-AP patients received apheresis.

According to the modified Atlanta Criteria, the AP patients were classified into mild acute pancreatitis (MAP), mild severe acute pancreatitis (MSAP), and severe acute pancreatitis (SAP). The percentages of MAP, MSAP, SAP were respectively 24, 19.8 56.2% in BAP, and 17.7, 28.9 and 53.4% in HTG-AP (Fig. 2).

Systemic complications and laboratory data

The laboratory data were displayed in Table 2, and systemic complications in Table 3. The results suggested that more ARDS ($p = 0.039$), AKI ($p<0.001$)and MODS($p = 0.032$) occurred in HTG-AP, together with significantly higher CRP ($p<0.01$) and creatinine ($p = 0.031$). Also, there were more deep venous thrombosis (DVT) (27 (6.4%) vs 37 (12.1%), $p = 0.008$) in HTG-AP than BAP. However, the other data were similar in two groups, as coagulation indexes of each group, hemoglobin, blood platelet, prothrombin time, activated partial thromboplastin time, and D-Dimer. 6(1.4%) BAP patients, but no HTG-AP patient, had suffered chylous fistula.

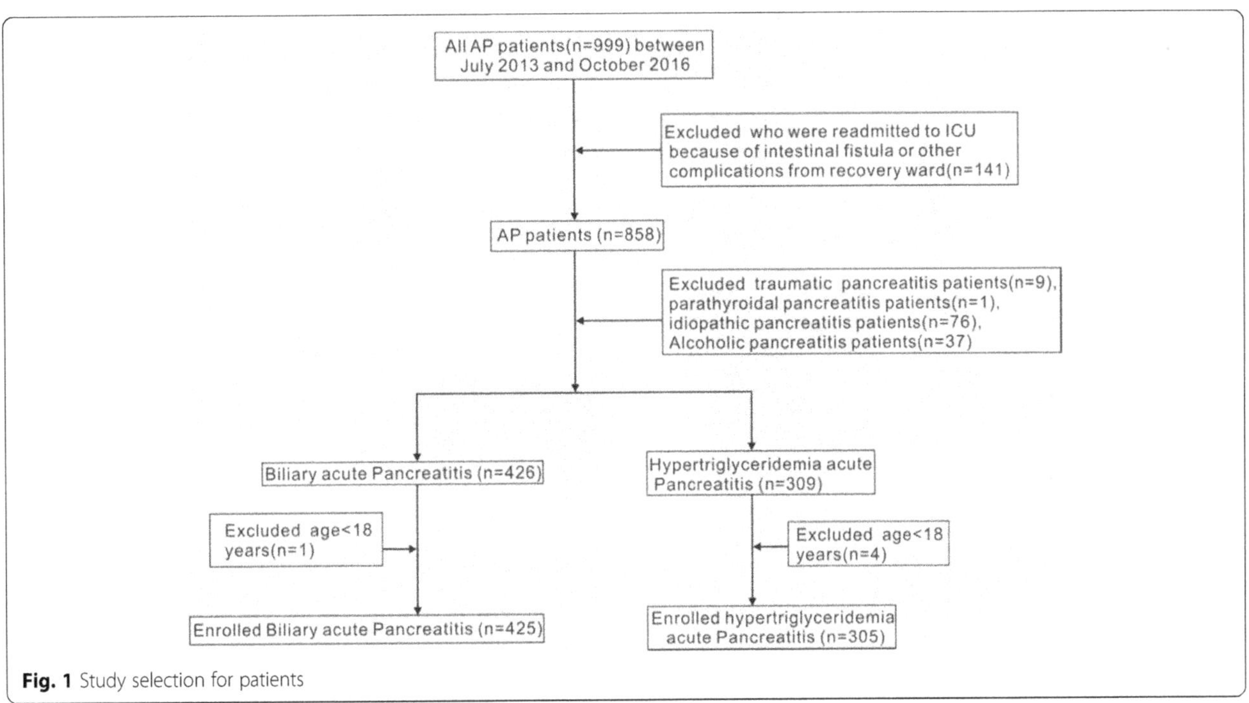

Fig. 1 Study selection for patients

Table 1 Demographic data and baseline characteristics of the patients

Characteristic	Biliary acute Pancreatitis (n = 425)	Hypertriglyceridemia acute Pancreatitis (n = 305)	P value
Age, year	51(43,64)	40(33,47)	$P < 0.01$
Gender, male/female	242/183	214/91	$P < 0.01$
BMI	22.7(20.1,25.2)	27(24.9,30.4)	$P < 0.01$
APACHE II score	8(6,12.5)	11(7,18)	$P < 0.01$
Hypertension	120(28.2%)	81(26.6%)	0.675
Diabetes mellitus	55(12.9%)	98(32.1%)	$P < 0.01$
Fatty liver	64(15.1%)	134(43.9%)	$P < 0.01$
High fat diet	62(14.6%)	130(42.6%)	$P < 0.01$
Transfer from other hospitals	406(95.5%)	295(96.7%)	0.449
Time taken for the patients transfer to our center after onset of symptoms, Days	10(4,30)	6(3,17)	0.541

BMI body mass index, *APACHE II* Acute Physiology and Chronic Health Evaluation II

Then, we wonder if the significantly higher incidence of ARDS, AKI and DVT in HTG-AP was affected by only the etiology or other factors, such as age, gender, body mass index, diabetic mellitus, fatty liver and high-fat diet. So, we did the multivariate analysis to determine the association of ARDS/AKI/DVT with the etiology (Table 4). On multivariate logistic regression of ARDS/AKI/DVT adjusting for etiology, age, gender, body mass index, diabetic mellitus, fatty liver and high-fat diet, HTG-AP was found to be independently associated with more AKI, and higher BMI with more AKI, ARDS and DVT.

Then, we divided HTG-AP patients into three groups according to their TG level (peak TG level within 72 h of hospital admission with AP): group A:≤10.2 mg/dl (less than the first quartile), group B: 10.3–21.9 mg/dl (between the first and third quartiles), and group C:≥22 mg/dl (more than the third quartile). The Cochran-Armitage trend test have been done to compare characteristics among three groups, results are displayed in Additional file 2: Table S1 and Additional file 3: Figure S2. However, higher TG level was not related with the incidence of systemic complication.

Local complications

The analysis of local complications, include acute peripancreatic fluid collection, pancreatic pseudocyst, acute necrotic collection, walled-off necrosis, and IPN, as shown in Table 5. The results in Table 5 showed that, more IPN were found in the BAP patients (193 (45.4%), 106 (34.8%), (p = 0.005)), although similarity in acute necrotic collection (292 (68.7%), 213 (69.8%), (p = 0.807)).

Outcome

The outcome comparison was shown in Table 6. The two groups were not statistically different in terms of in-hospital mortality. Thanks to our four-step drainage strategy [6], the amount of patients who need surgery was less than 11%.The length of hospital stay or ICU

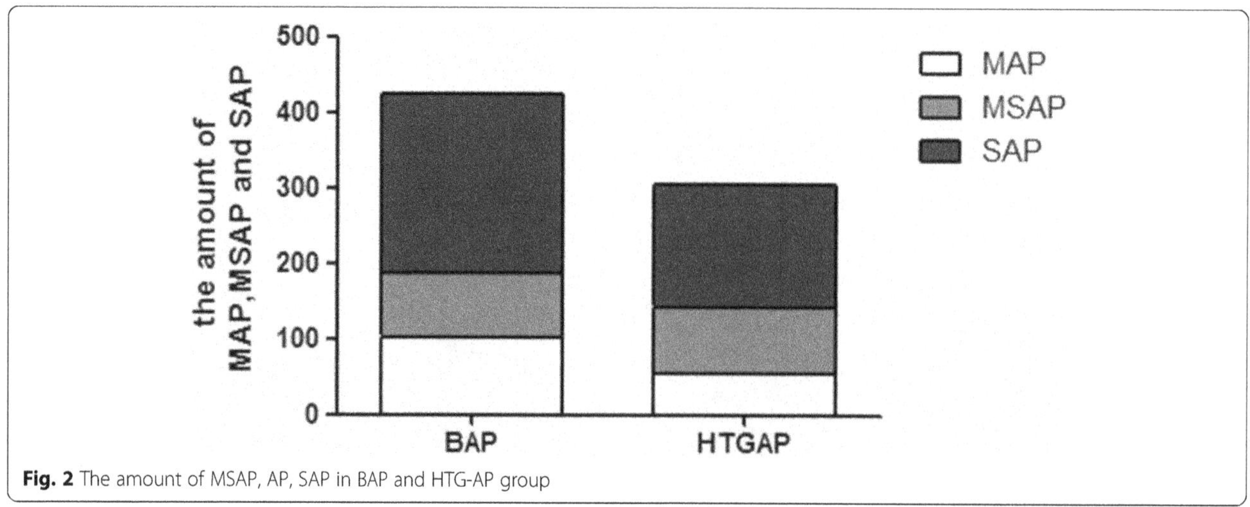

Fig. 2 The amount of MSAP, AP, SAP in BAP and HTG-AP group

Table 2 Initial Laboratory data of the patients

Physiological Indexes	Biliary acute Pancreatitis (n = 425)	Hypertriglyceridemia acute Pancreatitis (n = 305)	P value
Amylase	86(41,219)	69(34,159.5)	0.13
Lipase	295(107,706)	355(127.5778.5)	0.599
WBC	11(7.5,14.9)	10.4(7.7,13.6)	0.306
CRP	114(47.4173.1)	152.1(87.6210.3)	$P < 0.01$
IL-6	60(30.4135.9)	98(51.7174.1)	0.282
Procalcitonin(PCT)	0.3(0.15,1.2)	1(0.2,3.4)	0.128
Urine toxic nitrogen	4.9(3.4,7.6)	5.1(3.7,8.8)	0.07
Creatinine	55(42,72)	60(46,84)	0.031
Total bilirubin (TBil)	19.4(13.1,31.1)	19.4(13.2,29.4)	0.381
Conjugated bilirubin(DBil)	13(4,36)	13(4,28)	0.365
Alanine aminotransferase(ALT)	37(23,73)	25(19,39)	$P < 0.01$
Aspartate transaminase(AST)	30(21,52)	31(20,50)	0.408
Hemoglobin	107(91.5127)	106(85,133)	0.709
Blood platelet	194(134,269)	178(119,244.5)	0.058
Prothrombin time(PT)	13.4(12.5,14.5)	13.1(12.5,14.3)	0.58
Activated partial thromboplastin time(APTT)	34(29.9,39.7)	32(28,36.4)	0.147
D-Dimer	3.3(1.5,5.9)	3.6(2.0,7.1)	0.141

WBC white blood cell, *CRP* C-reactive protein

stay between two group was similar and nearly 60% needed to be admitted to ICU.

Discussion

This retrospective study demonstrated significantly different clinical features between HTG-AP and BAP patients. The results indicated that HTG-AP patients were younger, more male, more ratio of high fat diet, higher BMI and higher prevalence of AKI/ARDS/DVT/MODS, but, the BAP patients had higher incidence of IPN and chylous fistula. Moreover, the multivariate analysis showed that HTG-AP was independently associated with more AKI as adjusting by age, gender, body mass index, diabetic mellitus, fatty liver and high-fat diet, but not with ARDS and DVT. However, BMI was found to be independently associated with AKI, ARDS and DVT.

Table 3 Systemic complications between the patients

Variable	Biliary acute Pancreatitis (n = 425)	Hypertriglyceridemia acute Pancreatitis (n = 305)	P value
ARDS	130(30.6%)	116(38.0%)	0.039
AKI	91(21.4%)	105(34.4%)	$P < 0.01$
Intra-abdominal hypertension	23(5.4%)	28(9.2%)	0.056
Shock	66(15.5%)	49(16.1%)	0.838
Intra-abdominal hemorrhage	56(13.2%)	34(11.1%)	0.427
Sepsis	39(9.2%)	21(6.9%)	0.278
Portal vein thrombosis	47(11.1%)	26(8.5%)	0.317
Deep venous thrombosis	27(6.4%)	37(12.1%)	0.008
Acute hepatic injury	45(10.6%)	21(6.9%)	0.090
Gastrointestinal fistula	75(17.6%)	44(14.4%)	0.265
Digestive tract hemorrhage	11(2.6%)	8(2.6%)	1
Chylous fistula	6(1.4%)	0(0.0%)	0.044
Diarrhea	9(2.1%)	9(3.0%)	0.479
Ileus	7(1.6%)	11(3.6%)	0.144
MODS	96(22.6%)	91(29.8%)	0.032

ARDS acute respiratory distress syndrome, *AKI* acute kidney injury, *MODS* multiple organ dysfunction syndrome

Table 4 Multivariate analysis showing association of proposed risk factors with ARDS/AKI/DVT

Multivariate analysis	ARDS		AKI		DVT	
	OR(95% CI)	*P* value	OR(95% CI)	*P* value	OR(95% CI)	*P* value
Etiology	0.88(0.58,1,32)	0.52	0.62(0.40,0.96)	0.03	1.03(0.53,2.00)	0.93
Age	0.99(0.98,1.01)	0.25	0.99(0.98,1.00)	0.17	1.01(0.99,1.03)	0.36
Gender	0.93(0.67,1.29)	0.66	0.69(0.48,0.99)	0.04	1.45(0.84,2.50)	0.19
BMI	0.95(0.91,0.98)	0.004	0.96(0.92,1.00)	0.03	0.91(0.86,0.97)	0.002
Diabetes mellitus	1.38(0.92,2.07)	0.12	1.34(0.87,2.05)	0.18	0.85(0.46,1.57)	0.60
Fatty liver	0.99(0.68,1.45)	0.98	0.79(0.54,1.17)	0.24	0.67(0.38,1.19)	0.17
High fat diet	0.76(0.52,1.10)	0.14	0.88(0.59,1.31)	0.53	0.79(0.44,1.41)	0.42

ARDS acute respiratory distress syndrome, *AKI* acute kidney injury, *DVT* deep venous thrombosis

The results suggested that higher incidence of AKI in HTG-AP was significantly and independently associated with the etiology, but more ARDS and DVT were more due to higher BMI.

HTG-AP is a rare but well-documented type of AP in Western countries (1.3–5%) [7, 8]. Recently, accumulating data have shown that HTG-AP has become the second common cause of AP in China, with a reported incidence up to12.3% in 2003 [9], 18.1% in 2007 [10], and 25.6% in 2013 [11], much higher than that in Western countries. In our center, which is the largest AP referral center in China, HTG-AP accounted for about 30% from 2013 to 2016, being also the second leading cause of AP. Previous studies had compared HTG-AP with other common etiologies, but the results vary. Linares et al. [12] reported that patients with HTG-AP suffered a more severe clinical course than those with alcohol or gallstone-induced based on the index such as ICU admission, CRP, and Balthazar scores and similar findings were repeatedly reported in the literature [13]. Tai et al. [14] reported no significant difference in specific complications like ARDS, AKI, gastrointestinal bleeding and sepsis. Besides, clinical studies assessing the impact of the TG level on the severity of AP also showed conflicting results. Zhang et al. [15], S. Balachandra et al. [16] and Fortson MR et al. [7] showed no difference detected in severity, based on APACHE II scores or complications in patients with the level of TG. While some reports demonstrated that patients with high level of triglyceride may suffer worse clinical outcome. A previous study showed that the level of TG in AP patients are independently and proportionally correlated with persistent organ failure regardless of etiology [17], in another study, AP patients with HTG (> 500 mg/dL) had higher 24 h APACHE II scores, more systemic complications and higher mortality [18].

The underlying pathogenesis of HTG-AP is not fully understood and the most widely accepted explanation hitherto is the "free fatty acids (FFA)" theory. It is assumed that at the onset of pancreatitis, a large amount of pancreatic lipase releases into the systemic circulation hydrolyzing serum TGs and adipose tissue, which would consequently generate high concentrations of free fatty acids with detergent properties. Free fatty acid micelle complexes injure the vascular endothelium and acinar cells of the pancreas, making internal environment increasingly acidic and ischemic, which triggers further free fatty acid toxicity and accelerate systemic inflammatory response [19]. Furthermore, direct tissue injury and lipotoxicity via mitochondrial stress [20–22] may cause the up-regulation of cytokines and the inflammatory cascade, predisposing to systemic inflammatory response [22].

In the complications of AP, the incidence of AKI was also found to be higher in HTG-AP in other reports [23]. Wu et al. indicated that TG may do a direct damage to renal parenchyma as reacting with pancreatic lipase around kidney tubules. The pancreatic enzymes assembled in glomerulus aggravates the damage of renal function [23]. Also Scheuer et al. reported that, the infiltrated TG in glomerular and tubulointerstitial could make the glomerulosclerosis grow worse in mouse model [24].

Table 5 Local complications between BAP and HTG-AP

Variable	Biliary acute Pancreatitis (*n* = 425)	Hypertriglyceridemia acute Pancreatitis (*n* = 305)	*P* value
Acute peripancreatic fluid collection	120(28.2%)	104(34.1%)	0.104
Pancreatic pseudocyst	11(2.6%)	8(2.6%)	1
Acute necrotic collection	292(68.7%)	213(69.8%)	0.807
Walled-off necrosis	5(1.2%)	3(1.0%)	1
Infected pancreatitis necrosis	193(45.4%)	106(34.8%)	0.005

Table 6 Outcome comparisons between the patients

Variable	Biliary acute Pancreatitis (*n* = 425)	Hypertriglyceridemia acute Pancreatitis (*n* = 305)	*P* value
Hospital mortality, no.	36(8.5%)	24(7.9%)	0.787
Need of surgery, no.	39(9.2%)	33(10.8%)	0.529
ICU admission	260(61.2%)	186(61.0%)	1
Length of ICU stay, days	4(2,12)	4(2,10.5)	0.975
Length of hospital stay, days	9(4,22.5)	9(5,23)	0.58
Cost, Thousand CHY	48.7(22.8157.8)	51.0(27.9134.6)	0.623

ICU intensive care unit

Moreover, the results in this study also showed that higher BMI was independently associated with AKI, ARDS and DVT in multivariate analysis. Up to date, quite a few articles had showed that BMI may increase the severity of AP from clinical findings and animal models [25]. A possible explanation is that adipose tissue appears as chronic inflammation releasing pro-inflammatory cytokines and obese individuals are more likely to have lifestyle-related chronic diseases/ respiratory problems [25, 26]. Obesity has also been inferred associated with an increased risk of extrapancreatic complications such as shock, renal failure, respiratory insufficiency, and fatal outcome [27, 28].

Furthermore, the results found the BAP patients suffered more infected local complications than HTG-AP. In BAP patients, when the gallstones pass through the Vater ampulla, spasm, fibrosis and obstruction of the hepatopancreatic ampulla happens, resulting in biliopancreatic reflux and the exclusion of bile and pancreatic juices. Then the elevated levels of bile and pancreatic juices and activation of pancreatic enzymes are responsible for pancreatitis attacking ultimately in this abnormal physiological status [3]. The refluxing of infected bile transfer into the pancreatic duct may generate *Escherichia coli* and other bacteria leading to the infection [29].

Conclusions

In conclusion, this study showed significantly different clinical features between HTG-AP and BAP patients. HTG-AP patients suffered higher occurrence rates of AKI/ARDS/DVT/MODS, while IPN was more common in BAP patients. After the multivariate analysis adjusted by age, gender, BMI, diabetes, fatty liver and high fat diet, HTG-AP was found to be significantly and independently related with more incidence of AKI. However, higher BMI was found to be related with AKI, ARDS and DVT. Further, larger prospective studies should be performed to study the features between the different etiologies of AP and the effect of BMI on disease severity.

Additional files

Additional file 1: Figure S1. The standardized protocol for the fluid resuscitation treatment.

Additional file 2: Table S1. Characteristics in three groups divided by triglyceride levels.

Additional file 3: FigureS2. Proportion of systemic complication with three groups according to the value of TG level in patients with HTG-AP using the Cochran-Armitage trend test. A. Proportion of ARDS with three groups according to the value of TG level in patients with HTG-AP. B. Proportion of AKI with three groups according to the value of TG level in patients with HTG-AP. C. Proportion of DVT with three groups according to the value of TG level in patients with HTG-AP. Cochran-Armitage test for trend was analyzed.

Abbreviations

AKI: Acute kidney injury; ALT: Alanine aminotransferase; AP: Acute pancreatitis; APACHE II: Acute physiology and chronic health evaluation II; ARDS: Acute respiratory distress syndrome; BAP: Biliary acute pancreatitis; BMI: Body mass Index; CECT: Contrast-enhanced computed tomography; CRP: C-reactive protein; DVT: Deep vein thrombosis; EUS: Endoscopic ultrasonography; FFA: Free fatty acids; HTG: Hypertriglyceridemia; HTG-AP: Hypertriglyceridemia acute pancreatitis; ICU: Intensive Care Unit; IPN: Infected pancreatitis necrosis; IQR: Interquartile range; MAP: Mild acute pancreatitis;; MODS: Multiple organ dysfunction syndrome; MRCP: Magnetic resonance cholangiopancreatography; MRI: Magnetic resonance imaging; MSAP: Moderate severe acute pancreatitis; SAP: Severe acute pancreatitis.; SICU: Surgical Intensive Care Unit

Acknowledgements

The authors are indebted to all doctors and researchers for the follow-up assessment and data collection during the study from the severe acute pancreatitis care center of Jinling Hospital, Medical School of Nanjing University.

Funding

The article processing charge was funded by National Natural Science Foundation of China (No.81570584). The article publication charge was funded by Social development project of Jiangsu Province(BE2015685), Medical Research Funding of PLA(AWS14C003). The funding bodies did not participate in the study design, data collection, data analysis, results interpretation or writing of the manuscript.

Authors' contributions

XYL, LK: Study concept and design, JD, LM: Statistical analysis, BY, WJM: Acquisition of data, analysis and interpretation of data, XYL: Drafting of the manuscript, QY, WQL: Critical revision of the manuscript for important intellectual content, WQL and JSL: Study supervision. All authors have read and approved the final version of this manuscript, including the authorship.

Consent for publication
Not applicable.

Competing interests
The authors declare that they have no competing interests.

References

1. Banks PA, Bollen TL, Dervenis C, Gooszen HG, Johnson CD, Sarr MG, Tsiotos GG, Vege SS, Acute pancreatitis classification working G. Classification of acute pancreatitis–2012: revision of the Atlanta classification and definitions by international consensus. Gut. 2013;62(1):102–11.
2. Dellinger EP, Forsmark CE, Layer P, Levy P, Maravi-Poma E, Petrov MS, Shimosegawa T, Siriwardena AK, Uomo G, Whitcomb DC, et al. Determinant-based classification of acute pancreatitis severity: an international multidisciplinary consultation. Ann Surg. 2012;256(6):875–80.
3. van Geenen EJM, van der Peet DL, Bhagirath P, Mulder CJJ, Bruno MJ. Etiology and diagnosis of acute biliary pancreatitis. Nat Rev Gastroenterol Hepatol. 2010;7(9):495–502.
4. Scherer J, Singh VP, Pitchumoni CS, Yadav D. Issues in hypertriglyceridemic pancreatitis: an update. J Clin Gastroenterol. 2014;48(3):195–203.
5. Tenner S, Baillie J, De Witt J, Vege SS, American College of G. American College of Gastroenterology guideline: management of acute pancreatitis. Am J Gastroenterol. 2013;108(9):1400–15. 1416
6. Tong Z, Ke L, Li B, Li G, Zhou J, Shen X, Li W, Li N, Li J. Negative pressure irrigation and endoscopic necrosectomy through man-made sinus tract in infected necrotizing pancreatitis: a technical report. BMC Surg. 2016;16:1.
7. Fortson MR, Freedman SN, Webster PD 3rd. Clinical assessment of hyperlipidemic pancreatitis. Am J Gastroenterol. 1995;90(12):2134–9.
8. Ivanova R, Puerta S, Garrido A, Cueto I, Ferro A, Ariza MJ, Cobos A, Gonzalez-Santos P, Valdivielso P. Triglyceride levels and apolipoprotein E polymorphism in patients with acute pancreatitis. Hepatobiliary Pancreat Dis Int. 2012;11(1):96–101.
9. Chang MC, Su CH, Sun MS, Huang SC, Chiu CT, Chen MC, Lee KT, Lin CC, Lin JT. Etiology of acute pancreatitis–a multi-center study in Taiwan. Hepatogastroenterology. 2003;50(53):1655–7.
10. Qian JM. Reviewing the etiology, diagnosis and treatment of acute pancreatitis in China. Zhonghua Nei Ke Za Zhi. 2007;46(12):979–80.
11. Yin G, Cang X, Yu G, Hu G, Ni J, Xiong J, Hu Y, Xing M, Chen C, Huang Y, et al. Different clinical presentations of Hyperlipidemic acute pancreatitis: a retrospective study. Pancreas. 2015;44(7):1105–10.
12. Lloret Linares C, Pelletier AL, Czernichow S, Vergnaud AC, Bonnefont-Rousselot D, Levy P, Ruszniewski P, Bruckert E. Acute pancreatitis in a cohort of 129 patients referred for severe hypertriglyceridemia. Pancreas. 2008; 37(1):13–2.
13. Adiamah A, Psaltis E, Crook M, Lobo DN. A systematic review of the epidemiology, pathophysiology and current management of hyperlipidaemic pancreatitis. Clin Nutr. 2017;
14. Tai WP, Lin XC, Liu H, Wang CH, Wu J, Zhang NW, Chen W. A retrospective research of the characteristic of Hypertriglyceridemic pancreatitis in Beijing, China. Gastroenterol Res Pract. 2016;2016:6263095.
15. Zhang XL, Li F, Zhen YM, Li A, Fang Y. Clinical study of 224 patients with hypertriglyceridemia pancreatitis. Chin Med J. 2015;128(15):2045–9.
16. Balachandra S, Virlos IT, King NK, Siriwardana HP, France MW, Siriwardena AK. Hyperlipidaemia and outcome in acute pancreatitis. Int J Clin Pract. 2006;60(2):156–9.
17. Nawaz H, Koutroumpakis E, Easler J, Slivka A, Whitcomb DC, Singh VP, Yadav D, Papachristou GI. Elevated serum triglycerides are independently associated with persistent organ failure in acute pancreatitis. Am J Gastroenterol. 2015;110(10):1497–503.
18. Deng LH, Xue P, Xia Q, Yang XN, Wan MH. Effect of admission hypertriglyceridemia on the episodes of severe acute pancreatitis. World J Gastroenterol. 2008;14(28):4558–61.
19. Samuel I, Zaheer S, Zaheer A. Bile-pancreatic juice exclusion increases p38MAPK activation and TNF-alpha production in ligation-induced acute pancreatitis in rats. Pancreatology. 2005;5(1):20–6.
20. Zeng Y, Wang X, Zhang W, Wu K, Ma J. Hypertriglyceridemia aggravates ER stress and pathogenesis of acute pancreatitis. Hepatogastroenterology. 2012;59(119):2318–26.
21. Chang YT, Chang MC, Su TC, Liang PC, Su YN, Kuo CH, Wei SC, Wong JM. Association of cystic fibrosis transmembrane conductance regulator (CFTR) mutation/variant/haplotype and tumor necrosis factor (TNF) promoter polymorphism in hyperlipidemic pancreatitis. Clin Chem. 2008;54(1):131–8.
22. Chang YT, Chang MC, Su TC, Liang PC, Su YN, Kuo CH, Wei SC, Wong JM. Lipoprotein lipase mutation S447X associated with pancreatic calcification and steatorrhea in hyperlipidemic pancreatitis. J Clin Gastroenterol. 2009; 43(6):591–6.
23. Wu C, Ke L, Tong Z, Li B, Zou L, Li W, Li N, Li J. Hypertriglyceridemia is a risk factor for acute kidney injury in the early phase of acute pancreatitis. Pancreas. 2014;43(8):1312–6.
24. Scheuer H, Gwinner W, Hohbach J, Grone EF, Brandes RP, Malle E, Olbricht CJ, Walli AK, Grone HJ. Oxidant stress in hyperlipidemia-induced renal damage. Am J Physiol Renal Physiol. 2000;278(1):F63–74.
25. Ikeura T, Kato K, Takaoka M, Shimatani M, Kishimoto M, Nishi K, Kariya S, Okazaki K. A body mass index >/=25 kg/m(2) is associated with a poor prognosis in patients with acute pancreatitis: a study of Japanese patients. Hepatobiliary Pancreat Dis Int. 2017;16(6):645–51.
26. Hersoug LG, Moller P, Loft S. Gut microbiota-derived lipopolysaccharide uptake and trafficking to adipose tissue: implications for inflammation and obesity. Obes Rev. 2016;17(4):297–312.
27. Lankisch PG, Schirren CA. Increased body weight as a prognostic parameter for complications in the course of acute pancreatitis. Pancreas. 1990;5(5): 626–9.
28. Blomgren KB, Sundstrom A, Steineck G, Wiholm BE. Obesity and treatment of diabetes with glyburide may both be risk factors for acute pancreatitis. Diabetes Care. 2002;25(2):298–302.
29. Arendt R, Liebe S, Erdmann K. Biliary pancreatitis–pathogenesis, therapy, results. Z Gesamte Inn Med. 1989;44(13):401–4.

15

Expanding laparoscopic pancreaticoduodenectomy to pancreatic-head and periampullary malignancy

Ke Chen[1], Xiao-long Liu[1], Yu Pan[1], Hendi Maher[2] and Xian-fa Wang[1*]

Abstract

Background: Laparoscopic pancreaticoduodenectomy (LPD) remains to be established as a safe and effective alternative to open pancreaticoduodenectomy (OPD) for pancreatic-head and periampullary malignancy. The purpose of this meta-analysis was to compare LPD with OPD for these malignancies regarding short-term surgical and long-term survival outcomes.

Methods: A literature search was conducted before March 2018 to identify comparative studies in regard to outcomes of both LPD and OPD for the treatment of pancreatic-head and periampullary malignancies. Morbidity, postoperative pancreatic fistula (POPF), mortality, operative time, estimated blood loss, hospitalization, retrieved lymph nodes, and survival outcomes were compared.

Results: Among eleven identified studies, 1196 underwent LPD, and 8247 were operated through OPD. The pooled data showed that LPD was associated with less morbidity (OR = 0.57, 95%CI: 0.41~ 0.78, $P < 0.01$), less blood loss (WMD = – 372.96 ml, 95% CI, – 507.83~ – 238.09 ml, $P < 0.01$), shorter hospital stays (WMD = – 197.49 ml, 95% CI, – 304.62~ – 90.37 ml, $P < 0.01$), and comparable POPF (OR = 0.85, 95%CI: 0.59~ 1.24, $P = 0.40$), and overall survival (HR = 1.03, 95%CI: 0.93~ 1.14, $P = 0.54$) compared to OPD. Operative time was longer in LPD (WMD = 87.68 min; 95%CI: 27.05~ 148.32, $P < 0.01$), whereas R0 rate tended to be higher in LPD (OR = 1.17; 95%CI: 1.00~ 1.37, $P = 0.05$) and there tended to be more retrieved lymph nodes in LPD (WMD = 1.15, 95%CI: -0.16~ 2.47, $P = 0.08$), but these differences failed to reach statistical significance.

Conclusions: LPD can be performed as safe and effective as OPD for pancreatic-head and periampullary malignancy with respect to both surgical and oncological outcomes. LPD is associated with less intraoperative blood loss and postoperative morbidity and may serve as a promising alternative to OPD in selected individuals in the future.

Keywords: Laparoscopy, Pancreaticoduodenectomy, Adenocarcinoma, Morbidity, Meta-analysis

* Correspondence: 3195011@zju.edu.cn
[1]Department of General Surgery, Sir Run Run Shaw Hospital, School of Medicine, Zhejiang University, 3 East Qingchun Road, Hangzhou 310016, Zhejiang Province, China
Full list of author information is available at the end of the article

Background

Pancreatic-head and periampullary malignancy mainly include pancreatic duct adenocarcinoma (PDAC) and periampullary adenocarcinoma (PAAC). PDAC causes a considerable amount of cancer-related death worldwide. In fact, PDAC is the fourth deadliest malignancy in developed countries and is predicted to become the second one within several years [1, 2]. PAAC, defined as malignancy located in the distal common bile duct, ampulla of Vater or adjacent duodenum, are uncommon cancers compared to PDAC. However, despite its relatively higher resectability rates compared with PDAC, the long-term survival outcomes of PAAC patients are poor [3]. These cancers represent great challenges for healthcare providers and require a multidisciplinary approach in which pancreaticoduodenectomy (PD) with lymphadenectomy remains the primary curative treatment for patients without distant metastasis.

Minimally invasive surgery, typically characterized by laparoscopic approach, is one of the main surgical advances in the twenty-first Century [4]. It has been applied to complex pancreatic procedures including laparoscopic PD (LPD) for neoplasms on the pancreatic head and periampullar region or laparoscopic distal pancreatectomy (LDP) for these on the pancreatic body or tail. LDP represents a technique, which is technically less demanding, without any reconstruction, whereas LPD is a demanding procedure, which should be performed only in referral centers by experienced surgeons. Now, several meta-analyses have been published regarding LDP for malignancy treatment [5, 6], there was still no meta-analysis on the potential advantages and disadvantages of LPD for cancers. This meta-analysis proposed to dig deeper into the surgical and oncologic outcomes of patients who suffered from pancreatic-head and periampullary malignancy and underwent LPD versus open PD (OPD).

Methods

Study selection

We systematically searched the relevant literature using PubMed, Embase, Cochrane Library, and EBSCO for articles published up to March 2018 The search terms “minimally invasive”, “laparoscopy”, “Whipple”, “pancreaticoduodenectomy”, “pancreatic ductal adenocarcinoma”, “pancreatic cancer”, “ampullary cancer”, “ampulla of Vater”, and “periampullary neoplasm” were utilized. All eligible studies were retrieved, and their bibliographies were further checked for other potential publications. The language of the publications was confined to English.

Inclusion criteria

Publications included in this study were based on the following criteria: (1) compared LPD and OPD in patients suffering from pancreatic-head and periampullary malignancy (PDAC and PAAC); (2) reported on at least one of the outcome measures mentioned below; and (3) if there was overlap between authors and/or institutions, the higher quality or more recent publication was selected.

Data extraction

Information was independently extracted from eligible studies by two authors (Chen K and Liu XL). The following information was collected: ① Primary outcomes: morbidity, mortality, postoperative pancreatic fistula (POPF), margin status, retrieved lymph nodes (RLNs), and long-term survival. ② Secondary outcomes: operative time, intraoperative blood loss, transfusion, and length of hospital stay. The postoperative morbidity was classified according to the Clavien-Dindo classification when possible [7]. POPF were diagnosed in accordance with the International Study Group for Pancreatic Fistula (ISGPF) criteria [8]. Clinically significant POPF was defined as ISGPF grade B/C. Resection margins were considered negative (R0) when no tumor was evident along the transection surface [9].

Quality assessment

The Newcastle-Ottawa Quality Assessment Scale (NOS) was used to evaluate the quality of non-randomized controlled trials (NRCTs). The quality of each study was scored by taking into account patient selection, comparability of the groups and assessment of the outcomes. The scale ranges from 0 to 9 stars: studies with a score ≥ 6 could be deemed as methodologically sound. Randomized controlled trials (RCTs) were assessed by the Jadad scale. High quality RCTs get more than 2 out of a maximum possible score of 5.

Statistical analysis

Statistical analysis was performed using the RevMan 5.1 software (Cochrane Collaboration, Oxford, UK). The odds ratio (OR) or weighted mean differences (WMD) with 95% confidence intervals (CI) were calculated for dichotomous and continuous results, respectively. Medians were converted to means by the method introduced by Hozo et al. [10]. The hazard ratio (HR) was used as a summary statistic for long-term survival. The log HR and its standard error (SE) were analyzed directly if the studies reported the HR and 95% CI. Otherwise, the log HR and its SE were estimated using the method described by Tierney et al. [11]. The fixed-effect model was firstly used for primary and secondary outcomes, and in case of significant heterogeneity (I^2>50% or Q test $P < 0.05$) the results were calculated using the random-effect model. Subgroup analysis was carried out according to the tumor primaries (PDAC or PAAC). Funnel plots were used to screen for publication bias based on the R0 rate. The statistical tests were two-sided, and $P < 0.05$ was considered statistically significant.

Results

Study characteristics and quality of included studies

The search strategy initially generated 668 relevant clinical trials. Of these, articles that did not compare LPD with OPD were excluded based on their titles and abstracts. Thus, 86 articles were selected and a full examination of the text was conducted. A further 73 papers were excluded because the surgical indications of these studies were not restricted to pancreatic-head and periampullary malignancy. Another two publications were then excluded due to overlapping patient cohorts [12, 13]. Finally, a total of 9443 patients [LPD 1196 (12.7%), OPD 8247 (87.3%)] from 11 studies were included [14–24]. Figure 1 illustrates the selection process. Only one RCR was found [22]. The indication of six studies was PDAC [14, 16–20], whereas two studies applied LPD only to PAAC [15, 24], the remaining three researches reported both PDAC and PAAC [21–23]. Table 1 lists the characteristics of these studies and details of the enrolled participants. The RCT conducted by Palanivelu et al. received a Jadad score of 3 [22]. The quality evaluation using NOS showed that the included NRCTs were methodologically sound with four studies receiving 9 stars, five studies receiving 8 stars, and the remaining study receiving 7 stars (Table 1).

Primary outcomes

POPF was described in 8 studies [14, 15, 18, 19, 21–24]. Pooling data indicated no significant difference in terms of overall POPF rates between two groups (OR = 0.85, 95%CI: 0.59~ 1.24, $P = 0.40$) (Fig. 2), as well as the clinically significant POPF rates (OR = 0.86, 95%CI: 0.53~ 1.41, $P = 0.56$). The morbidity was available from 7 studies [14, 15, 18, 19, 21–23]. The pooled data indicated that the overall postoperative morbidity was significantly decreased in LPD (OR = 0.57, 95%CI: 0.41~ 0.78, $P < 0.01$) (Fig. 3). Eight studies recorded postoperative mortality [14, 15, 19–24]. Mortality was similar in LPD and OPD for malignancies (OR = 0.88, 95%CI: 0.64~ 1.20, $P = 0.41$) (Fig. 4). Negative margin (R0) rate was reported in all studies. The difference in R0 rate was not significant in pooling results, but had a tendency to be higher in the LPD group than in the OPD group (OR = 1.17, 95%CI: 1.00~ 1.37, $P = 0.05$) (Fig. 5). The funnel plot for studies reporting the ORs of R0 was used to detect publication bias. Visual inspection of the funnel plot revealed symmetry, indicating no serious publication bias, as illustrated in Fig. 6. The RLNs were pooled from 10 studies [14–17, 19–24]. Pooled results revealed a tendency of more RLNs in the LPD group than in the OPD group with a marginal difference (WMD = 1.15, 95%CI: -0.16~ 2.47, $P = 0.08$) (Fig. 7). Six studies reported survival outcomes. The overall survival rate was not found to be different among the two groups (HR = 1.03, 95%CI: 0.93~ 1.14, $P = 0.54$) (Fig. 8). The primary outcomes of the quantitative meta-analysis were summarized in Table 2.

Secondary outcomes

Five studies reported operative time [14, 19, 22–24]. The operative time in LPD group was longer than that in OPD group (WMD = 87.68 min, 95%CI: 27.05~ 148.32, $P < 0.01$). Also five studies reported blood loss [14, 19, 22–24]. The estimated blood loss was significantly reduced in LPD group (WMD = – 197.49 ml, 95% CI, – 304.62~ – 90.37 ml, $P < 0.01$). A similar result was achieved in the field of blood transfusions (OR = 0.64, 95 %CI: 0.50~ 0.84, $P < 0.01$). Nine

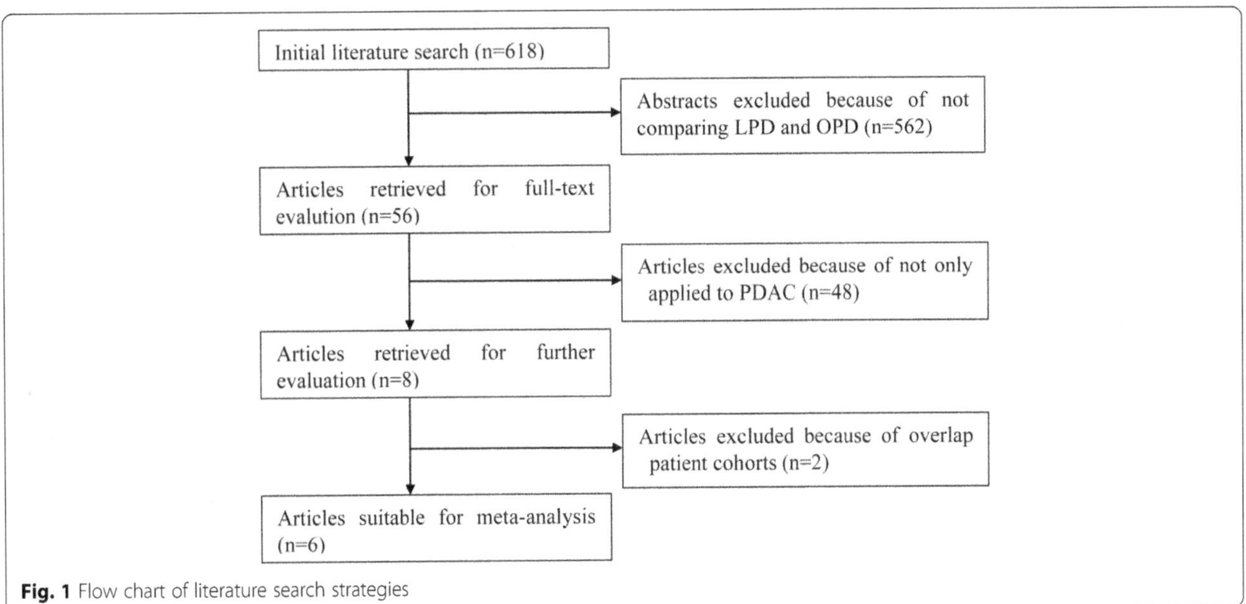

Fig. 1 Flow chart of literature search strategies

Table 1 Summary of studies included in the meta-analysis

Author	Region	Design	Year	Study Period	Sample size		Indications	Conversion n (%)	ITT	ISGPF	Clavien–Dindo	Mortality	Quality scores
					LPD	OPD							
Croome	USA	OCS (P,S)	2014	2008–2013	108	214	PDAC	7(6.5)	Yes	Yes	Yes	30d	8
Hakeem	UK	OCS (R,S)	2014	2005–2009	12	12	PAAC	NR	NR	NR	Yes	30d	9
Chen	China	OCS (P,S)	2015	2010–2013	19	38	PDAC	1(5.3)	Yes	Yes	Yes	NR	8
Song	Korea	OCS (R,S)	2015	2007–2012	11	261	PDAC	NR	No	Yes	Yes	30d	8
Dokmak	France	OCS (P,S)	2015	2011–2014	15	14	PDAC	NR	Yes	Yes	Yes	90d	7
Stauffer	USA	OCS (P,S)	2017	1995–2014	58	193	PDAC	14(24.1)	Yes	Yes	Yes	90d	8
Kantor	USA	OCS (R,M)	2017	2010–2013	828	7385	PDAC	E	NR	NR	NR	90d	8
Conrad	USA	OCS (P,S)	2017	2000–2010	40	25	Mixed	9(18.4)[a]	No	Yes	Yes	90d	9
Palanivelu	India	RCT	2017	2013–2015	32	32	Mixed	1(3.1)	Yes	Yes	Yes	90d	3[a]
Khaled	UK	OCS (R,S)	2017	2002–2015	15	15	Mixed	1(6.7)	Yes	Yes	Yes	30d	9
Meng	China	OCS (R,S)	2018	2010–2015	58	58	PAAC	NR	NR	Yes	Yes	30d	9

OCS observational clinical study, *RCT* randomized controlled trial, *P* prospectively collected data, *R* retrospectively collected data, *M* muti-centers, *S* single center, *DP* distal pancreatectomy, *PD* pancreatoduodenectomy, *L* laparoscopy, *O* open, *ITT* intention-to-treat analysis, *ISGPF* international study group of pancreatic fistula, *PJ* pancreaticojejunostomy, *DTM* duct-to-mucosa, *E* exclude, *NR* not reported

[a] Jadad score

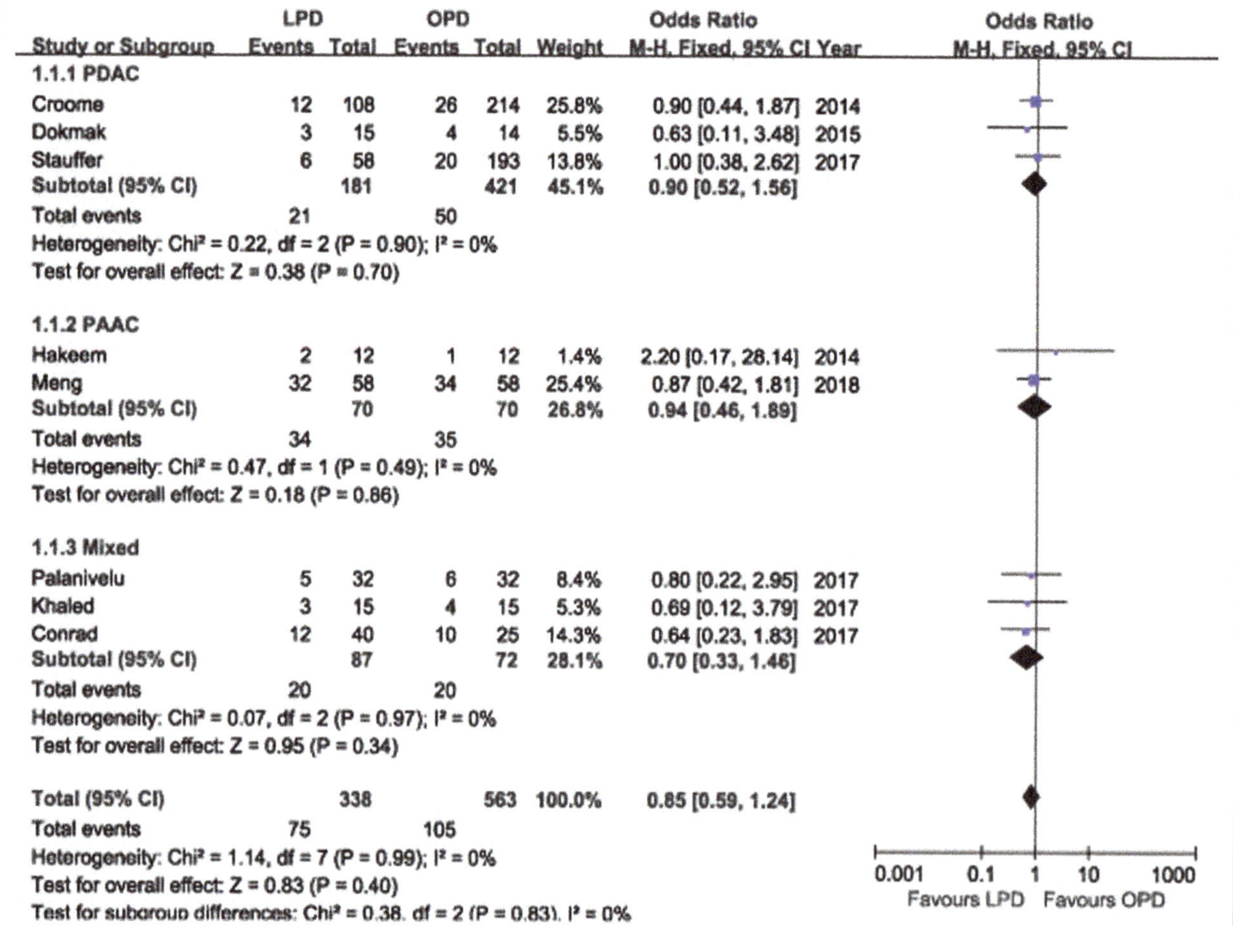

Study or Subgroup	LPD Events	LPD Total	OPD Events	OPD Total	Weight	Odds Ratio M-H, Fixed, 95% CI	Year
1.1.1 PDAC							
Croome	12	108	26	214	25.8%	0.90 [0.44, 1.87]	2014
Dokmak	3	15	4	14	5.5%	0.63 [0.11, 3.48]	2015
Stauffer	6	58	20	193	13.8%	1.00 [0.38, 2.62]	2017
Subtotal (95% CI)		181		421	45.1%	0.90 [0.52, 1.56]	
Total events	21		50				
Heterogeneity: Chi² = 0.22, df = 2 (P = 0.90); I² = 0%							
Test for overall effect: Z = 0.38 (P = 0.70)							
1.1.2 PAAC							
Hakeem	2	12	1	12	1.4%	2.20 [0.17, 28.14]	2014
Meng	32	58	34	58	25.4%	0.87 [0.42, 1.81]	2018
Subtotal (95% CI)		70		70	26.8%	0.94 [0.46, 1.89]	
Total events	34		35				
Heterogeneity: Chi² = 0.47, df = 1 (P = 0.49); I² = 0%							
Test for overall effect: Z = 0.18 (P = 0.86)							
1.1.3 Mixed							
Palanivelu	5	32	6	32	8.4%	0.80 [0.22, 2.95]	2017
Khaled	3	15	4	15	5.3%	0.69 [0.12, 3.79]	2017
Conrad	12	40	10	25	14.3%	0.64 [0.23, 1.83]	2017
Subtotal (95% CI)		87		72	28.1%	0.70 [0.33, 1.46]	
Total events	20		20				
Heterogeneity: Chi² = 0.07, df = 2 (P = 0.97); I² = 0%							
Test for overall effect: Z = 0.95 (P = 0.34)							
Total (95% CI)		338		563	100.0%	0.85 [0.59, 1.24]	
Total events	75		105				
Heterogeneity: Chi² = 1.14, df = 7 (P = 0.99); I² = 0%							
Test for overall effect: Z = 0.83 (P = 0.40)							
Test for subgroup differences: Chi² = 0.38, df = 2 (P = 0.83), I² = 0%							

Odds Ratio M-H, Fixed, 95% CI

0.001 0.1 1 10 1000

Favours LPD Favours OPD

Fig. 2 Forest plot of the meta-analysis: overall POPF

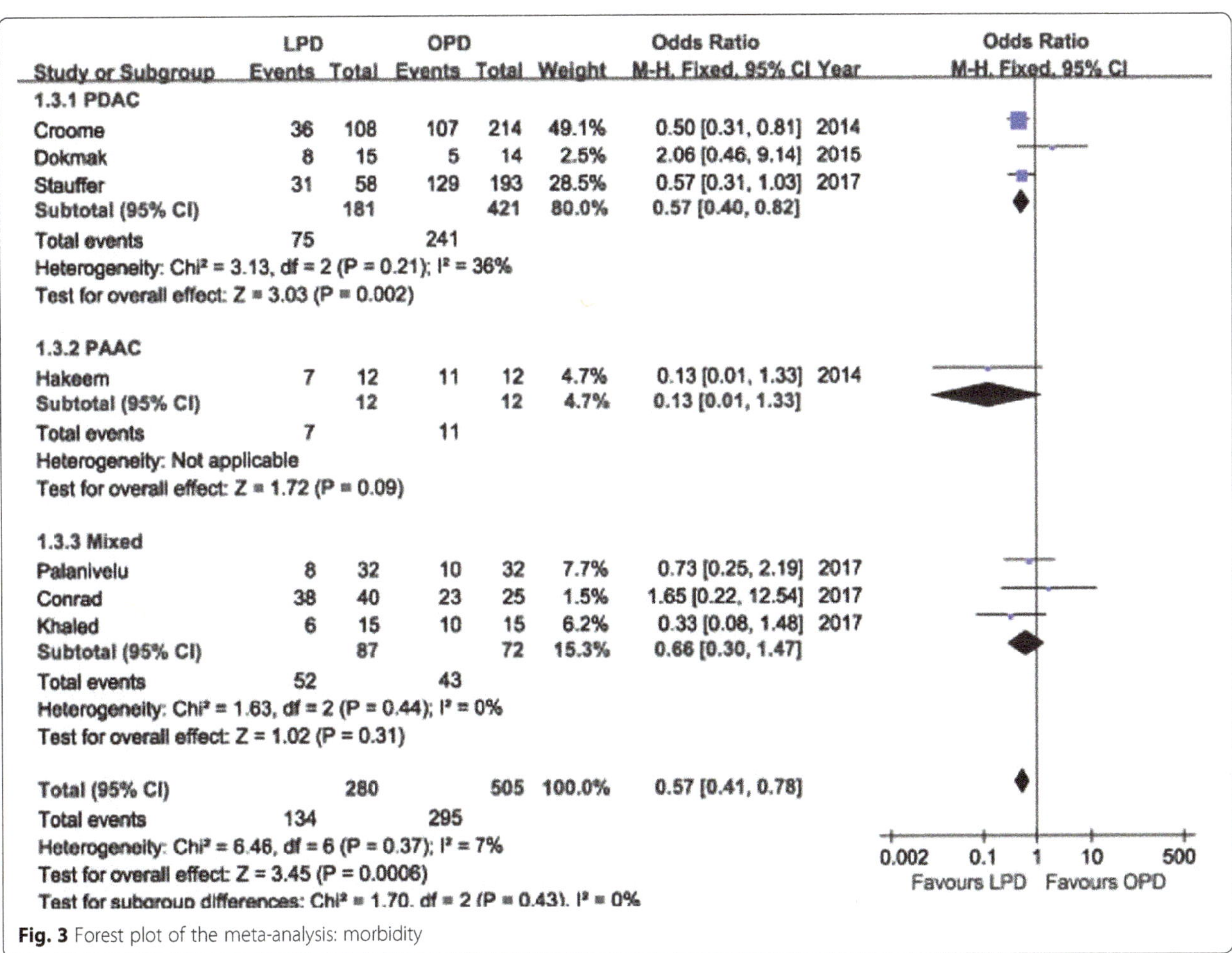

Fig. 3 Forest plot of the meta-analysis: morbidity

studies reported the length of hospital stay [14, 15, 18–24]. The pooled data indicated a comparable length of hospital stay between groups (WMD = – 1.07, 95%CI, – 3.05~ – 0.92, $P = 0.29$). Tumor size was available except in one study [20]. The tumor size of OPD was larger than that of LPD (WMD = – 0.16, 95%CI, – 0.31~ – 0.02, $P = 0.03$). The secondary outcomes of the quantitative meta-analysis are outlined in Table 2.

Sensitivity analysis

One retrospectively muti-institutional study conducted by Kantor et al. [20], in which only PDAC were included, provided the vast majority of cases. The study offered outcomes of mortality, R0 rate, RLNs, overall survival, and length of hospital stay. We investigated the influence of this study on the overall estimated risk by sequentially removing it from the pooled outcomes. We found only the pooling data of R0 rate changed from marginal difference (OR = 1.17, 95%CI: 1.00~ 1.37, $P = 0.05$) to no significant difference (OR = 1.28, 95%CI: 0.89~ 1.84, $P = 0.19$), whereas the main results presented no obvious changes.

Discussion

Minimally invasive PD (MIPD), a laparoscopic surgery, was first described by Gagner and Pompin in 1994, and there has been a recent surge of interest for this demanding technique [25, 26]. PD is a complex procedure and the advantages of minimally invasive approaches used to be closely scrutinized. Although several meta-analyses have confirmed the advantages of MIPD over open surgery, there has been no analysis restricted to malignancy. Moreover, effects of oncologic results were not well evaluated due to insufficient data. In Table 3, we present several previous meta-analyses comparing MIPD to OPD for benign and malignant periampullary disease [27–34].

This meta-analysis selected and summarized the available literature that compared the short-term surgical and long-term survival results of LPD and OPD for malignant periampullary disease. To the best of our knowledge, this is the first meta-analysis comparing LPD versus OPD for the treatment of pancreatic-head and periampullary cancer. No statistically significant differences were identified between the two groups regarding POPF, mortality, overall survival rate, and hospital stay.

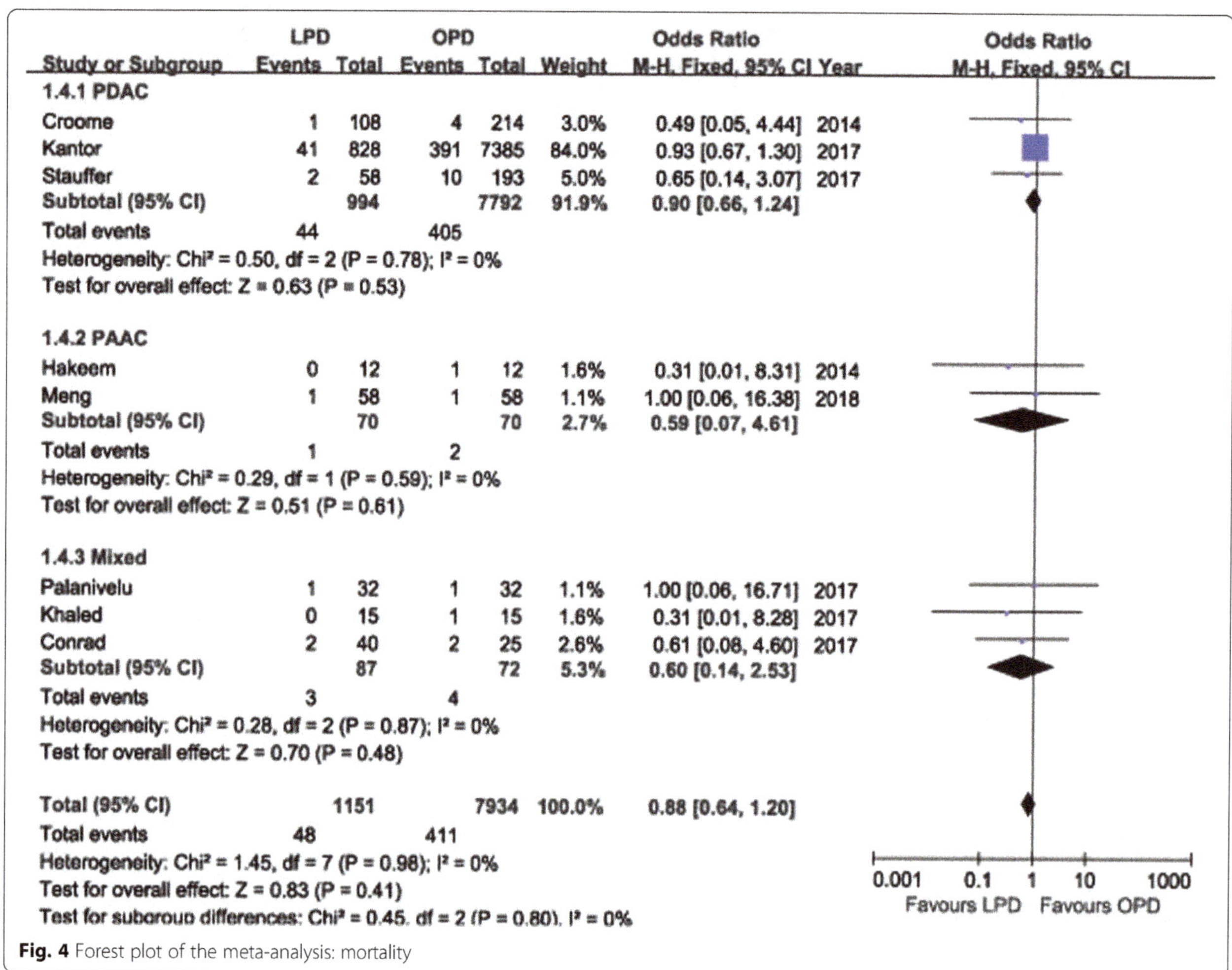

Fig. 4 Forest plot of the meta-analysis: mortality

Operative time was significantly longer in the LPD group. The differences of R0 rate, and RLNs did not reach statistical significance, but tended to be superior in the LPD group. Moreover, LPD exhibited statistically significant benefits in terms of blood loss, and overall postoperative complications.

The progress of LPD was slow due to the threatening complication of POPF. High rates ranging from 4 to 33% for conventional open surgery were previously reported for both benign and malignant lesions [35, 36]. POPF rates range from 11.8 to 55.2% in LPD for malignancy as reported seemed to somewhat higher than the results above (Table 4). It was also reported that LPD for resection of periampullary tumors was associated with higher morbidity, mainly due to severe POPF [18]. However, our pooling data demonstrated comparable rates, regardless of overall POPFs or clinically significant POPFs between LPD and OPD for malignancy. The approaches which could reduce POPFs also can be completed under laparoscope [37]. The end-to-side, duct-to-mucosa pancreaticojejunostomy (PJ) was now the most commonly performed pancreatic anastomosis approach under laparoscopy just as the conventional open approach [38]. Importantly, our results have shown improved overall morbidity of LPD. Since surgical complications, mainly POPFs, were comparable between the two groups because of the same organ and lymphatic resection area of LPD and OPD, the reduced overall complications may be the result of fewer medical complications. PD involves multiple systems and the complexity of performing three anastomoses can result in enormous surgical trauma, which would result in high risks of medical complications. Pulmonary, cardiovascular, and cerebrovascular morbidities were the most frequent systemic complications in major abdominal surgery. Less bleeding and use of transfusion contribute to preserve stable pulmonary and cardiovascular functions [39]. In addition, less pain and earlier ambulation allows patients to restore physiological homeostasis.

The pooling results show that LPD is linked with a tendency of lower positive margin rate ($P = 0.05$) and more retrieved lymph nodes ($P = 0.08$), two of the oncologic outcomes. Appropriate lymphadenectomy is crucial because elimination of a sufficient quantity of lymphadens could help to strengthen the staging accuracy and

Study or Subgroup	LPD Events	LPD Total	OPD Events	OPD Total	Weight	Odds Ratio M-H, Fixed, 95% CI	Year
1.5.1 PDAC							
Croome	84	108	164	214	8.3%	1.07 [0.61, 1.86]	2014
Chen	18	19	35	38	0.4%	1.54 [0.15, 15.91]	2015
Song	8	11	209	261	1.6%	0.66 [0.17, 2.59]	2015
Dokmak	9	15	7	14	1.0%	1.50 [0.34, 6.53]	2015
Kantor	651	828	5623	7385	82.2%	1.15 [0.97, 1.37]	2017
Stauffer	49	58	154	193	3.7%	1.38 [0.62, 3.05]	2017
Subtotal (95% CI)		1039		8105	97.2%	1.15 [0.98, 1.35]	
Total events	819		6192				
Heterogeneity: Chi² = 1.09, df = 5 (P = 0.96); I² = 0%							
Test for overall effect: Z = 1.72 (P = 0.09)							
1.5.2 PAAC							
Hakeem	9	12	8	12	0.7%	1.50 [0.25, 8.84]	2014
Meng	58	58	55	58	0.2%	7.38 [0.37, 146.12]	2018
Subtotal (95% CI)		70		70	0.8%	2.62 [0.62, 11.08]	
Total events	67		63				
Heterogeneity: Chi² = 0.84, df = 1 (P = 0.36); I² = 0%							
Test for overall effect: Z = 1.31 (P = 0.19)							
1.5.3 Mixed							
Conrad	35	40	21	25	1.1%	1.33 [0.32, 5.53]	2017
Khaled	13	15	11	15	0.5%	2.36 [0.36, 15.45]	2017
Palanivelu	31	32	30	32	0.3%	2.07 [0.18, 24.01]	2017
Subtotal (95% CI)		87		72	1.9%	1.72 [0.62, 4.77]	
Total events	79		62				
Heterogeneity: Chi² = 0.25, df = 2 (P = 0.88); I² = 0%							
Test for overall effect: Z = 1.05 (P = 0.29)							
Total (95% CI)		1196		8247	100.0%	1.17 [1.00, 1.37]	
Total events	965		6317				
Heterogeneity: Chi² = 3.45, df = 10 (P = 0.97); I² = 0%							
Test for overall effect: Z = 2.00 (P = 0.05)							
Test for subgroup differences: Chi² = 1.79, df = 2 (P = 0.41), I² = 0%							

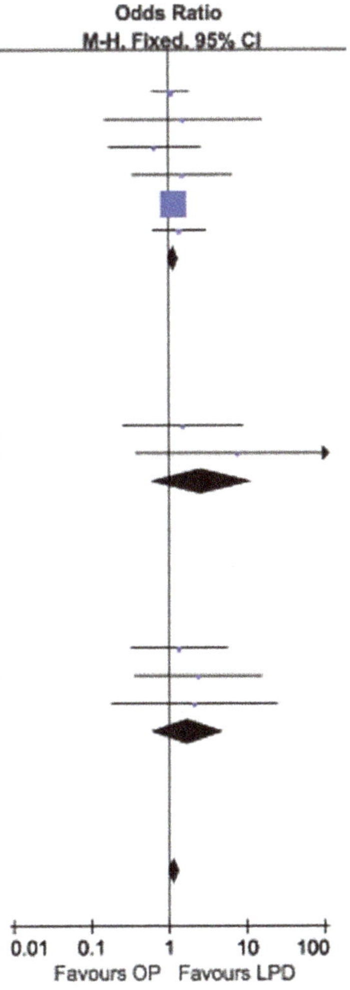

Odds Ratio M-H, Fixed, 95% CI

0.01 0.1 1 10 100

Favours OP Favours LPD

Fig. 5 Forest plot of the meta-analysis: R0 rate

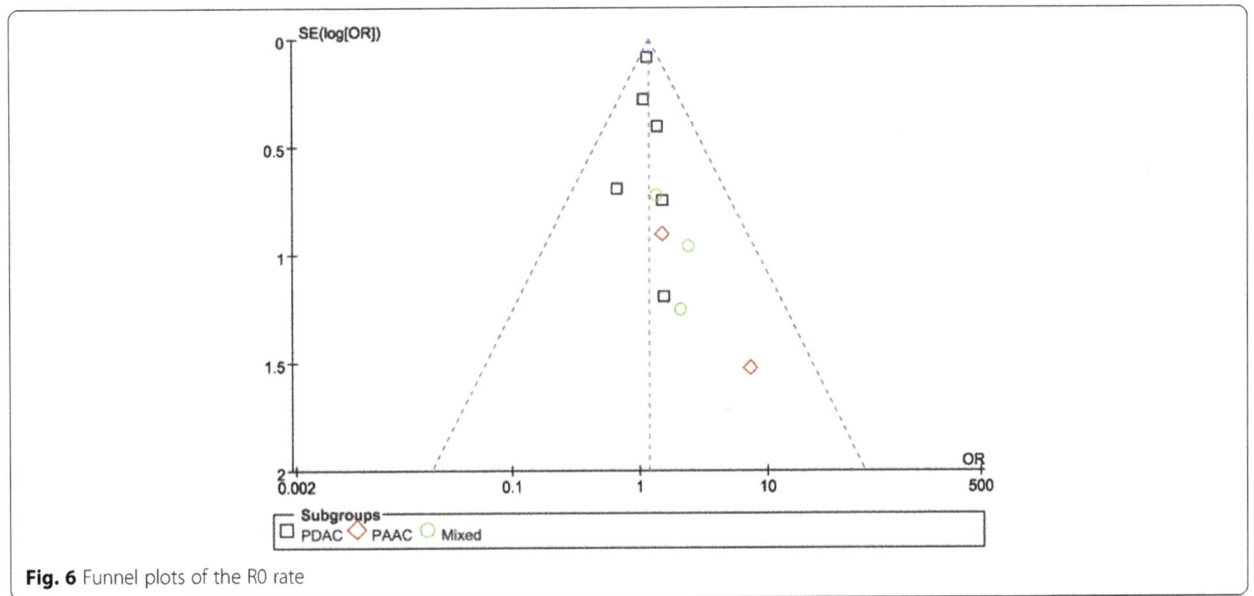

Fig. 6 Funnel plots of the R0 rate

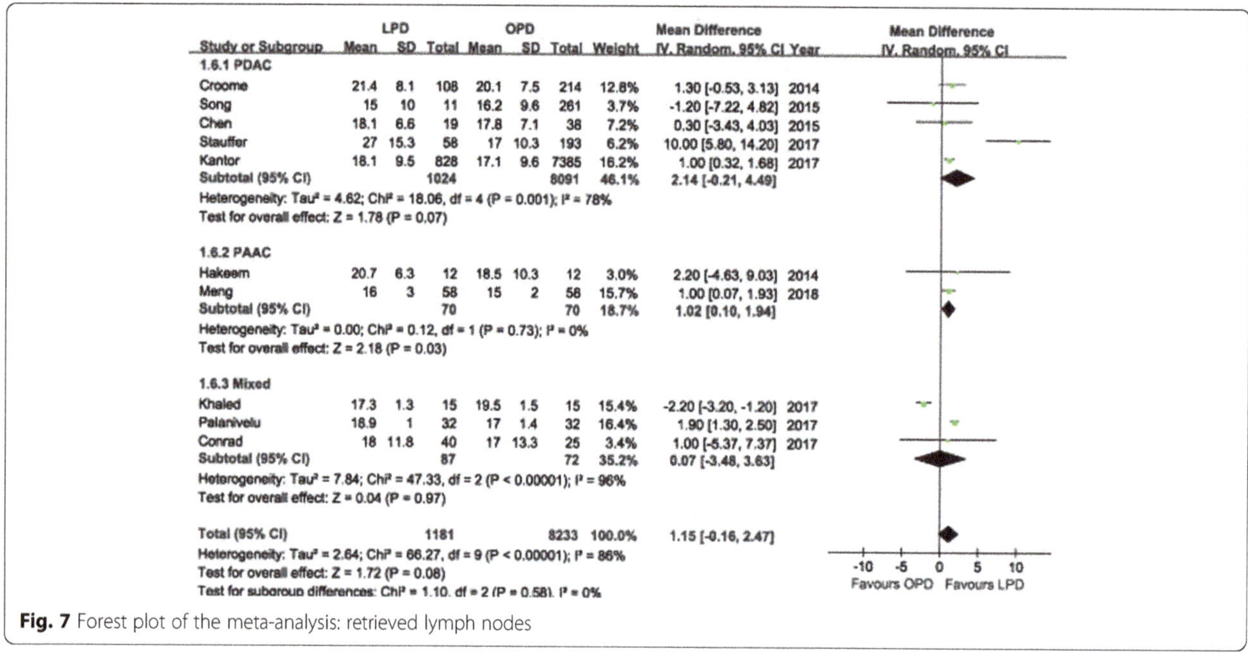

Study or Subgroup	LPD Mean	LPD SD	LPD Total	OPD Mean	OPD SD	OPD Total	Weight	Mean Difference IV, Random, 95% CI	Year
1.6.1 PDAC									
Croome	21.4	8.1	108	20.1	7.5	214	12.8%	1.30 [-0.53, 3.13]	2014
Song	15	10	11	16.2	9.6	261	3.7%	-1.20 [-7.22, 4.82]	2015
Chen	18.1	6.6	19	17.8	7.1	38	7.2%	0.30 [-3.43, 4.03]	2015
Stauffer	27	15.3	58	17	10.3	193	6.2%	10.00 [5.80, 14.20]	2017
Kantor	18.1	9.5	828	17.1	9.6	7385	16.2%	1.00 [0.32, 1.68]	2017
Subtotal (95% CI)			1024			8091	46.1%	2.14 [-0.21, 4.49]	
Heterogeneity: Tau² = 4.62; Chi² = 18.06, df = 4 (P = 0.001); I² = 78%									
Test for overall effect: Z = 1.78 (P = 0.07)									
1.6.2 PAAC									
Hakeem	20.7	6.3	12	18.5	10.3	12	3.0%	2.20 [-4.63, 9.03]	2014
Meng	16	3	58	15	2	58	15.7%	1.00 [0.07, 1.93]	2018
Subtotal (95% CI)			70			70	18.7%	1.02 [0.10, 1.94]	
Heterogeneity: Tau² = 0.00; Chi² = 0.12, df = 1 (P = 0.73); I² = 0%									
Test for overall effect: Z = 2.18 (P = 0.03)									
1.6.3 Mixed									
Khaled	17.3	1.3	15	19.5	1.5	15	15.4%	-2.20 [-3.20, -1.20]	2017
Palanivelu	18.9	1	32	17	1.4	32	16.4%	1.90 [1.30, 2.50]	2017
Conrad	18	11.8	40	17	13.3	25	3.4%	1.00 [-5.37, 7.37]	2017
Subtotal (95% CI)			87			72	35.2%	0.07 [-3.48, 3.63]	
Heterogeneity: Tau² = 7.84; Chi² = 47.33, df = 2 (P < 0.00001); I² = 96%									
Test for overall effect: Z = 0.04 (P = 0.97)									
Total (95% CI)			1181			8233	100.0%	1.15 [-0.16, 2.47]	
Heterogeneity: Tau² = 2.64; Chi² = 66.27, df = 9 (P < 0.00001); I² = 86%									
Test for overall effect: Z = 1.72 (P = 0.08)									
Test for subgroup differences: Chi² = 1.10, df = 2 (P = 0.58), I² = 0%									

Fig. 7 Forest plot of the meta-analysis: retrieved lymph nodes

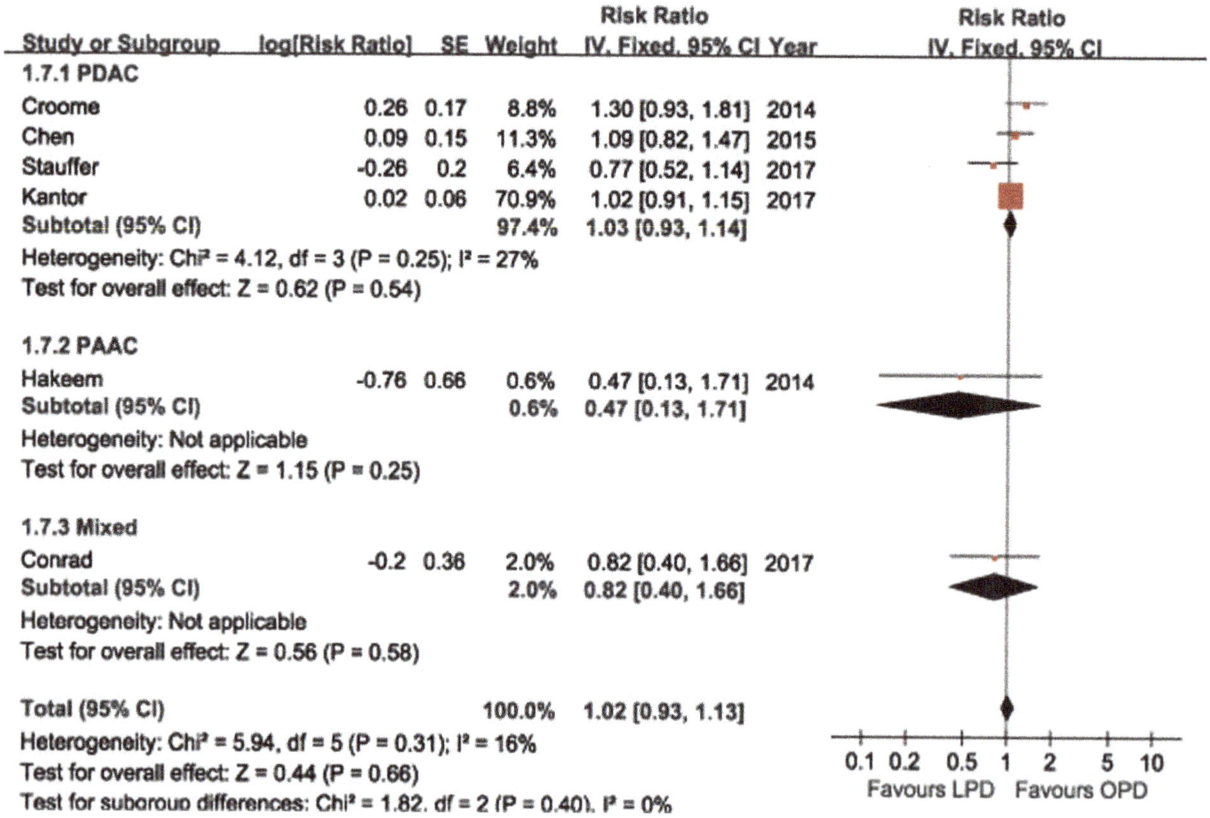

Study or Subgroup	log[Risk Ratio]	SE	Weight	Risk Ratio IV, Fixed, 95% CI	Year
1.7.1 PDAC					
Croome	0.26	0.17	8.8%	1.30 [0.93, 1.81]	2014
Chen	0.09	0.15	11.3%	1.09 [0.82, 1.47]	2015
Stauffer	-0.26	0.2	6.4%	0.77 [0.52, 1.14]	2017
Kantor	0.02	0.06	70.9%	1.02 [0.91, 1.15]	2017
Subtotal (95% CI)			97.4%	1.03 [0.93, 1.14]	
Heterogeneity: Chi² = 4.12, df = 3 (P = 0.25); I² = 27%					
Test for overall effect: Z = 0.62 (P = 0.54)					
1.7.2 PAAC					
Hakeem	-0.76	0.66	0.6%	0.47 [0.13, 1.71]	2014
Subtotal (95% CI)			0.6%	0.47 [0.13, 1.71]	
Heterogeneity: Not applicable					
Test for overall effect: Z = 1.15 (P = 0.25)					
1.7.3 Mixed					
Conrad	-0.2	0.36	2.0%	0.82 [0.40, 1.66]	2017
Subtotal (95% CI)			2.0%	0.82 [0.40, 1.66]	
Heterogeneity: Not applicable					
Test for overall effect: Z = 0.56 (P = 0.58)					
Total (95% CI)			100.0%	1.02 [0.93, 1.13]	
Heterogeneity: Chi² = 5.94, df = 5 (P = 0.31); I² = 16%					
Test for overall effect: Z = 0.44 (P = 0.66)					
Test for subgroup differences: Chi² = 1.82, df = 2 (P = 0.40), I² = 0%					

Risk Ratio IV, Fixed, 95% CI

0.1 0.2 0.5 1 2 5 10

Favours LPD Favours OPD

Fig. 8 Forest plot of the meta-analysis: overall survival rate

Table 2 Results of the meta-analysis

Outcomes	No. Studies	Sample size		Heterogeneity (P, I^2)	Model	Overall effect size	95% CI of overall effect	P
		LPD	OPD					
Primary Outcomes								
POPF	8	338	563	0.99, 0%	F	OR = 0.85	0.59~ 1.24	0.40
Significant POPF	5	271	512	0.96, 0%	F	OR = 0.86	0.53~ 1.41	0.56
Morbidity	7	280	505	0.37, 7%	F	OR = 0.57	0.41~ 0.78	< 0.01
Mortality	8	1151	7934	0.98, 0%	F	OR = 0.88	0.64~ 1.20	0.41
R0 rate	11	1196	8247	0.97, 0%	F	OR = 1.17	1.00~ 1.37	0.05
Retrieved lymph nodes	10	1181	8233	< 0.01, 86%	R	WMD = 1.15	-0.16~ 2.47	0.08
Overall survival	6	1065	7867	0.31, 16%	R	HR = 1.02	0.93~ 1.13	0.66
Secondary Outcomes								
Operation time (min)	5	271	512	< 0.01, 99%	R	WMD = 87.68	27.05~ 148.32	< 0.01
Blood loss (mL)	5	271	512	< 0.01, 96%	R	WMD = −197.49	− 304.62~ − 90.37	< 0.01
Transfusion	5	296	522	0.36, 7%	F	OR = 0.64	0.50~ 0.84	< 0.01
Hospital stay (days)	9	1166	7948	< 0.01, 85%	R	WMD = −1.07	−3.05~ 0.92	0.29
Tumor size	10	368	862	0.46, 0%	F	WMD = −0.16	−0.31~ − 0.02	0.03

regional tumor control. In addition, curative R0 resection is referred as the most important factor determining, which is deemed the only chance to survival [40], and the prognostic validity of margin status may be primarily confined to pancreatic head cancers rather than neoplasms in body or tail [41]. Elaborate manipulation and better visualization of critical anatomy could explain our outcomes. However, as our results also indicated a shorter tumor size in LPD group, some researches may include LPD cases of small, easily resectable tumors that would be partial to LPD, the benefit of LPD for margin status and lymph nodes harvesting cannot be confirmed, but at least not inferior to open surgery. Long-term survival rate is crucial the outcome for evaluating surgical interventions in oncological therapy. Periampullary cancer, especially PDAC, has significantly more aggressive inherent tumor biology, for which there are hardly any effect of adjuvant therapy [42, 43]. Large series on PDAC reported 5-year survival rates only around 20% [44, 45], and estimated at only 20–50% for PAAC [3, 46]. None of the previous studies on LPD identify survival advantages of the laparoscopic approach, and our analysis

Table 3 Previous meta-analyses comparing MIPD with OPD for benign and malignant periampullary disease

Variables	Correa	Nigri	Lei	Qin	de Rooij	Zhang	Peng	Shin[b]	Shin[b]
Year	2014	2014	2014	2014	2016	2016	2017	2017	2017
Included studies	6	8	9	11	19	22	9	8	5
Minimally invasive method	MIPD	MIPD	MIPD	MIPD	MIPD	MIPD	RPD	LPD	RPD
Total MIPD numbers	169	204	209	327	710	1018	245	450	160
POPF	NS	NS	NS	NS	NS	NS	NS	NS	NS
Morbidity	NS	NS	NS	NS[a]	N/A	NS	Favor RPD	NS	NS[a]
Mortality	N/A	NS	NS	NS	NS	NS	NS	N/A	N/A
R0 rate	Favor MIPD	NS	Favor MIPD	NS[a]	Favor MIPD	Favor MIPD	Favor RPD	NS	NS
Retrieved lymph nodes	Favor MIPD	NS[a]	NS	NS	NS	NS[a]	NS	NS	NS
Survival	N/A	N/A	N/A	N/A	N/A	N/A	N/A	N/A	N/A
Operation time	Favor OPD	Favor OPD	Favor OPD	Favor OPD	Favor OPD	Favor OPD	NS	Favor OPD	Favor OPD
Blood loss	Favor MIPD	Favor MIPD	Favor MIPD	Favor MIPD	Favor MIPD	Favor MIPD	N/A	NS	Favor RPD
Transfusion	N/A	NS	Favor MIPD	N/A	N/A	Favor MIPD	N/A	N/A	N/A
Hospital stay (days)	Favor MIPD	Favor MIPD	Favor MIPD	Favor MIPD	Favor MIPD	Favor MIPD	Favor RPD	Favor LPD	Favor RPD

NS not significant, *N/A* not available
[a] not significant but tended to favor MIPD
[b] one separate study

Table 4 Studies on LPD for pancreatic cancer

	Croome	Hakeem	Chen	Song	Dokmak	Stauffer	Kantor	Conrad	Palanivelu	Khaled	Meng
Age (years)	66.6 ± 9.6	67.0 ± 10.2	–	68.1 ± 7	–	69.9(40.6–84.8)	65.9 ± 10.7	68(45–83)	57.8 ± 2.0	65 (35–78)	60.0 ± 9.1
Sex (M/F)	57/51	8/4	–	–	–	32/26	–	26/14	18/14	8/7	32/26
BMI	27.4 ± 5.4	25.8 ± 3.7	–	–	–	25.9(17.7–49.6)	–	23.9 (14.9–34.1)	24.9 ± 0.7	23.4 (18–26)	22.3 ± 3.0
Tumor size (cm)	3.3 ± 1.0	2.0 ± 1.0	3.0 ± 0.9	2.8 ± 0.6	2.4(1.5–4)	2.5(0.3–10.0)	–	2.5 (0.3–8.0)	3.3 ± 0.7	2.0 (0.7–8.0)	1.9 (1.5–2.6)
Retrieved LNs	21.4 ± 8.1	20.7 ± 6.3	18.1 ± 6.6	15 ± 10	20(8–59)	27(9–70)	18.1 ± 9.5	18(6–53)	18.9 ± 1.0	18 (14–19)	16(15–18)
R0 rate	77.8%	75.0%	94.7%	72.7%	60%	84.5%	79.1%	87.5%	96.9%	86.7%	100%
Operative time (min)	379.4 ± 93.5	–	–	–	–	518(313–761)	–	–	359 ± 14	470 (280–660)	475 (420–546)
Blood loss (mL)	492.4 ± 519.3	–	–	–	–	250(50–8500)	–	–	250 ± 22	300 (50–600)	200 (100–325)
POPF	–	16.7%	–	–	20%	11.8%	–	30%	15.6%	20.0%	55.2%
Significant POPF	11%	–	–	–	–	7.8%	–	–	6.3%	20.0%	13.8%
Morbidity	5.6% CD>2	58.3%	–	–	53%	53.4%	–	95%	25.0%	40.0%	15.5% CD>2
Hospital stay (days)	6 (4–118)	14.9 ± 6.6	–	–	15(6–53)	6(4–68)	10.2 ± 8.5	24.5 (9–311)	7(5–52)	9.0(7–20)	14.0 (11.0–17.3)
Readmission	–	–	–	–	–	22.4% 90d	6.8% 30d	–	6.3% 90d	–	–
Mortality	0.9% 30d	0% 30d	–	0% 30d	0% 90d	3.4% 90d	6.9% 90d	5% 90d	3.1% 90d	0% 30d	1.7% 30d
Survival	MS: 25.3 m	1,3,5y-DFS:100, 92,83%; 1,3,5y-OS:100, 92,75%.	–	5y-OS: 53.6%	–	1,2,3,4,5y-OS: 66.5,43.3,43.3%, 38.5,32.1%	MS: 20.7 m	MS: 35.5 m; 1,3,5y-DFS: 62.3, 37.9, 25.7%; 1,3,5y-OS: 80.5, 49.2, 39.7%	–	1,3,5y-OS: 100, 80, 67%	MS: 45 m

OS overall survival rate, *MS* median survival time, *m* month

revealed the HR of overall survival rate was comparable between LPD and OPD. We agree with the viewpoint of Croome et al. that neither the laparoscopic or open procedure was technically superior would largely depend on the technique of surgeon and on pathologic analytic variability. Thus, a technically similar oncologic resection could be performed regardless of whether the open or laparoscopic approach was meticulously used [14].

Regarding the operative time and blood loss, our pooled data indicated similar outcomes to the previous studies (Table 3). Because of the intricate dissection and complicated gastrointestinal, LPD present a more demanding and challenging approach for pancreatic surgeons. Kendrick and Cusati report their initial duration of LPD to be approximately 8 h, which improved to 5 h after approximately 50 cases [47]. Therefore, adequate training and optimizing surgical potency to reduce the operative time is required before LPD becomes a generally accepted and sustainable procedure. Another benefit of laparoscopic surgery lies in the enhanced postoperative recovery. Reduced use of analgesic drugs, shortened time of abdominal cavity exposure, and earlier postoperative activities are considered to be the main reasons.

This systematic review and meta-analysis of LDP versus ODP for pancreatic-head and periampullary malignancy represents the most comprehensive collection of evidence available within this field. However, the results should still be explained with caution for several limitations. First, only one study was RCT, while others were NRCTs. Selection biases necessarily consist in surgeons' or patients' decision on operation and adjuvant therapy. Moreover, various biases are real concerns because hardly any of the included studies employed standardized appraisal for the end points. Second, clinical heterogeneity needs significant attention. The surgical techniques, take the different the extension of lymph node dissection for example, and histopathological protocols were variable in both open and laparoscopic groups. Third, there are biological differences between PDAC and PAAC. Although a subgroup analysis was conducted, we should still admit various histologies unpowered our outcomes because several studies did not differentiate PDAC and PAAC in their studies, and even in PAAC, there are several different histologies. Last but not least, it should be kept in mind that these studies were on behalf of the best centers' experience on LPD around the world. The literature showed that specialization in pancreatic surgery results in both better short- and long-term survival [48]. Obtained conclusions might not be feasible in less specialized centers.

Conclusions

Our meta-analysis demonstrated that in contrasted to OPD, LPD could achieve short-term advantages within blood loss, and postoperative morbidity for pancreatic-head and periampullary malignancy. Moreover, both procedures have comparable oncological and long-term survival outcomes. LPD may serve as a promising alternative to OPD in selected individuals suffered pancreatic-head and periampullary malignancy. However, taking into account all the limitations of the study, methodologically high-quality controlled clinical trials are necessary for further evaluation. Anyway, we believe our study could serve as a useful background for future researches.

Abbreviations

CI: Confidence intervals; HR: Hazard ratio; ISGPF: International Study Group for Pancreatic Fistula; LDP: Laparoscopic distal pancreatectomy; LPD: Laparoscopic pancreaticoduodenectomy; MIPD: Minimally invasive pancreaticoduodenectomy; NOS: Newcastle-Ottawa Quality Assessment Scale; NRCT: Nonrandomized comparative study; OPD: Open pancreaticoduodenectomy; OR: Odds ratio; PAAC: Periampullary adenocarcinoma; PD: Pancreaticoduodenectomy; PDAC: Pancreatic duct adenocarcinoma; RCT: Randomized controlled trial; RLN: Retrieved lymph nodes; RPD: Robotic pancreaticoduodenectomy; SD: Standard deviation; SE: Standard error; WMD: Weighted mean difference

Authors' contributions

KC and YP designed the study; XLL collected relevant literature and conducted the analysis of pooled data; KC and HM wrote the manuscript; XFW proofread and revised the manuscript. All authors have approved the version to be published.

Consent for publication

Not applicable.

Competing interests

The authors declare that they have no competing interests.

Author details

[1]Department of General Surgery, Sir Run Run Shaw Hospital, School of Medicine, Zhejiang University, 3 East Qingchun Road, Hangzhou 310016, Zhejiang Province, China. [2]School of Medicine, Zhejiang University, 866 Yuhangtang Road, Hangzhou 310058, Zhejiang Province, China.

References

1. Torre LA, Bray F, Siegel RL, Ferlay J, Lortet-Tieulent J, Jemal A. Global cancer statistics, 2012. CA Cancer J Clin. 2015;65(2):87–108.
2. Rahib L, Smith BD, Aizenberg R, Rosenzweig AB, Fleshman JM, Matrisian LM. Projecting cancer incidence and deaths to 2030: the unexpected burden of thyroid, liver, and pancreas cancers in the United States. Cancer Res. 2014; 74(11):2913–21.
3. Neoptolemos JP, Moore MJ, Cox TF, Valle JW, Palmer DH, McDonald AC, Carter R, Tebbutt NC, Dervenis C, Smith D, et al. Effect of adjuvant chemotherapy with fluorouracil plus folinic acid or gemcitabine vs observation on survival in patients with resected periampullary adenocarcinoma: the ESPAC-3 periampullary cancer randomized trial. Jama. 2012;308(2):147–56.
4. Gawande A. Two hundred years of surgery. N Engl J Med. 2012;366(18):1716–23.
5. Ricci C, Casadei R, Taffurelli G, Toscano F, Pacilio CA, Bogoni S, D'Ambra M, Pagano N, Di Marco MC, Minni F. Laparoscopic versus open distal pancreatectomy for ductal adenocarcinoma: a systematic review and meta-analysis. J Gastrointest Surg. 2015;19(4):770–81.
6. Riviere D, Gurusamy KS, Kooby DA, Vollmer CM, Besselink MG, Davidson BR, van Laarhoven CJ. Laparoscopic versus open distal pancreatectomy for pancreatic cancer. Cochrane Database syst Rev. 2016;4:CD011391.
7. Clavien PA, Barkun J, de Oliveira ML, Vauthey JN, Dindo D, Schulick RD, de Santibanes E, Pekolj J, Slankamenac K, Bassi C, et al. The Clavien-Dindo classification of surgical complications: five-year experience. Ann Surg. 2009; 250(2):187–96.
8. Bassi C, Dervenis C, Butturini G, Fingerhut A, Yeo C, Izbicki J, Neoptolemos J, Sarr M, Traverso W, Buchler M. Postoperative pancreatic fistula: an international study group (ISGPF) definition. Surgery. 2005;138(1):8–13.
9. Wittekind C, Compton C, Quirke P, Nagtegaal I, Merkel S, Hermanek P, Sobin LH. A uniform residual tumor (R) classification: integration of the R classification and the circumferential margin status. Cancer. 2009;115(15):3483–8.
10. Hozo SP, Djulbegovic B, Hozo I. Estimating the mean and variance from the median, range, and the size of a sample. BMC Med Res Methodol. 2005;5:13.
11. Tierney JF, Stewart LA, Ghersi D, Burdett S, Sydes MR. Practical methods for incorporating summary time-to-event data into meta-analysis. Trials. 2007;8:16.
12. Sharpe SM, Talamonti MS, Wang CE, Prinz RA, Roggin KK, Bentrem DJ, Winchester DJ, Marsh RD, Stocker SJ, Baker MS. Early National Experience with laparoscopic Pancreaticoduodenectomy for ductal adenocarcinoma: a comparison of laparoscopic Pancreaticoduodenectomy and open Pancreaticoduodenectomy from the National Cancer Data Base. J Am Coll Surg. 2015;221(1):175–84.
13. Nussbaum DP, Adam MA, Youngwirth LM, Ganapathi AM, Roman SA, Tyler DS, Sosa JA, Blazer DG 3rd. Minimally invasive Pancreaticoduodenectomy does not improve use or time to initiation of adjuvant chemotherapy for patients with pancreatic adenocarcinoma. Ann Surg Oncol. 2016;23(3):1026–33.
14. Croome KP, Farnell MB, Que FG, Reid-Lombardo KM, Truty MJ, Nagorney DM, Kendrick ML. Total laparoscopic pancreaticoduodenectomy for pancreatic ductal adenocarcinoma: oncologic advantages over open approaches? Ann Surg. 2014;260(4):633–8.
15. Hakeem AR, Verbeke CS, Cairns A, Aldouri A, Smith AM, Menon KV. A matched-pair analysis of laparoscopic versus open pancreaticoduodenectomy: oncological outcomes using Leeds pathology protocol. Hepatobiliary Pancreat Dis Int. 2014;13(4):435–41.
16. Chen S, Chen JZ, Zhan Q, Deng XX, Shen BY, Peng CH, Li HW. Robot-assisted laparoscopic versus open pancreaticoduodenectomy: a prospective, matched, mid-term follow-up study. Surg Endosc. 2015;29(12):3698–711.
17. Song KB, Kim SC, Hwang DW, Lee JH, Lee DJ, Lee JW, Park KM, Lee YJ. Matched case-control analysis comparing laparoscopic and open pylorus-preserving Pancreaticoduodenectomy in patients with Periampullary tumors. Ann Surg. 2015;262(1):146–55.
18. Dokmak S, Fteriche FS, Aussilhou B, Bensafta Y, Levy P, Ruszniewski P, Belghiti J, Sauvanet A. Laparoscopic pancreaticoduodenectomy should not be routine for resection of periampullary tumors. J Am Coll Surg. 2015; 220(5):831–8.

19. Stauffer JA, Coppola A, Villacreses D, Mody K, Johnson E, Li Z, Asbun HJ. Laparoscopic versus open pancreaticoduodenectomy for pancreatic adenocarcinoma: long-term results at a single institution. Surg Endosc. 2017; 31(5):2233–41.
20. Kantor O, Talamonti MS, Sharpe S, Lutfi W, Winchester DJ, Roggin KK, Bentrem DJ, Prinz RA, Baker MS. Laparoscopic pancreaticoduodenectomy for adenocarcinoma provides short-term oncologic outcomes and long-term overall survival rates similar to those for open pancreaticoduodenectomy. Am J Surg. 2017;213(3):512–5.
21. Conrad C, Basso V, Passot G, Zorzi D, Li L, Chen HC, Fuks D, Gayet B. Comparable long-term oncologic outcomes of laparoscopic versus open pancreaticoduodenectomy for adenocarcinoma: a propensity score weighting analysis. Surg Endosc. 2017;31(10):3970–8.
22. Palanivelu C, Senthilnathan P, Sabnis SC, Babu NS, Srivatsan Gurumurthy S, Anand Vijai N, Nalankilli VP, Praveen Raj P, Parthasarathy R, Rajapandian S. Randomized clinical trial of laparoscopic versus open pancreatoduodenectomy for periampullary tumours. Br J Surg. 2017;104(11):1443–50.
23. Khaled YS, Fatania K, Barrie J, De Liguori N, Deshpande R, O'Reilly DA, Ammori BJ. Matched case-control comparative study of laparoscopic versus open Pancreaticoduodenectomy for malignant lesions. Surg laparosc Endosc Percutan Tech. 2017;28:47–51.
24. Meng LW, Cai YQ, Li YB, Cai H, Peng B. Comparison of laparoscopic and open Pancreaticoduodenectomy for the treatment of nonpancreatic Periampullary adenocarcinomas. Surg Laparosc Endosc Percutan Tech. 2018;28:56.
25. Gagner M, Pomp A. Laparoscopic pylorus-preserving pancreatoduodenectomy. Surg Endosc. 1994;8(5):408–10.
26. de Rooij T, Klompmaker S, Abu Hilal M, Kendrick ML, Busch OR, Besselink MG. Laparoscopic pancreatic surgery for benign and malignant disease. Nat Rev Gastroenterol Hepatol. 2016;13(4):227–38.
27. Correa-Gallego C, Dinkelspiel HE, Sulimanoff I, Fisher S, Vinuela EF, Kingham TP, Fong Y, DeMatteo RP, D'Angelica MI, Jarnagin WR, et al. Minimally-invasive vs open pancreaticoduodenectomy: systematic review and meta-analysis. J Am Coll Surg. 2014;218(1):129–39.
28. Lei P, Wei B, Guo W, Wei H. Minimally invasive surgical approach compared with open pancreaticoduodenectomy: a systematic review and meta-analysis on the feasibility and safety. Surg Laparosc Endosc Percutan Tech. 2014;24(4):296–305.
29. Nigri G, Petrucciani N, La Torre M, Magistri P, Valabrega S, Aurello P, Ramacciato G. Duodenopancreatectomy: open or minimally invasive approach? Surgeon. 2014;12(4):227–34.
30. Qin H, Qiu J, Zhao Y, Pan G, Zeng Y. Does minimally-invasive pancreaticoduodenectomy have advantages over its open method? A meta-analysis of retrospective studies. PLoS One. 2014;9(8):e104274.
31. de Rooij T, Lu MZ, Steen MW, Gerhards MF, Dijkgraaf MG, Busch OR, Lips DJ, Festen S, Besselink MG. Minimally invasive versus open Pancreatoduodenectomy: systematic review and meta-analysis of comparative cohort and registry studies. Ann Surg. 2016;264(2):257–67.
32. Zhang H, Wu X, Zhu F, Shen M, Tian R, Shi C, Wang X, Xiao G, Guo X, Wang M, et al. Systematic review and meta-analysis of minimally invasive versus open approach for pancreaticoduodenectomy. Surg Endosc. 2016;30(12):5173–84.
33. Peng L, Lin S, Li Y, Xiao W. Systematic review and meta-analysis of robotic versus open pancreaticoduodenectomy. Surg Endosc. 2017;31(8):3085–97.
34. Shin SH, Kim YJ, Song KB, Kim SR, Hwang DW, Lee JH, Park KM, Lee YJ, Jun E, Kim SC. Totally laparoscopic or robot-assisted pancreaticoduodenectomy versus open surgery for periampullary neoplasms: separate systematic reviews and meta-analyses. Surg Endosc. 2017;31(9):3459–74.
35. Xiong JJ, Tan CL, Szatmary P, Huang W, Ke NW, Hu WM, Nunes QM, Sutton R, Liu XB. Meta-analysis of pancreaticogastrostomy versus pancreaticojejunostomy after pancreaticoduodenectomy. Br J Surg. 2014; 101(10):1196–208.
36. Zhou W, Lv R, Wang X, Mou Y, Cai X, Herr I. Stapler vs suture closure of pancreatic remnant after distal pancreatectomy: a meta-analysis. Am J Surg. 2010;200(4):529–36.
37. Ecker BL, McMillan MT, Asbun HJ, Ball CG, Bassi C, Beane JD, Behrman SW, Berger AC, Dickson EJ, Bloomston M, et al. Characterization and optimal Management of High-Risk Pancreatic Anastomoses during Pancreatoduodenectomy. Ann Surg. 2017;267:608–16.
38. Sun YL, Zhao YL, Li WQ, Zhu RT, Wang WJ, Li J, Huang S, Ma XX. Total closure of pancreatic section for end-to-side pancreaticojejunostomy decreases incidence of pancreatic fistula in pancreaticoduodenectomy. Hepatobiliary Pancreat Dis Int. 2017;16(3):310–4.
39. Ramana CV, DeBerge MP, Kumar A, Alia CS, Durbin JE, Enelow RI. Inflammatory impact of IFN-gamma in CD8+ T cell-mediated lung injury is mediated by both Stat1-dependent and -independent pathways. Am J Physiol Lung Cell Mol Physiol. 2015;308(7):L650–7.
40. Howard TJ, Krug JE, Yu J, Zyromski NJ, Schmidt CM, Jacobson LE, Madura JA, Wiebke EA, Lillemoe KD. A margin-negative R0 resection accomplished with minimal postoperative complications is the surgeon's contribution to long-term survival in pancreatic cancer. J Gastrointest Surg. 2006;10(10): 1338–45. discussion 1345-1336
41. Demir IE, Jager C, Schlitter AM, Konukiewitz B, Stecher L, Schorn S, Tieftrunk E, Scheufele F, Calavrezos L, Schirren R, et al. R0 versus R1 resection matters after Pancreaticoduodenectomy, and less after distal or Total Pancreatectomy for pancreatic Cancer. Ann Surg. 2017;267:608–16.
42. Youngwirth LM, Nussbaum DP, Thomas S, Adam MA, Blazer DG 3rd, Roman SA, Sosa JA. Nationwide trends and outcomes associated with neoadjuvant therapy in pancreatic cancer: an analysis of 18 243 patients. J Surg Oncol. 2017;116(2):127–32.
43. Acharya A, Markar SR, Sodergren MH, Malietzis G, Darzi A, Athanasiou T, Khan AZ. Meta-analysis of adjuvant therapy following curative surgery for periampullary adenocarcinoma. Br J Surg. 2017;104(7):814–22.
44. Luo J, Xiao L, Wu C, Zheng Y, Zhao N. The incidence and survival rate of population-based pancreatic cancer patients: shanghai Cancer registry 2004-2009. PLoS One. 2013;8(10):e76052.
45. Distler M, Ruckert F, Hunger M, Kersting S, Pilarsky C, Saeger HD, Grutzmann R. Evaluation of survival in patients after pancreatic head resection for ductal adenocarcinoma. BMC Surg. 2013;13:12.
46. Kim K, Chie EK, Jang JY, Kim SW, Oh DY, Im SA, Kim TY, Bang YJ, Ha SW. Role of adjuvant chemoradiotherapy for ampulla of Vater cancer. Int J Radiat Oncol Biol Phys. 2009;75(2):436–41.
47. Kendrick ML, Cusati D. Total laparoscopic pancreaticoduodenectomy: feasibility and outcome in an early experience. Arch Surg. 2010;145(1):19–23.
48. Ahola R, Siiki A, Vasama K, Vornanen M, Sand J, Laukkarinen J. Effect of centralization on long-term survival after resection of pancreatic ductal adenocarcinoma. Br J Surg. 2017;104(11):1532–8.

16

Amoxicillin/clavulanic acid-induced pancreatitis

Sana Chams*, Skye El Sayegh, Mulham Hamdon, Sarwan Kumar and Vesna Tegeltija

Abstract

Background: Acute pancreatitis is an acute inflammation of the pancreas that varies in severity from mild to life threatening usually requiring hospitalization. The true incidence of drug-induced pancreatitis (DIP) is indeterminate due to the inadequate documentation of case reports of DIP. Here we present the case of amoxicillin/clavulanic acid-induced pancreatitis in a previously healthy male after excluding all other causes of pancreatitis.

Case presentation: A 58-year-old Caucasian man presenting for acute sharp abdominal pain with associated nausea and heaves. Pain was non-radiating and worsening with movement. Patient had no constitutional symptoms. The only medication he received prior to presentation was amoxicillin/clavulanic acid as prophylaxis for a dental procedure with his symptoms starting on day 9th of therapy. Laboratory studies revealed mild leukocytosis, increased levels of serum lipase, amylase, and C-reactive protein (CRP). Abdominal computed tomography (CT) was notable for acute pancreatitis with no pseudocyst formation. Hence, patient was diagnosed with mild acute pancreatitis that was treated with aggressive intravenous (IV) hydration and pain management with bowel rest of 2 days duration and significant improvement being noticed within 72 h. On further questioning, patient recalled that several years ago he had similar abdominal pain that developed after taking amoxicillin/clavulanic acid but did not seek medical attention at that time and the pain resolved within few days while abstaining from food intake. All other causes of pancreatitis were ruled out in this patient who is non-alcoholic, non-smoker, and never had gallstones. Abdominal ultrasound and magnetic resonance cholangiopancreatography (MRCP) eliminated out the possibility of gallstones, biliary ductal dilatation, or choledocholithiasis. Patient had no hypertriglyceridemia nor hypercalcemia, never had endoscopic retrograde cholangiopancreatography (ERCP), never took steroids, has no known malignancy, infection, trauma, or exposure to scorpions.

Conclusion: This case describes a patient with DIP after the intake of amoxicillin/clavulanic acid and when all other common causes of acute pancreatitis were excluded. Only two other case reports were available through literature review regarding amoxicillin/clavulanic acid- induced pancreatitis.
We again stress on the importance of identifying and reporting cases of DIP to raise awareness among physicians and clinicians.

Keywords: Amoxicillin/clavulanic acid, Amoxicillin, Pancreatitis, Drug-induced pancreatitis

Background

Acute pancreatitis is an acute inflammation of the pancreas that varies in severity from mild to life threatening usually requiring hospitalization. The predominant symptom is severe abdominal pain and diagnosis can be made through blood tests and imaging studies such as x-rays, ultrasound, and computed tomography (CT) scan. The major causes of acute pancreatitis are gallstones (30–60%) and heavy alcohol use (15–30%) in addition to other common causes: hypertriglyceridemia, hyperparathyroidism, endoscopic retrograde cholangiopancreatography (ERCP), trauma, pancreatic tumors, surgery, infections, and medications [1]. Of increasing interest is the drug-induced pancreatitis (DIP) which is less common (1–2%) even though true incidence is indeterminate due to the inadequate documentation of case reports of DIP where DIP is often undiagnosed, misdiagnosed, or underdiagnosed [1–4]. Here lies the importance of identifying cases of DIP in medical practice and the need for documenting and publishing such cases to increase the awareness among physicians regarding the side effects of most commonly used drugs and also to aid scientists and

* Correspondence: schams@med.wayne.edu
Department of Internal Medicine, Wayne State University School of Medicine, Rochester Hills, MI, USA

researchers in identifying the mechanism behind DIP. Here we present the case of amoxicillin/clavulanic acid-induced pancreatitis in a previously healthy male after excluding all other causes of pancreatitis.

We followed CARE reporting guidelines in publishing our case report.

Case presentation

A 58-year-old Caucasian man presented to the emergency department for acute abdominal pain. The abdominal pain was mainly in the epigastric area, was sharp in nature, with severity of 8/10, non-radiating, worsens with movement, and mildly improves with rest. The pain was associated with nausea and heaves. On review of systems he denied any constitutional symptoms (weight loss, fever, chills, weakness or fatigue), no cardiovascular, respiratory, neurological, musculoskeletal, hematological or endocrinological problems. Past medical history is only significant for hypothyroidism for which he takes levothyroxine. No previous surgeries done. Patient was not taking any medications except for Levothyroxine for hypothyroidism for the past 10 years. The only medication he received prior to presentation was amoxicillin/clavulanic acid as prophylaxis for a dental procedure (even though not indicated at that time) with dosage of 875 mg twice daily for a total of 10 days with his symptoms starting on day 9th of therapy and amoxicillin/clavulanic acid was discontinued on admission to hospital. On further questioning, patient recalled that several years ago he had similar abdominal pain that developed after taking amoxicillin/clavulanic acid but did not seek medical attention at that time and the pain resolved within few days while abstaining from food intake. He is a non-smoker, has never used recreational drugs, drinks only socially on certain occasions not exceeding twice a month and not exceeding 2 beers, 5% alcohol based, in one sitting (a total of 24 oz), and denies binge drinking. On admission, he was hemodynamically stable. His physical examination was noticeable for epigastric tenderness only. Laboratory studies revealed mild leukocytosis (white blood count (WBC): 13.5 × 10^9/L), increased levels of serum lipase > 600 U/L, amylase: 1220 U/L, and CRP: 19.6 mg/dL. Abdominal CT was notable for acute pancreatitis with no pseudocyst formation (Fig. 1).

Based on clinical presentation and CT findings, patient was diagnosed with mild acute pancreatitis with Bedside Index of Severity in Acute Pancreatitis (BISAP) score of 0 (< 1% risk of mortality), which is characterized by the absence of organ failure and local or systemic complications. During his hospital stay, patient was managed with aggressive IV hydration and pain management with bowel rest of 2 days duration and significant improvement being noticed within 72 h after which patient was discharged home.

In order to identify the cause of his acute pancreatitis, extensive history and workup was done with the help of the gastroenterology team to eliminate the most common causes of pancreatitis. Magnetic resonance cholangiopancreatography (MRCP) and abdominal ultrasound and eliminated out the possibility of gallstones, biliary sludge, biliary ductal dilatation, or choledocholithiasis (Figs. 2 and 3).

Endoscopic ultrasonography was done as outpatient by the gastroenterologist on the case and ruled out biliary

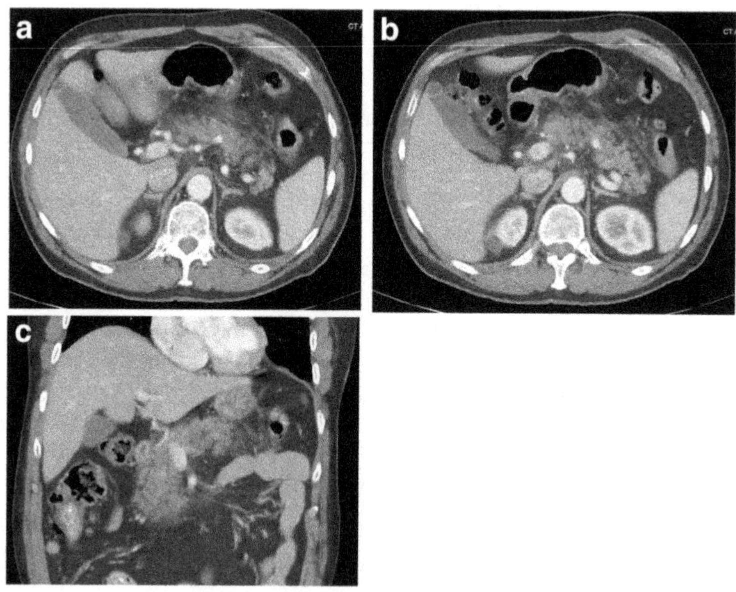

Fig. 1 CT of the abdomen and pelvis. **a** and **b** Axial plane showing infiltration of the peripancreatic fat planes by soft tissue attenuation complicated with inflammation. No pancreatic ductal dilatation or discrete peripancreatic fluid collections observed. No stones in adjacent gall bladder. **c** Similar findings in coronal plane

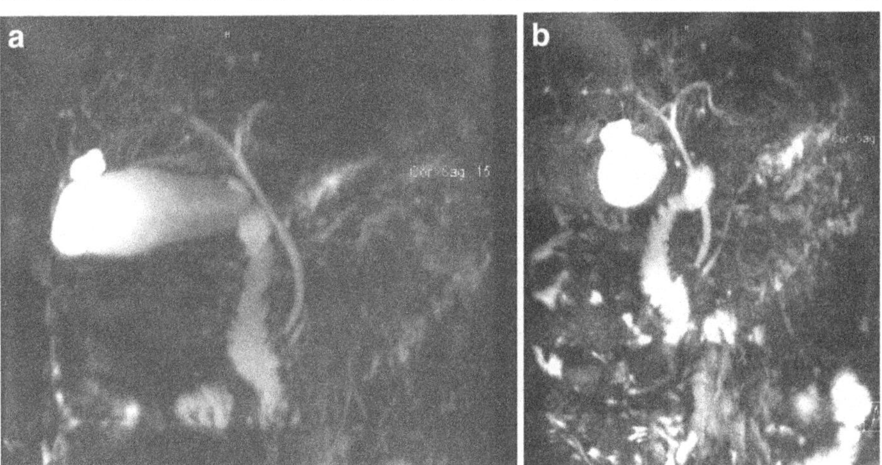

Fig. 2 MRCP images. **a** Normal caliber CBD (common bile duct). **b** Normal caliber main pancreatic duct

microlithiasis. Patient had no hypertriglyceridemia (his triglyceride (TG): 142 mg/dL), never had endoscopic retrograde cholangiopancreatography (ERCP), no hypercalcemia (his corrected calcium (Ca): 9.3 mg/dL), no steroids taken, no known malignancy, no infection, no trauma, no exposure to scorpions. The most plausible link for his pancreatitis was his use of amoxicillin/clavulanic acid prior to presentation given that he had a similar presentation when he took the same antibiotic several years ago but was not diagnosed with pancreatitis since he did not seek medical attention at that time. Additionally, patient denied intake of any other penicillin agents. Table 1 summarizes our case's timeline.

Discussion and conclusions

Identifying the cause of acute pancreatitis can be somewhat challenging especially when trying to identify a certain drug as the causative agent. Drugs are responsible for approximately 0.1–2% of acute pancreatitis incidents with most information about drug-induced pancreatitis being collected from case reports and case series which means that true incidence can be even higher [1–4]. There is no one main mechanism behind drug-induced acute pancreatitis, but several potential mechanisms are currently based on theories. Of the proposed mechanisms include: pancreatic duct constriction with localized angioedema and arteriolar thrombosis, cytotoxic and metabolic effects, and hypersensitivity reactions [2]. As well as drugs with side effects of hypertriglyceridemia and chronic hypercalcemia that are considered risk factors for acute pancreatitis [2]. The diagnosis of drug-induced acute pancreatitis requires a diagnosis of acute pancreatitis and ruling out all other etiologies. Etiologies that were ruled out in this case comprise all possible causes of pancreatitis: gallstones, biliary sludge and microlithiasis, alcohol, smoking, hypertriglyceridemia, scorpion venom, post endoscopic retrograde cholangiopancreatography (ERCP), hypercalcemia, steroids intake, malignancy, infection, trauma, vascular disease [1–4]. Based on American College of Gastroenterology guidelines, consideration for genetic testing for hereditary pancreatitis is based on expert opinion and warranted for

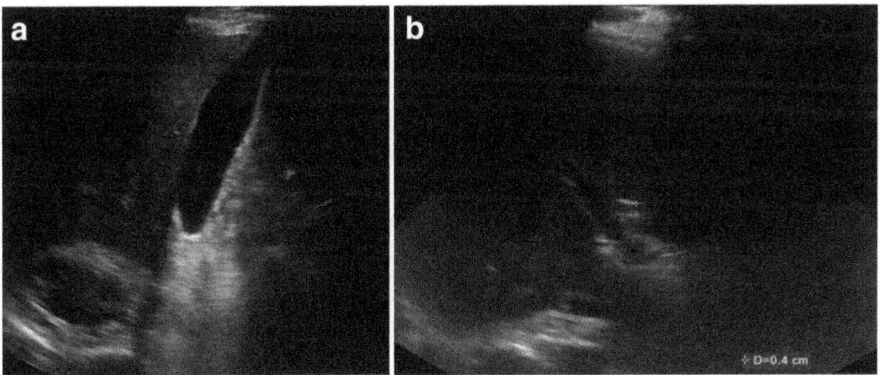

Fig. 3 Abdominal ultrasound images. **a** Gallbladder without any stones. **b** Normal caliber common bile duct ≤ 7 mm demonstrated

Table 1 Timeline Table

Relevant Past Medical History and Interventions		
Past medical history significant for hypothyroidism. Patient received amoxicillin/clavulanic acid as prophylaxis for a dental procedure (even though not indicated at that time) with dosage of 875 mg twice daily for a total of 10 days with his symptoms starting on day 9th of therapy prior to presentation. Several years ago, he had similar abdominal pain that developed after taking amoxicillin/clavulanic acid but did not seek medical attention at that time and the pain resolved within few days while abstaining from food intake.		
Summaries from Initial and Follow-up Visits	Diagnostic Testing	Interventions
Based on clinical presentation and CT findings, patient was diagnosed with mild acute pancreatitis with Bedside Index of Severity in Acute Pancreatitis (BISAP) score of 0 (< 1% risk of mortality), which is characterized by the absence of organ failure and local or systemic complications. During his hospital stay, patient was managed with aggressive IV hydration and pain management with bowel rest of 2 days duration and significant improvement being noticed within 72 h after which patient was discharged home.	Laboratory studies: WBC, amylase, lipase, and CRP.	Discontinuation of offending drug (amoxicillin/clavulanic acid); aggressive IV hydration and pain management with bowel rest of 2 days duration.
No follow-up visits needed	Imaging: Abdominal CT, MRCP, abdominal ultrasound, and endoscopic ultrasonography.	

pancreatic cancer patients with a personal history of at least 2 attacks of acute pancreatitis of unknown etiology, a family history of pancreatitis, or early-age onset chronic pancreatitis [5]; therefore, the decision was made by the primary and gastroenterology teams on the case not to forgo with genetic testing to rule out hereditary pancreatitis. Immunoglobulin G4 level was 24 mg/dL (reference range: 1–100 mg/dL) which ruled out autoimmune pancreatitis. The evidence found to implicate a certain drug to the development of acute pancreatitis is often inadequate especially when the mechanism is unknown. Badalov N. et al. proposed a classification system of drug-induced acute pancreatitis. This system was based on the number of case reports found in the literature, the available rechallenge data, latency period and ability to exclude other causes of acute pancreatitis [6]. After reviewing summary of drug induced acute pancreatitis based on drug class, we found that ampicillin and penicillin are considered class IV (single case report published, but neither a rechallenge nor a consistent latency period documented) [6]. If the pancreatitis resolves after discontinuation of the drug, suspicion for drug-induced pancreatitis increases. A firm diagnosis can be reasonably established with

Table 2 Comparing the case of our patient with published data

Case	Patient	Findings	Drug	Delay between introduction of the drug and pancreatitis	Re-challenge	Outcome
Chams et al. 2018 (our case)	58-year-old male	Elevated amylase, lipase with CT abdomen showing pancreatitis	Amoxicillin-clavulanic acid	On day 9th of antibiotic treatment	Not performed	Clinical improvement with fluid hydration and cessation of antibiotic
Campo et al. 2015 [7]	42-year-old woman	Elevated lipase with CT abdomen showing pancreatitis	Amoxicillin-clavulanic acid	While on antibiotic treatment; unknown duration	Not performed	Clinical improvement with fluid hydration and cessation of antibiotic
Cerezo Ruiz et al. 2015 [8]	48-year-old female	Elevated lipase with US abdomen showing pancreatitis	Amoxicillin-clavulanic acid	*Data unavailable*	*Data unavailable*	Spontaneous resolution
Sammett et al. 1998 [9]	7-year-old male	Elevated amylase, lipase with US abdomen showing pancreatitis	Penicillin	3 weeks prior to diagnosis was treated with 10 days of oral penicillin	Not performed	Clinical improvement with fluid hydration and food restriction
Galindo et al.; 1995 [10]	25-year-old male	Acute pancreatitis and cholestatic cute hepatitis	Amoxicillin-clavulanic acid	After 4 weeks of an antibiotic treatment	Not performed	Clinical improvement with fluid hydration and food restriction
Hanlien 1987 [11]	73-year-old woman	Elevated serum amylase, lipase and urine amylase	Ampicillin	On day 6th of antibiotic treatment	Re-exposure 2 weeks later for treatment of pneumonia, with repeat elevated enzymes on the 4th day	Clinical improvement after discontinuation of antibiotic treatment

a rechallenge of the offending drug that results in the recurrence of pancreatitis symptoms [1–4]. Rechallenge was not done in this case. Very few cases, less than 5 total cases, were documented in the literature regarding ampicillin, penicillin, and amoxicillin/clavulanic acid induced acute pancreatitis with true mechanism still being unidentified [7–11]. Table 2 shows the comparison between our patient's case with published data in the literature.

Drug-induced acute pancreatitis remains rare but should not be disregarded when medical practitioners are faced with a patient presenting with acute pancreatitis with no obvious cause. Being familiar with reports of drugs causing acute pancreatitis can be helpful in identifying the causality and association with a certain drug. Despite the fact that DIP can have a benign course with good prognosis, fatal outcomes still occur and thus DIP should not be overlooked. This case describes a patient with DIP after the intake of amoxicillin/clavulanic acid and when all other common causes of acute pancreatitis were excluded. We again stress on the importance of identifying and reporting cases of DIP to raise awareness among physicians and clinicians. We also stress on the importance of encouraging scientists and researchers to better understand the mechanism of developing drug-induced acute pancreatitis.

Abbreviations

BISAP: Bedside Index of Severity in Acute Pancreatitis; Ca: Calcium; CRP: C-reactive protein; CT: Computed tomography; DIP: Drug-induced pancreatitis; ERCP: Endoscopic retrograde cholangiopancreatography; IV: Intravenous; MRCP: Magnetic resonance cholangiopancreatography; TG: Triglyceride; WBC: White blood count

Funding

The authors declare that they received no specific grant from any funding agency in the public, commercial or not-for-profit sectors.

Authors' contributions

SC and SE assembled, analyzed and interpreted the patient's data and case presentation of drug-induced pancreatitis. MH reviewed the literature. SK and VT edited and critically revised the manuscript for intellectual content. All authors contributed to writing the manuscript. All authors read and approved the final manuscript.

Consent for publication

Written informed consent was obtained from the patient for publication of this case report and accompanying images. A copy of the written consent is available for review by the Editor-in-Chief of this journal.

Competing interests

The authors declare that they have no competing interests.

References

1. Książyna D. Drug-induced acute pancreatitis related to medications commonly used in gastroenterology. European Journal of Internal Medicine. 2011;22(1):20–5. https://doi.org/10.1016/j.ejim.2010.09.004.
2. Jones MR, Hall OM, Kaye AM, Kaye AD. Drug-induced acute pancreatitis: a review. Ochsner J. 2015;15(1):45–51.
3. Nitsche C, Maertin S, Scheiber J, Ritter C, Lerch M, Mayerle J. Drug-induced pancreatitis. Current Gastroenterology Reports. 2012;14(2):131–8.
4. Eltookhy A, Pearson NL. Drug-induced pancreatitis. Canadian Pharmacists Journal. 2006;139(6):58–60.
5. Syngal S, Brand R, Church J, Giardiello F, Hampel H, Burt R. ACG clinical guideline: genetic testing and Management of Hereditary Gastrointestinal Cancer Syndromes. Am J Gastroenterol. 2015;110(2):223–62. https://doi.org/10.1038/ajg.2014.435.
6. Badalov N, Baradarian R, Kadirawel I, et al. Drug-induced acute pancreatitis: an evidence-based review. Clin Gastroenterol Hepatol. 2007;5:648.
7. Campo L, Halak A, Olivo R, Changela K, Culliford A, Babich J. Amoxicillin-clavulanic acid induced pancreatitis: a case report. Am J Gastroenterol. 2015; 110(S1):S89.
8. Cerezo Ruiz A, Domínguez Jiménez J, Cortez Quiroga G, García QJ. Acute pancreatitis associated with amoxycillin-clavulanic acid. Gastroenterol Hepatol. 2015;38(6):410–1. https://doi.org/10.1016/j.gastrohep.2014.08.004.
9. Sammett D, Greben C, Sayeed-Shah U. Acute pancreatitis caused by penicillin. Dig Dis Sci. 1998;43(8):1778–83.
10. Galindo C, Buenestado J, Reñé J, Piñol M. Acute pancreatitis associated with hepatotoxicity induced by amoxicillin-clavulanic acid. Rev Esp Enferm Dig. 1995;87(8):597–600.
11. Hanlien MH. Acute pancreatitis caused by ampicillin. South Med J. 1987;80:1069.

Risk factors for post-ERCP cholecystitis: a single-center retrospective study

Jun Cao[1], Chunyan Peng[1], Xiwei Ding[1], Yonghua Shen[1], Han Wu[1], Ruhua Zheng[1], Lei Wang[1,2*] and Xiaoping Zou[1,2*]

Abstract

Background: The risk factors for post-ERCP cholecystitis (PEC) have not been characterized. Hence, this study aimed to identify the potential risk factors for PEC.

Methods: The medical records of 4238 patients undergoing the first ERCP in a single center from January 2012 to December 2016 were analyzed in this study. A multivariate analysis was used to identify the risk factors.

Results: This study included 2672 patients who met the enrollment criteria. Of these, 36 patients (incidence rate of 1.35%) developed PEC within 2 weeks of the procedure. Univariate and multivariate analyses identified the following factors associated with PEC: history of acute pancreatitis [odds ratio (OR) = 2.60; 95% confidence interval (CI): 1.29–5.23], history of chronic cholecystitis (OR = 8.47; 95% CI: 2.54–28.24), gallbladder opacification (OR = 2.79; 95% CI: 1.37–5.70), biliary duct metallic stent placement (OR = 3.66; 95% CI: 1.78–7.54), and high leukocyte count before ERCP (OR = 1.10; 95% CI: 1.04–1.17). The prediction model incorporating these factors demonstrated an area under the receiver operating characteristic curve of 0.85 (95% CI, 0.80–0.91). A prognostic nomogram was developed using the aforementioned variables to estimate the probability of PEC.

Conclusions: The risk factors, including the history of acute pancreatitis, history of chronic cholecystitis, gallbladder opacification, biliary duct metallic stent placement, and high leucocyte counts before ERCP, increased the occurrence of PEC and were positive predictors for PEC. The constructed nomogram was used to estimate the risk of PEC, guiding the implementation of prophylactic measures to prevent PEC in clinical practice.

Keywords: ERCP, Cholecystitis, Nomogram, Risk factors, Success prediction

Background

Endoscopic retrograde cholangiopancreatography (ERCP) is an endoscopic procedure performed under visual and fluoroscopic guidance. It is widely used in diagnosing and treating of biliary and pancreatic diseases. ERCP is a technically challenging endoscopic procedure that can cause serious adverse events and occasionally even death. Possible ERCP-related adverse events include acute pancreatitis, hemorrhage, perforation, cholangitis, and acute cholecystitis. Of these, post-ERCP pancreatitis (PEP) is the most common one with 9.7% incidence and 0.7% mortality rate [1]. Due to its high incidence, numerous studies have investigated the risk factors of PEP. The risk factors of PEP include suspected sphincter of Oddi dysfunction, major papilla pancreatogram, needle-knife precut, and female gender [2, 3].

In contrast, post-ERCP cholecystitis (PEC) gained much less attention. Freemen et al. reported cholecystitis in 0.5% (11/2347) of patients 16 days after biliary sphincterotomy [4]. In this study, no predictors of cholecystitis were identified other than the presence of stones in the gallbladder. Most studies reporting the adverse events of ERCP did not investigate the risk factors and predictors of PEC alone, which might be due to its relatively low incidence. However, most PECs require emergency cholecystectomy and extended hospitalization time. In addition, some PECs are severe and potentially fatal. Identifying the risk factors for PEC may help prevent this adverse event. The aim of this study was to assess the risk factors for PEC in patients with

* Correspondence: 867152094@qq.com; 13770771661@163.com
[1]Department of Gastroenterology, Nanjing Drum Tower Hospital, The Affiliated Hospital of Nanjing University Medical School, Nanjing, China
Full list of author information is available at the end of the article

gallbladder in situ within 2 weeks of procedure in a single large-volume center.

Methods

The study was approved by the Ethical Committee at Nanjing Drum Tower Hospital Affiliated to Nanjing University Medical School (study number 2017–167-01). All subjects were anonymized; hence, informed consent was not required. This study conformed to Strengthening the Reporting of Observational Studies in Epidemiology guidelines.

Patients

The medical records of patients with gallbladder in situ who underwent ERCP for the first time in the hospital from January 2012 to December 2016 were reviewed and analyzed retrospectively. Patients who had concomitant acute cholecystitis at the time of ERCP or had a previous ERCP history were excluded from the study. The medical records of eligible patients were reviewed retrospectively to identify any occurrence of acute cholecystitis within 2 weeks after ERCP.

Risk factors

The following predefined parameters were analyzed for PEC within 2 weeks. The demographic information included the following: age and sex. The past history included the following: acute pancreatitis, chronic cholecystitis, acute cholangitis, hypertension, hyperlipidemia, and diabetes mellitus. The laboratory examination indexes before ERCP were as follows: alanine aminotransferase, aspartate aminotransferase, alkaline phosphatase, gamma-glutamyltranspeptidase, total bilirubin, direct bilirubin, leukocyte count, hemoglobin, and platelet count. The indexes during ERCP were as follows: gallbladder opacification, biliary duct stent, and common bile duct (CBD) diameter. Other factors before ERCP included temperature and antibiotics. During the bile duct opacification, we recorded gallbladder opacification if contrast medium entered into gallbladder and the outline of gallbladder could be seen. No additional efforts were made to get the entire gallbladder outlined by contrast medium if this had not been accomplished simultaneously with bile duct opacification.

Endoscopy protocol

Duodenal side-viewing endoscopes (JF-260, TJF-240, or TJF-260; Olympus, Tokyo, Japan) were used to perform the ERCP procedure. The patients were under midazolam sedation. Sphincterotomy was performed using a standard sphincterotome and/or a needle knife. Balloon sphincteroplasty was performed using a Boston Scientific controlled radial expansion balloon with a diameter range of 12–15 mm, 15–18 mm or 18–20 mm). Stones were extracted using retrieval baskets and/or balloon-tipped catheters. An endoscopic mechanical lithotripsy or laser lithotripsy was attempted to crush down the stones if the stones were too big to remove. Obstructive jaundice resulting from malignant bile duct stenosis was treated by placing nasobiliary drainage (ENBD), plastic stents, or self-expandable biliary metal stents. The benign biliary stricture was treated by dilation or placement of plastic stents or fully covered self-expandable biliary metal stents. Pancreaticobiliary maljunction or pancreas divisum was treated by placing ENBD or plastic stents.

Diagnostic criteria of acute cholecystitis

Acute cholecystitis was diagnosed according to the 2018 Tokyo guidelines of acute cholecystitis [5]. The diagnostic criteria were based on the following three aspects: (A) local signs of inflammation, including (1) Murphy's sign and (2) right upper abdominal quadrant mass/pain/tenderness; (B) systemic signs of inflammation, including (1) fever, (2) elevated CRP, and (3) elevated WBC count; and (C) imaging finding characteristic of acute cholecystitis. A definite diagnosis was as follows: one item in A + one item in B + C.

Statistical analysis

Mean ± standard deviation was used to describe deviation of the data with the normal distribution of the variables. Median (quartile spacing) was used to describe the data that did not meet the normal distribution of the variables. Frequency (percentage) was used to describe the classification of variables. The differences between groups were compared using *t*-test, chi-square test, or rank-sum test [6]. Logistic regression was used to analyze the findings of a multivariate analysis of acute cholecystitis after ERCP [7]. The nomogram was used to visualize the logistic regression model [8]. The Bonferroni method was used to calibrate the adjusted test level for pairwise comparison of the findings of the chi-square test. Binned Scatterplot was used to describe the relationship between preoperative leukocytes and the risk of acute cholecystitis within 2 weeks after ERCP. SPSS 13.0 was used for statistical analysis. pROC and rms package in R 3.3.3 software were used to construct receiver operating characteristic (ROC) curve and nomogram. A two-tailed value of $P < 0.05$ was established as the threshold of statistical significance.

Results

Patient population

A total of 4238 patients who underwent the first ERCP procedure between January 1, 2012, and December 31, 2016, in the hospital were included. Of these, 1352 patients were excluded from the study due to concomitant acute cholecystitis ($n = 182$) or a history of cholecystectomy ($n = 1170$)

before ERCP. Further, 214 patients with more than 15% of missing data were also excluded. Finally, 2672 patients with intact gallbladder were included in the retrospective analysis to analyze the incidence of acute cholecystitis within 2 weeks after the initial ERCP. The mean age of the patients was 62.4 ± 16.2 years (range, 1–106 years); 1166 patients (43.6%) were female (Table 1). Also, 36 patients (incidence rate of 1.35%) finally developed acute cholecystitis within 2 weeks after the first ERCP (Fig. 1).

Risk factors for acute cholecystitis within 2 weeks after the first ERCP

The results of univariate analysis of potential risk factors for the development of acute cholecystitis within 2 weeks after ERCP are shown in Table 1. The following parameters were found to be closely correlated with PEC in the univariate analysis: history of acute pancreatitis ($\chi^2 = 17.754$, $P < 0.001$), chronic cholecystitis ($\chi^2 = 20.815$, $P < 0.001$), gallbladder opacification ($\chi^2 = 11.816$, $P = 0.001$), bile duct stents ($\chi^2 = 15.805$, $P = 0.001$), leukocyte count before ERCP ($Z = -3.610$, $P < 0.001$). The multiple logistic regression analysis identified the following variables significantly correlated with post-ERCP acute cholecystitis (Table 2): history of acute pancreatitis (OR = 2.60; 95% CI: 1.29–5.23; $P = 0.007$); history of chronic cholecystitis (OR = 8.47; 95% CI: 2.54–28.24; $P = 0.001$), gallbladder opacification (OR = 2.79; 95% CI: 1.37–5.70; $P = 0.005$), biliary duct metallic stent placement (OR = 3.66;

Table 1 Univariate analysis of potential risk factors for the development of acute cholecystitis after ERCP

Variable	Acute Cholecystitis		Statistic	*P*
	No ($n = 2636$)	Yes ($n = 36$)		
Age (y), Mean ± SD	62.4 ± 16.28	62.2 ± 12.90	$t = 0.097$	0.923
Female	1145 (43.4%)	21 (58.3%)	$\chi^2 = 2.627$	0.105
Past history				
Hypertension	976 (37.0%)	13 (36.1%)	$\chi^2 = 0.013$	0.910
Hyperlipemia	70 (2.7%)	1 (2.9%)	$\chi^2 = 0.005$	0.942
Diabetes mellitus	473 (18.0%)	7 (20.0%)	$\chi^2 = 0.098$	0.755
Acute pancreatitis	459 (17.4%)	16 (44.4%)	$\chi^2 = 17.754$	< 0.001
Acute cholangitis	532 (20.2%)	6 (16.7%)	$\chi^2 = 0.273$	0.601
Chronic cholecystitis	1427 (54.1%)	33 (91.7%)	$\chi^2 = 20.185$	< 0.001
Antibiotics before ERCP	948 (36.0%)	11 (30.6%)	$\chi^2 = 0.451$	0.601
Gallbladder opacification	1016 (38.5%)	24 (66.7%)	$\chi^2 = 11.816$	0.001
Diameter of CBD(cm)	1.2 ± 0.48	1.1 ± 0.42	$t = 1.237$	0.216
Temperature before ERCP (℃)	36.6 ± 0.58	36.8 ± 0.84	$t = -1.891$	0.059
Bile duct stents			$\chi^2 = 15.805$	0.001
No stent	1174 (66.2%)	19 (52.8%)		
Metallic stent	414 (15.7%)	14 (38.9%)		
Plastic stent	436 (16.5%)	2 (5.6%)		
Metallic+plastic stent	42 (1.6%)	1 (2.8%)		
Laboratory index before ERCP (Median,P_{25},P_{75})				
ALT	83.0 (37.3, 193.3)	58.7 (37.5, 191.0)	$Z = -0.027$	0.979
AST	54.9 (27.9, 119.0)	53.5 (28.7, 83.8)	$Z = -0.143$	0.886
AKP	198.1 (114.9, 359.8)	196.3 (94.2, 321.2)	$Z = -0.414$	0.679
GGT	292.5 (125.7, 550.2)	246.9 (91.9, 543.8)	$Z = -0.181$	0.856
TB	34.9 (15.5, 126.8)	23.7 (13.7, 83.3)	$Z = -0.845$	0.391
DB	21.2 (6.7, 98.8)	12.8 (7.1, 73.4)	$Z = -0.641$	0.522
WBC	6.1 (4.8, 8.2)	7.9 (5.9, 11.0)	$Z = -3.610$	< 0.001
Hemoglobin	125.0 (111.0, 136.0)	131.0 (121.0, 138.0)	$Z = -1.413$	0.158
Platelet count	192.0 (148.0, 245.0)	192.0 (146.0, 276.0)	$Z = -0.210$	0.833

CBD common bile duct, *ALT* alanine aminotransferase, *AST* aspartate anminotransferase, *AKP* alkaline phosphatase, *GGT* gamma-glutamyltranspeptidase, *TB* total bilirubin, *DB* direct bilirubin, *WBC* white blood cell

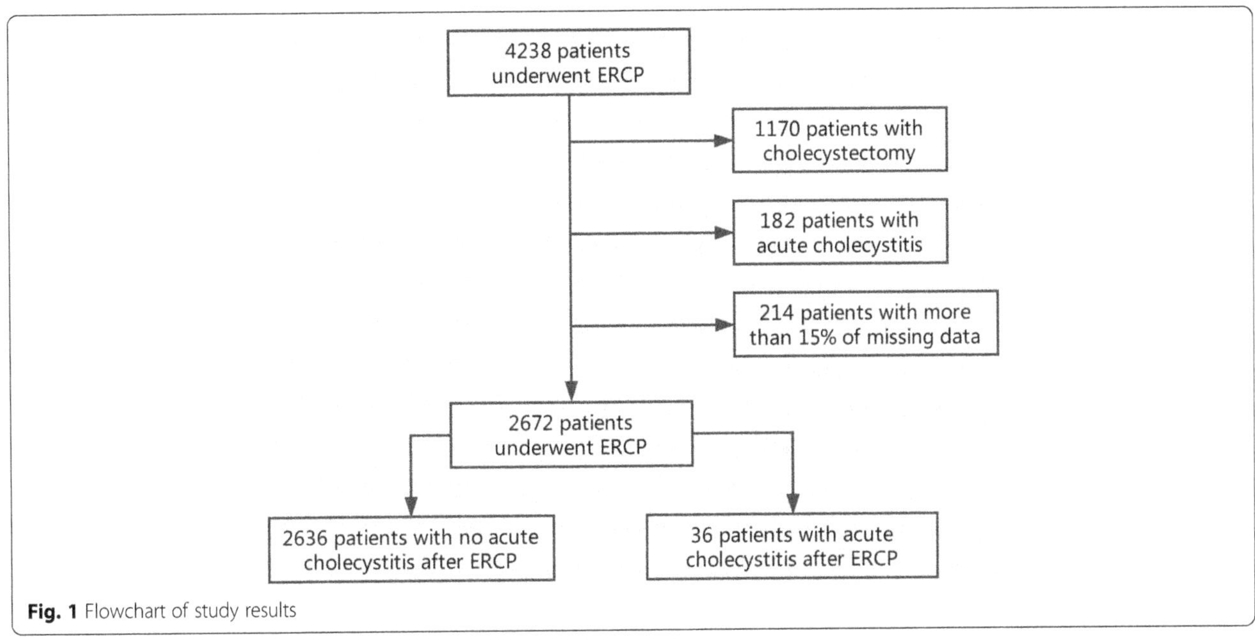

Fig. 1 Flowchart of study results

95% CI: 1.78–7.54; $P<0.001$) and leukocyte count before ERCP (OR = 1.10; 95% CI: 1.04–1.17; $P = 0.001$). In the 36 patients who developed PEC, 29 had gallstones.

The multivariate models were built to predict the incidence of acute cholecystitis after ERCP within 2 weeks. According to the ROC of the multivariate model, the area under the curve (AUC) was 0.852; the sensitivity and specificity were 82.3% and 73.3%, respectively (Fig. 2). The result revealed a good concordance and a good predictive ability.

Finally, the correlation between white blood cell counts before ERCP and PEC was estimated using a binned scatterplot diagram (Fig. 3). The results indicated a curvilinear relationship; also, the risk of PEC increased with the increase in preoperative WBC.

Discussion

Although PEC is not as common as PEP, it can lead to purulent cholecystitis and result in emergency operation or percutaneous transhepatic gallbladder drainage. Therefore, PEC should be recognized early. The present study, included 2666 patients with intact gallbladder who underwent the first ERCP, and the incidence of acute cholecystitis was 1.35% (36/2672) within 2 weeks after ERCP. The univariate and multivariate analyses indicated that the history of chronic cholecystitis, previous acute pancreatitis, gallbladder opacification, biliary stent placement, and high leukocyte count before ERCP were risk factors for the occurrence of PEC within 2 weeks of the procedure. Of note, biliary metallic stent placement significantly increased the occurrence of PEC.

As a risk factor for PEC, chronic cholecystitis may increase PEC perhaps owing to gallbladder contamination by nonsterile contrast or intestinal reflux. The diameter of the biliary duct metallic stent was greater than that of the plastic stent. Therefore, metallic stent placement during ERCP greatly increased duodenal biliary reflux,

Table 2 Multivariate logistic regression analysis of potential risk factors for subsequent post-ERCP cholecystitis

Variable	*B*	*S.E*	*P*	*OR (95% CI)*
WBC before ERCP	0.099	0.029	0.001	1.10 (1.04, 1.17)
History of acute pancreatitis	0.955	0.357	0.007	2.60 (1.29, 5.23)
History of chronic cholecystitis	2.137	0.614	0.001	8.47 (2.54, 28.24)
Gallbladder opacification	1.026	0.364	0.005	2.79 (1.37, 5.70)
Stent types	–	–	0.001	–
No	reference	reference	reference	reference
Metallic stent	1.298	0.369	< 0.001	3.66 (1.78, 7.54)
Plastic stent	−0.578	0.759	0.446	0.56 (0.13, 2.48)
Metallic +plastic stent	1.735	1.077	0.107	5.67 (0.69, 46.78)
Constant	reference	reference	reference	reference

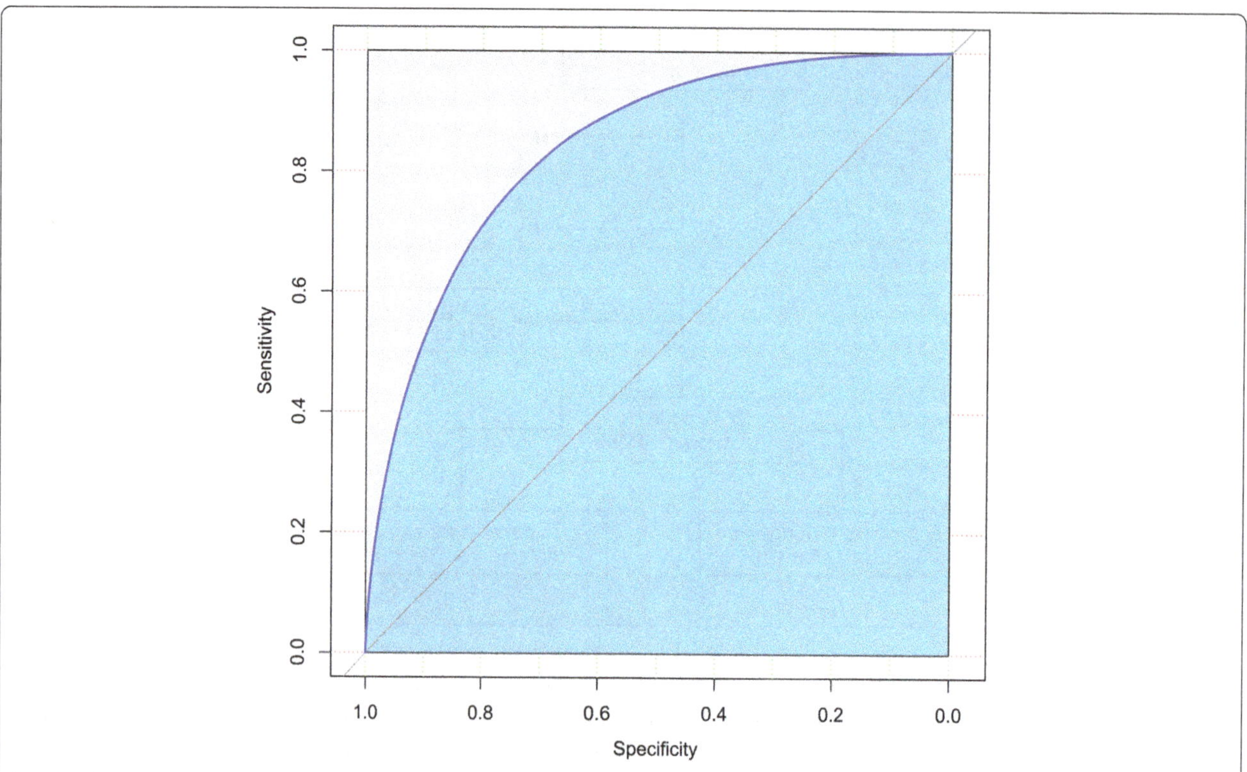

Fig. 2 ROC curve for logistic regression model predicting post-ERCP cholecystitis. It included a history of chronic cholecystitis, history of pancreatitis, gallbladder opacification, leukocyte count, and biliary metallic duct stent. AUC = 0.85; 95% CI: 0.80–0.91

further increasing the possibility of PEC. Obstructions of the cystic duct by the stent may also contribute to the development of PEC. An interesting finding in the study was that the biliary duct plastic stent did not increase the risk of PEC. The patients with high leukocyte count before ERCP were predisposed to PEC. The correlations between white blood cell counts before ERCP and PEC were estimated using a binned scatterplot diagram. The results indicated that the risk of acute cholecystitis had a positive correlation with preoperative WBC. However, the association was not strong because the OR was low (OR = 1.1).

The present study, analyzed whether serum total bilirubin level and CBD diameter were risk factors for PEC. The result suggested no correlation between them. The result was

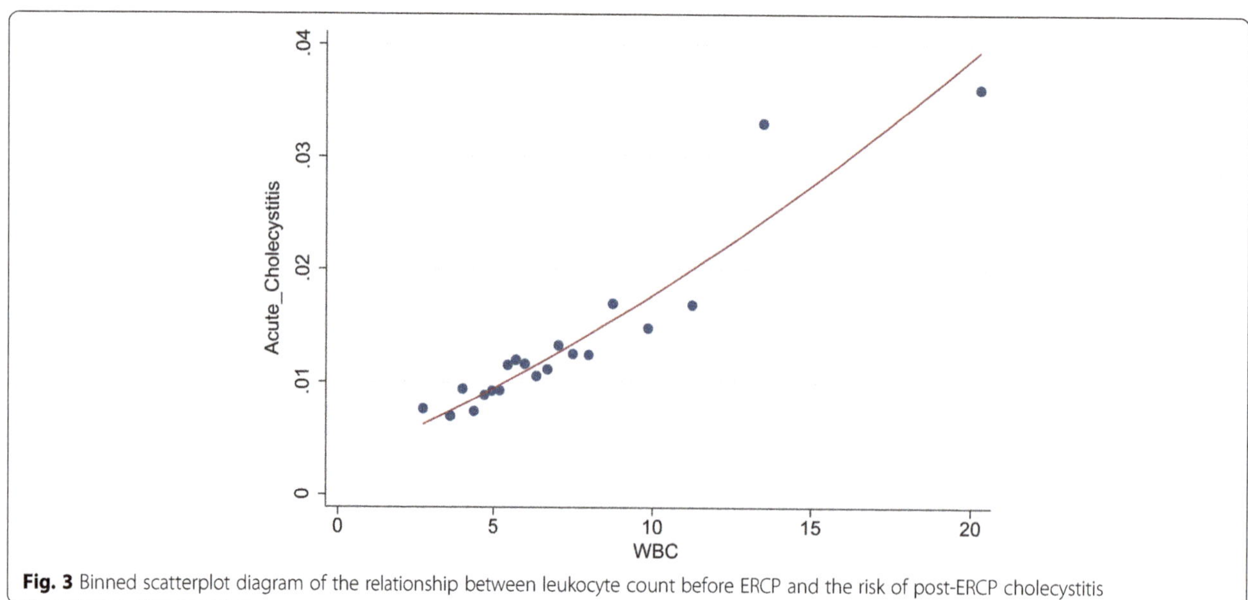

Fig. 3 Binned scatterplot diagram of the relationship between leukocyte count before ERCP and the risk of post-ERCP cholecystitis

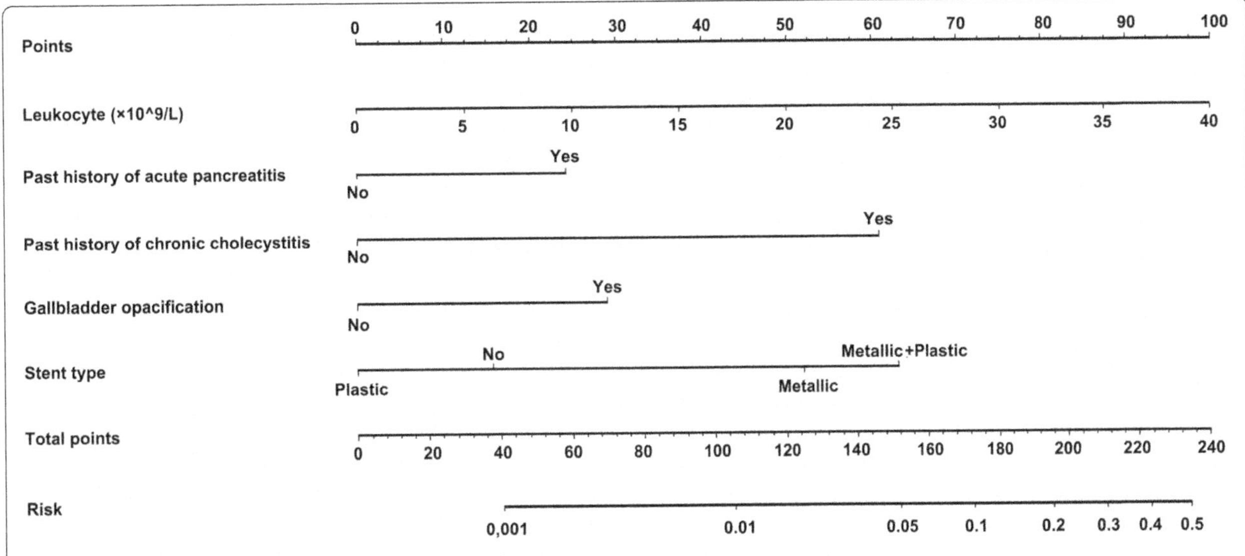

Fig. 4 The Nomogram to predict the risk of post-ERCP cholecystitis. The behavioral variables are presented in rows 2–6, and points for each variable correspond to the scale in row 1. The points of five variables are added to the total points presented on the scale in row 7, which corresponds to the risk predictor of post-ERCP acute cholecystitis within 2 weeks in rows 8

different from those of previous studies. Lee et al. assessed the risk factors for acute cholecystitis after endoscopic CBD stone removal during a mean 18-month follow-up [9]. They reported that a serum total bilirubin level < 1.3 mg/dL and a CBD diameter < 11 mm at the time of endoscopic CBD stone removal were the risk factors for the development of PEC; the incidence of PEC was 17%. However, the follow-up time of their study on the occurrence of PEC was much longer than that in the present study.

The past history of acute pancreatitis was a risk factor of PEC in this study. The causes for previous acute pancreatitis in medical records for most patients were unclear and indefinite. It was difficult to explain why previous acute pancreatitis was associated with PEC. However, according to published endoscopic ultrasonography studies, a number of patients with past "idiopathic" acute pancreatitis might have suffered from acute pancreatitis due to microlithiasis and sludge.

In the present study, a practical nomogram was established to predict PEC with a good sensitivity and specificity (Fig. 4). According to the ROC of multivariate model, the AUC was 0.85 (95% CI 0.80–0.91), and the sensitivity and specificity were 82.3% and 73.3%, respectively. The nomogram revealed a good concordance and a good predictive ability for PEC. The present study reported the first nomogram for predicting PEC. External validation of this nomogram is needed in further studies.

Identifying the risk factors related to PEC is important for taking precautions to reduce the occurrence of PEC. When patients with these risk factors undergo ERCP, prophylactic measures should be taken to prevent PEC. Endoscopic gallbladder drainage, as a safe and efficacious internal drainage, improved patient pain and decreased the likelihood of the drain being dislodged [10]. Therefore, endoscopic gallbladder drainage has been used for elderly patients with multiple comorbidities at high risk for cholecystectomy to decompress the gallbladder as a temporary measure prior to surgery or as the definitive treatment [10–13]. Briefly, patients at high risk of PEC may undergo drainage with an endoscopically placed nasocholecystic tube or plastic stents.

The present study had several limitations. First, it was a single-center retrospective study with a possibility of accumulation of inappropriate data. Moreover, cholecystitis was not classified as acalculous or calculous because of the small number of patients with PEC. Prospective studies should be performed to further establish the risk factors for PEC.

Conclusions

A history of acute pancreatitis, history of chronic cholecystitis, gallbladder opacification, biliary metal stent placement, and high leukocyte counts before ERCP were established as potential risk factors for the occurrence of PEC within 2 weeks by univariate and multivariate analyses. When patients with these risk factors undergo ERCP, prophylactic measures should be taken to prevent PEC.

Abbreviations

AUC: Area under the curve; CBD: Common bile duct; CI: Confidence interval; ENBD: Nasobiliary drainage; ERCP: Endoscopic retrograde cholangiopancreatography; PEC: Post-ERCP cholecystitis; PEP: Post-ERCP pancreatitis; ROC: Receiver operating characteristic curve

Funding
This study was supported by Nanjing Medical Science and Technique Development Foundation (QRX17037).

Authors' contributions
XZ and LW contributed to conception and design of the study and have been involved in revising the manuscript critically. CP and YS contributed to analysis and interpretation of data. JC contributed to the study design, analysis of data and drafting the manuscript. RZ and HW contributed to the acquisition of data. XD contributed to critically revising the manuscript and interpretation of data. All authors read and approved the final version of the manuscript.

Consent for publication
Not applicable.

Competing interests
The authors declare that they have no competing interests.

Author details
[1]Department of Gastroenterology, Nanjing Drum Tower Hospital, The Affiliated Hospital of Nanjing University Medical School, Nanjing, China. [2]Zhongshan Road 321, Department of Gastroenterology, Nanjing Drum Tower Hospital, The Affiliated Hospital of Nanjing University Medical School, Nanjing 210008, Jiang Su Province, China.

References
1. Kochar B, Akshintala VS, Afghani E, Elmunzer BJ, Kim KJ, Lennon AM, Khashab MA, Kalloo AN, Singh VK. Incidence, severity, and mortality of post-ERCP pancreatitis: a systematic review by using randomized, controlled trials. Gastrointest Endosc. 2015;81(1):143–9.
2. Cotton PB, Garrow DA, Gallagher J, Romagnuolo J. Risk factors for complications after ERCP: a multivariate analysis of 11,497 procedures over 12 years. Gastrointest Endosc. 2009;70(1):80–8.
3. Wang P, Li ZS, Liu F, Ren X, Lu NH, Fan ZN, Huang Q, Zhang X, He LP, Sun WS, et al. Risk factors for ERCP-related complications: a prospective multicenter study. Am J Gastroenterol. 2009;104(1):31–40.
4. Freeman ML, Nelson DB, Sherman S, Haber GB, Herman ME, Dorsher PJ, Moore JP, Fennerty MB, Ryan ME, Shaw MJ, et al. Complications of endoscopic biliary sphincterotomy. N Engl J Med. 1996;335(13):909–18.
5. Yokoe M, Hata J, Takada T, Strasberg SM, Asbun HJ, Wakabayashi G, Kozaka K, Endo I, Deziel DJ, Miura F, et al. Tokyo guidelines 2018: diagnostic criteria and severity grading of acute cholecystitis (with videos). J Hepatobiliary Pancreat Sci. 2018;25(1):41–54.
6. Zhang Z. Univariate description and bivariate statistical inference: the first step delving into data. Ann Transl Med. 2016;4(5):91.
7. Zhang Z. Variable selection with stepwise and best subset approaches. Ann Transl Med. 2016;4(7):136.
8. Zhang Z, Kattan MW. Drawing Nomograms with R: applications to categorical outcome and survival data. Ann Transl Med. 2017;5(10):211.
9. Lee JK, Ryu JK, Park JK, Yoon WJ, Lee SH, Lee KH, Kim YT, Yoon YB. Risk factors of acute cholecystitis after endoscopic common bile duct stone removal. World J Gastroenterol. 2006;12(6):956–60.
10. Itoi T, Kawakami H, Katanuma A, Irisawa A, Sofuni A, Itokawa F, Tsuchiya T, Tanaka R, Umeda J, Ryozawa S, et al. Endoscopic nasogallbladder tube or stent placement in acute cholecystitis: a preliminary prospective randomized trial in Japan (with videos). Gastrointest Endosc. 2015;81(1):111–8.
11. Kjaer DW, Kruse A, Funch-Jensen P. Endoscopic gallbladder drainage of patients with acute cholecystitis. Endoscopy. 2007;39(4):304–8.
12. Mutignani M, Iacopini F, Perri V, Familiari P, Tringali A, Spada C, Ingrosso M, Costamagna G. Endoscopic gallbladder drainage for acute cholecystitis: technical and clinical results. Endoscopy. 2009;41(6):539–46.
13. Widmer J, Alvarez P, Sharaiha RZ, Gossain S, Kedia P, Sarkaria S, Sethi A, Turner BG, Millman J, Lieberman M, et al. Endoscopic gallbladder drainage for acute Cholecystitis. Clin Endosc. 2015;48(5):411–20.

18

Risk factor for steatorrhea in pediatric chronic pancreatitis patients

Lu Hao[1,2†], Teng Wang[2,3†], Lin He[2†], Ya-Wei Bi[2], Di Zhang[2], Xiang-Peng Zeng[2], Lei Xin[2,3], Jun Pan[2], Dan Wang[2], Jun-Tao Ji[3], Ting-Ting Du[2], Jin-Huan Lin[2], Li-Sheng Wang[4], Wen-Bin Zou[2], Hui Chen[2,3], Ting Xie[5], Hong-Lei Guo[2], Bai-Rong Li[6], Zhuan Liao[2,3], Zheng-Lei Xu[4*], Zhao-Shen Li[2,3*] and Liang-Hao Hu[2,3*]

Abstract

Background: Pediatric patients always suffer from chronic pancreatitis (CP), especially those with steatorrhea. This study aimed to identify the incidence of and risk factors for steatorrhea in pediatric CP. To our best knowledge, there is no pediatric study to document the natural history of steatorrhea in CP.

Methods: CP patients admitted to our center from January 2000 to December 2013 were enrolled. Patients were assigned to the pediatric (< 18 years old) and adult group according to their age at onset of CP. Cumulative rates of steatorrhea in both groups were calculated. Risk factors for both groups were identified, respectively.

Results: The median follow-up duration for the whole cohort was 7.6 years. In a total of 2153 patients, 13.5% of them were pediatrics. The mean age at the onset and the diagnosis of CP in pediatrics were 11.622 and 19.727, respectively. Steatorrhea was detected in 46 patients (46/291, 15.8%) in the pediatric group and in 447 patients (447/1862, 24.0%) in the adult group. Age at the onset of CP (hazard ratio [HR], 1.121), diabetes mellitus (DM, HR, 51.140), and severe acute pancreatitis (SAP, HR, 13.946) was identified risk factor for steatorrhea in the pediatric group.

Conclusions: Age at the onset of CP, DM and SAP were identified risk factors for the development of steatorrhea in pediatric CP patients. The high-risk populations were suggested to be followed up closely. They may benefit from a full adequate pancreatic exocrine replacement therapy.

Keywords: Chronic pancreatitis, Pediatric, Steatorrhea, Risk factors

Background

Chronic pancreatitis (CP) is a rare disease in children. Recent studies have estimated that the incidence of CP in children is approximately 0.5 per 100,000 per year [1–3]. The essence of this disease is the destruction of the organ's parenchyma by a progressive inflammation process [4]. Pediatric patients with CP always suffer from the severe pain and progressive loss of both exocrine and endocrine function. The irreversible damage of pancreatic exocrine function in CP patients will result in pancreatic enzyme insufficiency (PEI). Severe PEI, or pancreatic exocrine failure, is considered to be clinical steatorrhea, and is a common adverse event of CP. PEI usually manifests as malnutrition, which resulting in vitamin and micronutrient deficiency and weight loss [5, 6], and is at risk of developing premature atherosclerosis, cardiovascular events, osteoporosis, fracture, immune deficiency, and infection [7–9]. PEI is extremely harmful for children. It is well known that malnutrition caused by reduced dietary intake and malabsorption delays the growth and development of these children [10], which also seriously impairs their childhood and mental health [11].

However, in CP patients, a significant proportion of PEI did not show dominant steatorrhea. Functional testing directly for PEI is difficult in clinical practice.

* Correspondence: 78249073@qq.com; zhaoshen-li@hotmail.com; lianghao-hu@hotmail.com
†Lu Hao, Teng Wang and Lin He contributed equally to this work.
[4]Department of Gastroenterology, The Second Clinical Medical College (Shenzhen People's Hospital), Jinan University, Guangdong, China
[2]Department of Gastroenterology, Gongli Hospital, The Second Military Medical University, Shanghai, China
Full list of author information is available at the end of the article

Therefore, patients with PEI were rarely confirmed at the early stage [12]. The detection of risk factors for PEI may be clinical important for pediatrics. Pancreatic exocrine replacement therapy (PERT) was recommended in pediatric CP patients according to Australasian Pancreatic Club recommendations [13], but it has a lower level of evidence, and more clinical data was needed. To our best knowledge, there is no pediatric study to document the natural history of steatorrhea in CP. Thus, we aimed to compare the profile of pediatric and adult CP patients. This study was based on a retrospective-prospective cohort of 2153 CP patients with a long duration of follow-up after the onset of CP. We compared the natural history, etiology, complications, and treatment of CP in pediatrics and adults. We also determined the incidence of steatorrhea, and identified the risk factors for this complication in pediatric and adult CP patients, respectively.

Methods

Patients and database

The subjects of this study were CP patients hospitalized in Shanghai Changhai Hospital from January 2000 to December 2013. From January 2000 to December 2004, a retrospective collection of patient data was made according to the medical record system, telephone, mail and e-mail follow-up. In order to follow up the patients with CP and facilitate the study of CP. The database system of CP (version 2.1, YINMA Information Technology Company, Shanghai, China) has been established in the Department of Gastroenterology of Changhai Hospital since January 2005 to collect the medical records of patients with CP. Data collected from January 2005 to December 2013 were prospectively collected [12, 14–23]. All patient information is first recorded in a paper-based case report form and then entered into an electronic document. The information collected includes basic information of patients, etiological characteristics (drinking, smoking, anatomic abnormalities, family history), natural course of CP (onset date, onset symptoms, diagnosis date, onset date of pain, pain classification, diagnosis date and treatment history of stones, diabetes mellitus, fatty diarrhea, pseudocysts, common bile duct stenosis); treatment strategy (conservative treatment, endoscopic treatment, surgical treatment).

The database system will remind researchers to notify patients for examination. Except for the examination

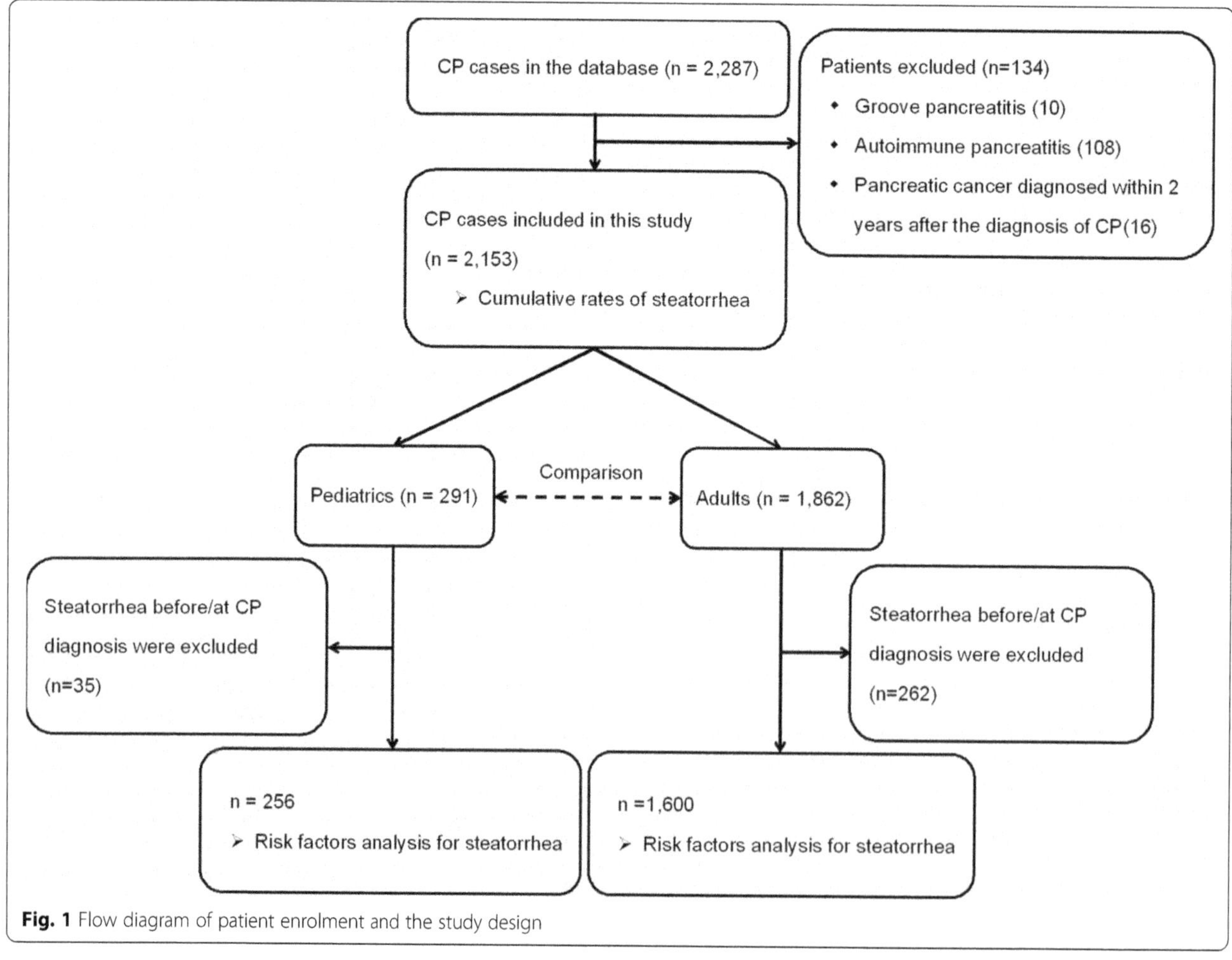

Fig. 1 Flow diagram of patient enrolment and the study design

Table 1 General Characteristics of 2153 patients with CP

Items	Overall ($n = 2153$) n (%)	Pediatrics ($n = 291$) n (%)	Adults ($n = 1862$) n (%)	*P* value
Gender (male)	1486 (69.0%)	143 (49.1%)	1343 (72.1%)	< 0.001
Age at the onset of CP, y[a]	38.230 ± 16.606	11.622 ± 4.652	42.388 ± 13.692	< 0.001
Age at the diagnosis of CP, y[a]	43.077 ± 15.548	19.727 ± 8.953	46.727 ± 12.980	< 0.001
Smoking history	723 (33.6%)	16 (5.5%)	707 (38.0%)	< 0.001
Alcohol consumption	–	–	–	< 0.001
0 g/d	1426 (66.2%)	272 (93.5%)	1154 (62.0%)	–
0-20 g/d	70 (3.3%)	8 (2.7%)	62 (3.3%)	–
20-80 g/d	237 (11.0%)	8 (2.7%)	229 (12.3%)	–
> 80 g/d	420 (19.5%)	3 (1.0%)	417 (22.4%)	–
Body mass index[a]	20.894 ± 3.354	19.380 ± 3.362	24.696 ± 88.765	0.338
Etiology	–	–	–	< 0.001
ICP	1633 (75.8%)	248 (85.2%)	1385 (74.4%)	–
ACP	404 (18.8%)	2 (0.7%)	402 (21.6%)	–
Abnormal anatomy of pancreatic duct	64 (3.0%)	24 (8.2%)	40 (2.1%)	–
HCP	30 (1.4%)	12 (4.1%)	18 (1.0%)	–
Post-traumatic CP	10 (0.5%)	3 (1.0%)	7 (0.4%)	–
Hyperlipidemic CP	12 (0.6%)	2 (0.7%)	10 (0.5%)	–
Initial manifestations	–	–	–	< 0.001
Abdominal pain	1796 (83.4%)	280 (96.2%)	1516 (81.4%)	–
Endocrine/Exocrine dysfunction	218 (10.1%)	9 (3.1%)	209 (11.2%)	–
Others	139 (6.5%)	2 (0.7%)	137 (7.4%)	–
Pancreatic stones[b]	1627 (75.6%)	269 (92.4%)	1358 (72.9%)	< 0.001
Age at pancreatic stones diagnosis	41.415 ± 15.323	20.443 ± 8.547	45.569 ± 12.746	< 0.001
Time between onset and pancreatic stone	5.762 ± 7.144	8.829 ± 9.174	5.154 ± 6.504	< 0.001
DM	616 (28.6%)	38 (13.1%)	578 (31.0%)	< 0.001
Age at DM diagnosis[a]	45.848 ± 11.812	28.578 ± 11.965	46.984 ± 10.890	< 0.001
Time between onset and DM[a]	5.136 ± 7.276	16.617 ± 13.447	4.381 ± 5.964	< 0.001
Steatorrhea	493 (22.9%)	46 (15.8%)	447 (24.0%)	0.002
Age at steatorrhea diagnosis[a]	42.563 ± 12.555	25.880 ± 9.358	44.279 ± 11.549	< 0.001
Time between onset and steatorrhea[a]	5.245 ± 8.485	13.929 ± 10.562	4.351 ± 7.719	< 0.001
Pancreatic pseudocyst	350 (16.3%)	30 (10.3%)	320 (17.2%)	0.003
Age at pancreatic pseudocyst diagnosis[a]	45.776 ± 15.077	16.232 ± 7.210	48.589 ± 12.365	< 0.001
Time between onset and pancreatic pseudocyst[a]	4.989 ± 6.954	5.640 ± 5.828	4.927 ± 7.058	0.605
Biliary stricture	340 (15.8%)	19 (6.5%)	321 (17.2%)	< 0.001
Age at biliary stricture diagnosis[a]	51.218 ± 13.169	31.548 ± 13.686	52.382 ± 12.200	< 0.001
Time between onset and biliary stricture[a]	5.592 ± 8.637	21.197 ± 17.565	4.668 ± 6.809	0.001
Pancreatic cancer	21 (1.0%)	1 (0.3%)	20 (1.1%)	0.238
Death	70 (3.3%)	2 (0.7%)	68 (3.7%)	0.008
Morphology of MPD	–	–	–	< 0.001
Pancreatic stone alone	590 (27.4%)	95 (32.6%)	495 (26.6%)	–
MPD stenosis alone	598 (27.8%)	57 (19.6%)	541 (29.1%)	–
MPD stenosis and stone	728 (33.8%)	128 (44.0%)	600 (32.2%)	–
Complex pathologic changes	237 (11.0%)	11 (3.8%)	226 (12.1%)	–

Table 1 General Characteristics of 2153 patients with CP *(Continued)*

Items	Overall ($n = 2153$) n (%)	Pediatrics ($n = 291$) n (%)	Adults ($n = 1862$) n (%)	*P* value
Type of pain	–	–	–	< 0.001
Recurrent acute pancreatitis	681 (31.6%)	102 (35.1%)	579 (31.3%)	–
Recurrent pain	638 (29.6%)	65 (22.3%)	573 (30.8%)	–
Recurrent acute pancreatitis and pain	570 (26.5%)	106 (36.4%)	464 (24.9%)	–
Chronic pain	106 (4.9%)	14 (4.8%)	92 (4.9%)	–
Without pain	158 (7.3%)	4 (1.4%)	154 (8.3%)	–
Severe acute pancreatitis	66 (3.1%)	7 (2.4%)	59 (3.2%)	0.482
Pancreatic duct successful drainage[c]	1930 (89.6%)	255 (87.6%)	1675 (90.0%)	0.216
Overall treatment	–	–	–	< 0.001
Endotherapy alone	1505 (69.9%)	247 (84.9%)	1258 (67.6%)	–
Surgery alone	244 (11.3%)	10 (3.4%)	234 (12.6%)	–
Both endotherapy and surgery	181 (8.4%)	20 (6.9%)	161 (8.6%)	–
Conservative treatment	223 (10.4%)	14 (4.8%)	209 (11.2%)	–
DM in first–/second–/third-degree relatives	135 (6.3%)	38 (13.1%)	97 (5.2%)	< 0.001
Pancreatic diseases in first–/second–/third-degree relatives (excluding hereditary CP)	37 (1.7%)	15 (5.2%)	22 (1.2%)	< 0.001

CP chronic pancreatitis, *DM* diabetes mellitus, *ICP* idiopathic chronic pancreatitis, *ACP* alcoholic chronic pancreatitis, *HCP* hereditary chronic pancreatitis, *MPD* main pancreatic duct

[a]Mean ± SD

[b]Pancreatic calcifications were also regarded as stones that are located in branch pancreatic duct or ductulus

[c]Patients with successful MPD drainage are those whose CP was established after ERCP or pancreatic surgery or those who underwent successful MPD drainage during administration when CP diagnosis was established

when patients feel unwell, all patients were checked regularly (at least once a year). Ultrasound, magnetic resonance imaging (MRI), or computed tomography (CT) examination was performed to assess the condition. Patients who did not return to our hospital were followed up by telephone and recorded in the database. The end point of the study was December 2013. In December 2013, we followed up all patients with CP in the database, with the exception of some lost visits and deaths [12]. Follow-up was defined from the onset of CP to the time of the last follow-up, death, or end of follow-up (December 2013), whichever came earliest.

The exclusion criteria for this study were as follows (Figure 1): CP patients diagnosed with pancreatic cancer within 2 years of CP diagnosis [24], grooved pancreatitis (GP) [25], and autoimmune pancreatitis (AIP). Patients were assigned into pediatric group (onset before 18 years of age) and adult group (onset after 18 years of age).

In the study of steatorrhea, patients with steatorrhea diagnosed before CP were excluded in both groups.

The CP database establishing was as mentioned in our previous study [12]. The study was approved by the Ethics Committee of Changhai Hospital. Written informed consent was obtained from all participating patients. All of the diagnostic and therapeutic modalities were carried out in accordance with the approved guidelines.

Definitions

The diagnosis of CP is based on the 2002 version of Asia Pacific consensus [26]. In the definition of etiologies, men with alcoholic intake of more than 80 g/d or women with alcoholic intake of more than 60 g/d for more than 2 years, excluding other causes, alcoholic CP could be diagnosed [27]. At least 2 first-degree relatives, or at least 3 s-degree relatives with CP and/or recurrent AP, excluding other causes, patients can be diagnosed as hereditary CP [28]. Patients with pancreatic divisum and abnormal pancreaticobiliary drainage are defined as abnormal anatomy of the pancreatic duct (although controversial) [29]. Patients with a clear history of pancreatic trauma and imaging findings suggesting secondary dilatation of the pancreatic duct may be diagnosed as traumatic CP. Hyperlipidemic CP was diagnosed in CP patients with plasma triglyceride > 1000 mg/dL [30]. When all the above causes are excluded, the patient can be diagnosed as idiopathic CP. The definition of severe acute pancreatitis (SAP) was based on the 1992 version of Atlanta classification [31].

Steatorrhea was diagnosed when one of the following two conditions was met: (1) stench, oily chronic diarrhea [32]; (2) positive result in quantification of fecal fat determination (fecal fat quantitation was performed within three days; patients with stool fat excretion over 14 g/day was diagnosed as steatorrhea).

Table 2 Predictive factors for steatorrhea development in pediatric patients after the diagnosis of CP (256 cases)

Predictors	n (%)	Univariate Analysis		Multivariate Analysis	
		P	HR (95% CI)	P	HR (95% CI)
Gender (male)	124 (48.4%)	0.411	0.353 (0.029–4.233)		
Age at the onset of CP, y[a]	11.573 ± 4.702	0.104	1.121 (0.977–1.286)	0.135	
Age at the diagnosis of CP, y[a]	18.141 ± 6.762	0.235	0.880 (0.712–1.087)		
Smoking history	14 (5.5%)	0.510	4.355 (0.055–346.356)		
Alcohol consumption		0.899			
0 g/d	241 (94.1%)	Control			
0-20 g/d	5 (2.0%)	0.447	0.036 (0.000–2.373E3)		
20-80 g/d	7 (2.7%)	0.716	0.043 (0.000–1.029E6)		
> 80 g/d	3 (1.2%)	0.735	0.042 (0.000–3.846E6)		
Body mass index[a]	19.304 ± 3.338	0.738	0.931 (0.611–1.419)		
Etiology		0.579			
ICP	220 (85.9%)	Control			
ACP	2 (0.8%)	0.710	2.081 (0.043–99.757)		
Abnormal anatomy of pancreatic duct	22 (8.6%)	0.690	2.271 (0.040–127.502)		
HCP	7 (2.7%)	0.912	1.375 (0.005–401.007)		
Post-traumatic CP	3 (1.2%)	1.000	1.008 (0.000–2.361E5)		
Hyperlipidemic CP	2 (0.8%)	0.065	208.297 (0.719–6.036E4)		
Initial manifestations		0.859			
Abdominal pain	249 (97.3%)	0.978	1.392E3 (0.000–9.416E228)		
Endocrine dysfunction	5 (2.0%)	0.972	1.175E4 (0.000–8.352E229)		
Others	2 (0.8%)				
Pancreatic stones[bc]	170 (66.4%)	0.582	1.540 (0.331–7.173)		
Biliary stricture[b]	9 (3.5%)	0.678	0.045 (0.000–1.013E5)		
DM[b]	8 (3.1%)	0.015	51.140 (2.172–1.203E3)	0.806	
Pancreatic pseudocyst[b]	26 (10.2%)	0.762	1.389 (0.165–11.705)		
Morphology of MPD		0.633			
Pancreatic stone alone	82 (32.0%)	0.329	0.082 (0.001–12.473)		
MPD stenosis alone	52 (20.3%)	0.350	0.060 (0.000–21.656)		
MPD stenosis and stone	113 (44.1%)	0.584	0.229 (0.001–44.967)		
Complex pathologic changes	9 (3.5%)	Control			
Type of pain[b]		0.845			
Recurrent acute pancreatitis	93 (36.3%)	0.571	0.218 (0.001–42.016)		
Recurrent pain	48 (18.8%)	0.950	1.167 (0.009–147.028)		
Recurrent acute pancreatitis and pain	92 (35.9%)	0.854	0.637 (0.005–78.045)		
Chronic pain	10 (3.9%)	0.670	0.123 (0.000–1.907E3)		
Without pain	13 (5.1%)	Control			
Severe acute pancreatitis[b]	7 (2.7%)	0.023	13.946 (1.442–134.909)	0.023	13.946 (1.442–134.909)
Pancreatic duct successful drainage[bd]	29 (11.3%)	0.904	0.774 (0.012–50.413)		
Treatment strategy		0.873			

Table 2 Predictive factors for steatorrhea development in pediatric patients after the diagnosis of CP (256 cases) *(Continued)*

Predictors	n (%)	Univariate Analysis		Multivariate Analysis	
		P	HR (95% CI)	P	HR (95% CI)
Endotherapy alone	44 (17.2%)	0.876	0.739 (0.017–32.985)		
Surgery alone	11 (4.3%)	0.621	0.231 (0.001–76.658)		
Both endotherapy and surgery	0	0.904	0.774 (0.012–51.413)		
Conservative treatment	201 (78.5%)	Control			
DM in first–/second–/third-degree relatives	29 (11.3%)	0.489	0.042 (0.000–327.986)		
Pancreatic diseases in first–/second–/third-degree relatives (excluding hereditary CP)	12 (4.7%)	0.572	0.278 (0.003–23.531)		

CP chronic pancreatitis, *DM* diabetes mellitus, *ICP* idiopathic chronic pancreatitis, *ACP* alcoholic chronic pancreatitis, *HCP* hereditary chronic pancreatitis, *MPD* main pancreatic duct, *HR* hazard ratio, *CI* confidence interval

[a]Mean ± SD

[b]Before or at the diagnosis of CP

[c]Pancreatic calcifications were also regarded as stones that are located in branch pancreatic duct or ductulus

[d]Patients with successful MPD drainage are those whose CP was established after ERCP or pancreatic surgery or those who underwent successful MPD drainage during administration when CP diagnosis was established

Treatment strategy

Endoscopic interventional therapy was the first choice for CP patients. Extracorporeal shock wave lithotripsy (ESWL) and endoscopic retrograde cholangiopancreatography (ERCP) were used to remove pancreatic duct stones and drain the main pancreatic duct successfully [15, 33–36]. The indications of surgery in CP patients include: endoscopic interventional therapy can not treat symptoms, combined with CBD stenosis but endoscopic treatment failed, cannot exclude malignant lesions or malignant diagnosed through biopsy, complex conditions and so on [37]. Surgical methods include surgical drainage, pancreaticoduodenectomy and distal pancreatectomy. In painless CP patients, endoscopic intervention or surgical treatment is indicated in patients with CBD stenosis or pancreatic portal hypertension [38].

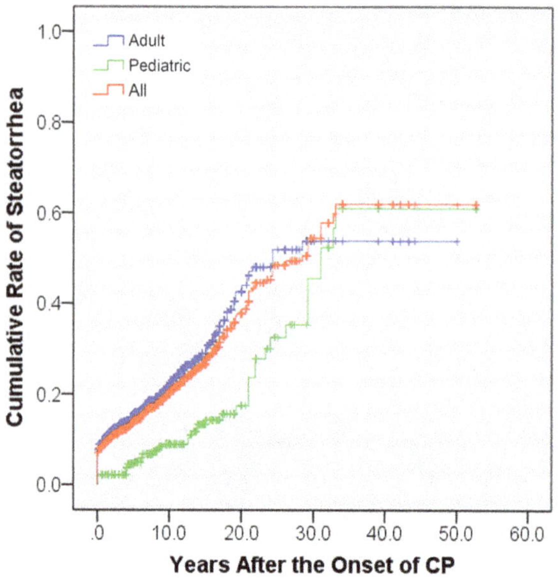

Fig. 2 The cumulative rates of steatorrhea after the onset of CP

Indications for endoscopic or surgical treatment did not include simple DM or steatorrhea. The treatment strategies of CP patients were as mentioned in our previous study [12].

Statistical analysis

In this study, continuous variables are represented in the form of mean ± standard deviation (SD) and compared with an unpaired, 2-tailed t test or the Mann-Whitney test. Categorical variables were expressed in the form of counting (percentage) and χ^2 test or the Fisher exact test were used to compare. CP patients who onset before 18 years of age were assigned into pediatric group and after 18 years of age were assigned into adult groups. The cumulative rates of steatorrhea in both groups after the onset of CP were calculated by Kaplan-Meier method [39]. The statistical analysis were as mentioned in our previous study [12].

Patients who had steatorrhea at/before the diagnosis of CP in pediatric and adult groups were excluded respectively. SPSS (version 21.0) was used to calculate the significance of each variable by multivariate Cox regression analysis in both groups.

Results

General characteristics of the subjects

As shown in Figure 1, from January 2000 to December 2013, a total of 2287 CP patients were entered into the Changhai CP Database. After the exclusion of 134 patients, including 10 patients diagnosed with GP, 108 patients diagnosed with AIP, and 16 patients diagnosed with pancreatic cancer within 2 years after the diagnosis of CP, a cohort of 2153 patients with CP was established. The median duration of follow-up was 7.6 years (range 0.0–52.7 years), with 10.4 years (range 0.0–52.7 years) in the pediatrics and 7.0 years (range 0.0–50.0 years) in the adults.

Table 3 Predictive factors for steatorrhea development in adult patients after the diagnosis of CP (1600 cases)

Predictors	n (%)	Univariate Analysis		Multivariate Analysis	
		P	HR (95%CI)	P	HR (95%CI)
Gender (male)	1161 (72.6%)	< 0.001	2.502 (1.639–3.820)	< 0.001	2.694 (1.756–4.133)
Age at the onset of CP, y[a]	42.777 ± 13.997	0.429	0.996 (0.984–1.007)		
Age at the diagnosis of CP, y[a]	46.798 ± 13.333	< 0.001	0.972 (0.961–0.984)	< 0.001	0.966 (0.953–0.978)
Smoking history	608 (38.0%)	0.188	1.222 (0.907–1.645)		
Alcohol consumption		0.098			
0 g/d	1000 (62.5%)	Control			
0-20 g/d	49 (3.1%)	0.481	0.661 (0.209–2.089)		
20-80 g/d	202 (12.6%)	0.129	1.386 (0.909–2.144)		
> 80 g/d	349 (21.8%)	0.036	1.437 (1.024–2.016)		
Body mass index[a]	25.316 ± 96.332	0.882	0.996 (0.942–1.052)		
Etiology		0.018		0.143	
ICP	1207 (75.4%)	Control		Control	
ACP	338 (21.1%)	0.037	1.414 (1.021–1.956)	0.219	
Abnormal anatomy of pancreatic duct	30 (1.9%)	0.373	0.530 (0.131–2.146)	0.658	
HCP	11 (0.7%)	0.962	0.000 (0.000–3.933E182)	0.345	
Post-traumatic CP	7 (0.4%)	0.003	8.514 (2.088–34.720)	0.041	
Hyperlipidemic CP	7 (0.4%)	0.952	0.000 (0.000–1.191E142)	0.178	
Initial manifestations		< 0.001		< 0.001	
Abdominal pain	1371 (85.7%)	< 0.001	0.401 (0.253–0.636)	< 0.001	0.308 (0.192–0.494)
Endocrine dysfunction	104 (6.5%)	0.130	0.604 (0.315–1.160)	0.059	0.491 (0.235–1.027)
Others	125 (7.8%)	Control		Control	
Pancreatic stones[bc]	1114 (69.6%)	0.830	0.966 (0.701–1.330)		
Biliary stricture[b]	124 (7.8%)	0.097	1.512 (0.928–2.463)		
DM[b]	265 (16.6%)	0.031	1.450 (1.034–2.035)	0.029	1.558 (1.047–2.319)
Pancreatic pseudocyst[b]	123 (7.7%)	0.355	1.284 (0.756–2.180)		
Morphology of MPD		0.063			
Pancreatic stone alone	394 (24.6%)	0.047	1.837 (1.009–3.343)		
MPD stenosis alone	495 (30.9%)	0.016	2.033 (1.144–3.613)		
MPD stenosis and stone	506 (31.6%)	0.194	1.483 (0.818–2.687)		
Complex pathologic changes	205 (12.8%)	Control			
Type of pain[b]		0.086			
Recurrent acute pancreatitis	472 (29.5%)	0.007	0.534 (0.339–0.843)		
Recurrent pain	438 (27.4%)	0.048	0.636 (0.406–0.996)		
Recurrent acute pancreatitis and pain	388 (24.3%)	0.021	0.578 (0.364–0.919)		
Chronic pain	62 (3.9%)	0.206	0.543 (0.211–1.398)		
Without pain	240 (15.0%)	Control			
Severe acute pancreatitis[b]	50 (3.1%)	0.061	0.153 (0.021–1.091)		
Pancreatic duct successful drainage[bd]	223 (13.9%)	0.987	1.004 (0.648–1.555)		
Treatment strategy		0.698			
Endotherapy alone	120 (7.5%)	0.657	0.871 (0.472–1.607)		
Surgery alone	87 (5.4%)	0.282	1.400 (0.758–2.585)		
Both endotherapy and surgery	14 (0.9%)	0.951	0.000 (0.000–3.013E148)		
Conservative treatment	1379 (86.2%)	Control			

Table 3 Predictive factors for steatorrhea development in adult patients after the diagnosis of CP (1600 cases) *(Continued)*

Predictors	n (%)	Univariate Analysis		Multivariate Analysis	
		P	HR (95%CI)	P	HR (95%CI)
DM in first–/second–/third-degree relatives	76 (4.8%)	0.241	0.587 (0.241–1.429)		
Pancreatic diseases in first–/second–/third-degree relatives (excluding hereditary CP)	16 (1.0%)	0.691	0.671 (0.094–4.793)		

CP chronic pancreatitis, *DM* diabetes mellitus, *ICP* idiopathic chronic pancreatitis, *ACP* alcoholic chronic pancreatitis, *HCP* hereditary chronic pancreatitis, *MPD* main pancreatic duct, *HR* hazard ratio, *CI* confidence interval
[a]Mean ± SD
[b]Before or at the diagnosis of CP
[c]Pancreatic calcifications were also regarded as stones that are located in branch pancreatic duct or ductulus
[d]Patients with successful MPD drainage are those whose CP was established after ERCP or pancreatic surgery or those who underwent successful MPD drainage during administration when CP diagnosis was established

The general characteristics of the patients with CP are presented in Table 1. The mean age at the onset and the diagnosis of CP were 11.622 and 19.727, respectively. The male-to-female ratio in pediatrics was approximately 1:1, while in adults was 3:1. Patients with smoking or drinking history were significantly less in pediatrics (both $P < 0.001$). DM, steatorrhea, pancreatic pseudocyst, and biliary stricture were significantly common in adults (all $P < 0.05$). The etiology and type of pain were also significantly different between the pediatric and the adult groups (both $P < 0.001$).

Cumulative rates of steatorrhea

Steatorrhea was found in 22.9% (493/2153) of patients after the onset of CP. The proportions were 15.8% (46/291) in pediatric patients and 24.0% (447/1862) in adult patients. The cumulative proportions of steatorrhea in pediatric patients were 2.1% (95% confidence interval [CI], 0.5–3.7%), 4.1% (95% CI, 1.6–6.6%) and 7.2% (95% CI, 3.5%-10.9) at 3, 5 and 10 years after the diagnosis of CP, respectively. The cumulative proportions of steatorrhea in adult patients were 12.8% (95% CI, 11.2–14.4%), 14.6% (95% CI, 12.8–16.4%) and 18.3% (95% CI, 16.1–20.5%) at 3, 5 and 10 years after the diagnosis of CP, respectively. Pediatric and adult patients showed significant difference in the rate of steatorrhea ($P = 0.002$, Figure 2).

Predictors for steatorrhea development in pediatric patients

After the exclusion of 35 patients diagnosed with steatorrhea before the diagnosis of CP in the pediatric patients, a total of 256 patients with CP were finally enrolled in the pediatric group. A univariate analysis for steatorrhea development among the 256 pediatric patients included in the study is shown in Table 2. Three variables showed a P value of less than 0.15: age at the onset of CP, DM, and SAP.

For the multivariate analysis, the 3 predictors above were included in the Cox proportional hazards regression model. Finally, 1 predictor for steatorrhea development in pediatric patients was identified. The risk of developing steatorrhea was significantly higher in pediatric patients with a history of SAP before the diagnosis of CP (Hazard ratio [HR], 13.946, 95% CI, 1.442–134.909).

Predictors for steatorrhea development in adult patients

After the exclusion of 262 patients diagnosed with steatorrhea before the diagnosis of CP in the adult patients, a total of 1600 patients with CP were finally enrolled in the adult group. A univariate analysis for steatorrhea development among the 1600 adult patients included in the study is shown in Table 3. Five variables showed a P value of less than 0.05: gender, age at the diagnosis of CP, etiology, initial manifestations, and DM.

For the multivariate analysis, the 5 predictors above were included in the Cox proportional hazards regression model. Finally, 4 predictors for steatorrhea development in adult patients were identified. The risk of developing steatorrhea was significantly higher in male patients (HR, 2.694, 95% CI, 1.756–4.133) and patients with a history of DM before the diagnosis of CP (HR, 1.558, 95% CI, 1.047–2.319). Adult patients with an older age at the diagnosis of CP (HR, 0.966, 95% CI, 0.953–0.978) were associated with decreased risk of developing steatorrhea. Initial manifestations were also identified risk factors for steatorrhea development in adult patients.

Discussion

We focused on CP in pediatrics in the present study. Presence of steatorrhea was set as the sign of severe PEI. To our knowledge, this is the first study to analyze the risk factors of steatorrhea in pediatric patients with CP.

In the present study, 15.8% (46/291) of pediatric patients with CP developed steatorrhea, and 24.0% (447/1862) of adult patients developed steatorrhea. A previous study showed that exocrine and endocrine insufficiency developed more slowly in early-onset CP than in late-onset CP [40]. This could be due to a better preservation of pancreatic function and better repair capacity after injury in pediatric CP patients. However, after a long term of follow-up for more than 30 years, the cumulative rate of steatorrhea in pediatrics was similar or even higher than in adults (Figure 2). Therefore, pediatric CP patients had a reduced risk of steatorrhea compared to adult CP patients in the early period of CP course, but the risk increased with longer-term of follow-up.

In the risk factor analysis, a history of SAP before the diagnosis of CP was identified significantly associated with steatorrhea development in pediatric CP patients. It is not exactly the same as risk factors in adult patients. In adult CP patients, genders, age at the diagnosis of CP, initial manifestations, and DM before the diagnosis of CP were identified risk factors for steatorrhea development. In the previous study, male gender, adults, DM, alcohol abuse and pancreaticoduodenectomy were identified risk factors for steatorrhea development in the general population [12], which are similar with the adult group in the present study.

The risk factor analysis of steatorrhea may help in the early diagnosis of PEI in pediatric patients. Pediatric CP patients with PEI suffer from decreased dietary intake and malabsorption. The malnutrition caused by PEI may retard their growth and development, even result in failure to thrive in these children. This may cause incredible suffering for the children and families who live with them [41]. However, steatorrhea and associated symptoms are not evident until duodenal lipase falls below 5–10% of normal postprandial levels [42]. Thus, PEI may have occurred even the children have no symptoms of steatorrhea. This study provided a relatively accurate risk factor analysis. Age at the onset of CP, DM and SAP were identified the risk factors for steatorrhea in pediatric CP patients. Therefore, these pediatric patient groups were suggested to be closely monitored.

These high-risk populations in pediatric CP patients may benefit from a full adequate PERT. Although PERT was recommended in all pediatric CP patients [13], closely follow-up and dosage adjustment was quite important for these high-risk populations. It can deliver sufficient enzymatic activity into the duodenal lumen simultaneously with the meal, in order to optimize digestion and absorption of nutrients. The PERT will improve the nutritional status for these children and help with their growth and development. This may help in the early treatment of PEI in pediatric patients and reduce the adverse events caused by PEI.

Our study has some limitations. First, clinical steatorrhea was a sign of severe PEI, regardless of dietary habits and steatorrhea associated with abdominal diseases. Second, data was retrospectively collected from 2000 to 2004, which may introduce a recall bias. However, statistical analysis showed that there was no significant difference in clinical characteristics between patients before and after January 2005. In this sense, the recall bias has the least impact on the results. Third, risk factors analysis did not include all potential factors associated with the development of steatorrhea. Fourth, 603 patients with CP were followed up for less than 2 years, which may introduce a misdiagnosis bias between CP and pancreatic cancer.

Conclusions

In conclusion, steatorrhea is extremely harmful for children. Age at the onset of CP. DM and SAP were identified risk factors for the development of steatorrhea in pediatric CP patients. Therefore, it is suggested that pediatric patients in these high-risk groups be closely followed and examined. They may benefit from adequate PERT.

Abbreviations

AIP: Autoimmune pancreatitis; CI: Confidence interval; CP: Chronic pancreatitis; CT: Computed tomography; DM: Diabetes mellitus; ERCP: Endoscopic retrograde cholangiopancreatography; ESWL: Extracorporeal shockwave lithotripsy; GP: Groove pancreatitis; HR: Hazard ratio; MRI: Magnetic resonance imaging; PEI: Pancreatic enzyme insufficiency; PERT: Pancreatic exocrine replacement therapy; SAP: Severe acute pancreatitis; SD: Standard deviation

Acknowledgements

Not applicable.

Authors' contributors

L Hao, TW and L He participated in the acquisition, analysis, and interpretation of data, as well as in the manuscript drafting. YWB, DZ, XPZ, LX, JP, DW, JTJ, TTD, JHL, LSW, WBZ, HC, TX, HLG, BRL and ZL participated in data acquisition and manuscript drafting. LHH, ZSL and ZLX contributed to the conception, design, and data interpretation, as well as revised the manuscript for important intellectual content. BRL, LHH, LX, and LSW provided the funding to this study. All authors read and approved the final manuscript. All authors have read and approved the manuscript, and ensure that this is the case.

Funding

This study was supported by the National Natural Science Foundation of China [Grant Nos. 81500490 (BRL), 81770635 (LHH), 81470883 (LHH) and 81770632(LX)] and Three engineering training funds in Shenzhen [Grant No. SYJY201713(LSW)] in data acquisition and manuscript drafting, Shanghai Rising-Star Program [Grant No. 17QA1405500 (LHH)], Shanghai Outstanding Youth Doctor Training Program [Grant No. AB83030002015034 (LHH)], and Shanghai Youth Top-notch Talent Program [Grant No. HZW2016FZ67 (LHH)], in conception design, data interpretation, and manuscript revise.

Consent for publication

Not applicable.

Competing interests
The authors declare that they have no competing interests.

Author details
[1]Department of Gastroenterology, Hainan Branch of Chinese PLA General Hospital, Hainan, China. [2]Department of Gastroenterology, Gongli Hospital, The Second Military Medical University, Shanghai, China. [3]Department of Gastroenterology, Changhai Hospital, The Second Military Medical University, Shanghai, China. [4]Department of Gastroenterology, The Second Clinical Medical College (Shenzhen People's Hospital), Jinan University, Guangdong, China. [5]Department of Gastroenterology, Zhongda Hospital, Southeast University, Nanjing, China. [6]Department of Gastroenterology, Air Force General Hospital, Beijing, China.

References

1. Yadav D, Timmons L, Benson JT, Dierkhising RA, Chari ST. Incidence, prevalence, and survival of chronic pancreatitis: a population-based study. Am J Gastroenterol. 2011;106:2192–9.
2. Spanier B, Bruno MJ, Dijkgraaf MG. Incidence and mortality of acute and chronic pancreatitis in the Netherlands: a nationwide record-linked cohort study for the years 1995-2005. World J Gastroenterol. 2013;19:3018–26.
3. Hirota M, Shimosegawa T, Masamune A, Kikuta K, Kume K, Hamada S, Kihara Y, Satoh A, Kimura K, Tsuji I, Kuriyama S. The sixth nationwide epidemiological survey of chronic pancreatitis in Japan. Pancreatology. 2012;12:79–84.
4. Braganza JM, Lee SH, McCloy RF, McMahon MJ. Chronic pancreatitis. Lancet. 2011;377:1184–97.
5. Dominguez-Munoz JE, Iglesias-Garcia J, Vilarino-Insua M, Iglesias-Rey M. 13C-mixed triglyceride breath test to assess oral enzyme substitution therapy in patients with chronic pancreatitis. Clin Gastroenterol Hepatol. 2007;5:484–8.
6. Dominguez-Munoz JE, Iglesias-Garcia J. Oral pancreatic enzyme substitution therapy in chronic pancreatitis: is clinical response an appropriate marker for evaluation of therapeutic efficacy? JOP. 2010;11:158–62.
7. Pongprasobchai S. Maldigestion from pancreatic exocrine insufficiency. J Gastroenterol Hepatol. 2013;28(Suppl 4):99–102.
8. Montalto G, Soresi M, Carroccio A, Scafidi E, Barbagallo CM, Ippolito S, Notarbartolo A. Lipoproteins and chronic pancreatitis. Pancreas. 1994;9:137–8.
9. Tignor AS, Wu BU, Whitlock TL, Lopez R, Repas K, Banks PA, Conwell D. High prevalence of low-trauma fracture in chronic pancreatitis. Am J Gastroenterol. 2010;105:2680–6.
10. Wang D, Bi Y-W, Ji J-T, Xin L, Pan J, Liao Z, Du T-T, Lin J-H, Zhang D, Zeng X-P, et al. Extracorporeal shock wave lithotripsy is safe and effective for pediatric patients with chronic pancreatitis. Endoscopy. 2017;49:447–55.
11. Schwarzenberg SJ, Bellin M, Husain SZ, Ahuja M, Barth B, Davis H, Durie PR, Fishman DS, Freedman SD, Gariepy CE, et al. Pediatric chronic pancreatitis is associated with genetic risk factors and substantial disease burden. J Pediatr. 2015;166:890–6 e891.
12. Li BR, Pan J, Du TT, Liao Z, Ye B, Zou WB, Chen H, Ji JT, Zheng ZH, Wang D, et al. Risk factors for steatorrhea in chronic pancreatitis: a cohort of 2,153 patients. Sci Rep. 2016;6:21381.
13. Toouli J, Biankin AV, Oliver MR, Pearce CB, Wilson JS, Wray NH, Australasian Pancreatic C. Management of pancreatic exocrine insufficiency: Australasian pancreatic Club recommendations. Med J Aust. 2010;193:461–7.
14. Wang W, Liao Z, Li ZS, Shi XG, Wang LW, Liu F, Wu RP, Zheng JM. Chronic pancreatitis in Chinese children: etiology, clinical presentation and imaging diagnosis. J Gastroenterol Hepatol. 2009;24:1862–8.
15. Li ZS, Wang W, Liao Z, Zou DW, Jin ZD, Chen J, Wu RP, Liu F, Wang LW, Shi XG, et al. A long-term follow-up study on endoscopic management of children and adolescents with chronic pancreatitis. Am J Gastroenterol. 2010;105:1884–92.
16. Wang W, Liao Z, Li G, Li ZS, Chen J, Zhan XB, Wang LW, Liu F, Hu LH, Guo Y, et al. Incidence of pancreatic cancer in chinese patients with chronic pancreatitis. Pancreatology. 2011;11:16–23.
17. Wang W, Guo Y, Liao Z, Zou DW, Jin ZD, Zou DJ, Jin G, Hu XG, Li ZS. Occurrence of and risk factors for diabetes mellitus in Chinese patients with chronic pancreatitis. Pancreas. 2011;40:206–12.
18. Xin L, He YX, Zhu XF, Zhang QH, Hu LH, Zou DW, Jin ZD, Chang XJ, Zheng JM, Zuo CJ, et al. Diagnosis and treatment of autoimmune pancreatitis: experience with 100 patients. Hepatobiliary Pancreat Dis Int. 2014;13:642–8.
19. Pan J, Xin L, Wang D, Liao Z, Lin JH, Li BR, Du TT, Ye B, Zou WB, Chen H, et al. Risk factors for diabetes mellitus in chronic pancreatitis: a cohort of 2011 patients. Medicine (Baltimore). 2016;95:e3251.
20. Yang YG, Hu LH, Chen H, Li B, Fan XH, Li JB, Wang JF, Deng XM. Target-controlled infusion of remifentanil with or without flurbiprofen axetil in sedation for extracorporeal shock wave lithotripsy of pancreatic stones: a prospective, open-label, randomized controlled trial. BMC Anesthesiol. 2015;15:161.
21. Hao L, Pan J, Wang D, Bi YW, Ji JT, Xin L, Liao Z, Du TT, Lin JH, Zhang D, et al. Risk factors and nomogram for pancreatic pseudocysts in chronic pancreatitis: a cohort of 1998 patients. J Gastroenterol Hepatol. 2017;32:1403–11.
22. Hao L, Bi YW, Zhang D, Zeng XP, Xin L, Pan J, Wang D, Ji JT, Du TT,Lin JH, et al. Risk factors and nomogram for common bile duct stricture inchronic pancreatitis: a cohort of 2153 patients. J ClinGastroenterol. 2017. https://doi.org/10.1097/MCG.0000000000000930.
23. Hao L, Zeng XP, Xin L, Wang D, Pan J, Bi YW, Ji JT, Du TT, Lin JH, Zhang D, et al. Incidence of and risk factors for pancreatic cancer in chronic pancreatitis: a cohort of 1656 patients. Dig Liver Dis. 2017;49(11):1249–56.
24. Li BR, Hu LH, Li ZS. Chronic pancreatitis and pancreatic cancer. Gastroenterology. 2014;147:541–2.
25. Malde DJ, Oliveira-Cunha M, Smith AM. Pancreatic carcinoma masquerading as groove pancreatitis: case report and review of literature. Jop. 2011;12: 598–602.
26. Tandon RK, Sato N, Garg PK. Chronic pancreatitis: Asia-Pacific consensus report. J Gastroenterol Hepatol. 2002;17:508–18.
27. Witt H, Sahin-Toth M, Landt O, Chen JM, Kahne T, Drenth JP, Kukor Z, Szepessy E, Halangk W, Dahm S, et al. A degradation-sensitive anionic trypsinogen (PRSS2) variant protects against chronic pancreatitis. Nat Genet. 2006;38:668–73.
28. Howes N, Lerch MM, Greenhalf W, Stocken DD, Ellis I, Simon P, Truninger K, Ammann R, Cavallini G, Charnley RM, et al. Clinical and genetic characteristics of hereditary pancreatitis in Europe. Clin Gastroenterol Hepatol. 2004;2:252–61.
29. Lu WF. ERCP and CT diagnosis of pancreas divisum and its relation to etiology of chronic pancreatitis. World J Gastroenterol. 1998;4:150–2.
30. Yadav D, Pitchumoni CS. Issues in hyperlipidemic pancreatitis. J Clin Gastroenterol. 2003;36:54–62.
31. Bradley EL, 3rd: A clinically based classification system for acute pancreatitis. Summary of the international symposium on acute pancreatitis, Atlanta, Ga, September 11 through 13, 1992. Arch Surg 1993, 128:586–590.
32. Affronti J. Chronic pancreatitis and exocrine insufficiency. Prim Care. 2011; 38:515–37 ix.
33. Li BR, Liao Z, Du TT, Ye B, Zou WB, Chen H, Ji JT, Zheng ZH, Hao JF, Jiang YY, et al. Risk factors for complications of pancreatic extracorporeal shock wave lithotripsy. Endoscopy. 2014;46:1092–100.
34. Sun XT, Hu LH, Xia T, Shi LL, Sun C, Du YQ, Wang W, Chen JM, Liao Z, Li ZS. Clinical features and endoscopic treatment of Chinese patients with hereditary pancreatitis. Pancreas. 2015;44:59–63.
35. Dumonceau JM, Delhaye M, Tringali A, Dominguez-Munoz JE, Poley JW, Arvanitaki M, Costamagna G, Costea F, Deviere J, Eisendrath P, et al. Endoscopic treatment of chronic pancreatitis: European Society of Gastrointestinal Endoscopy (ESGE) clinical guideline. Endoscopy. 2012;44:784–800.
36. Li BR, Liao Z, Du TT, Ye B, Chen H, Ji JT, Zheng ZH, Hao JF, Ning SB, Wang D, et al. Extracorporeal shock wave lithotripsy is a safe and effective treatment for pancreatic stones coexisting with pancreatic pseudocysts. Gastrointest Endosc. 2016;84:69–78.
37. Schreyer AG, Jung M, Riemann JF, Niessen C, Pregler B, Grenacher L, Hoffmeister A. S3 guideline for chronic pancreatitis - diagnosis, classification and therapy for the radiologist. Rofo. 2014;186:1002–8.
38. Ito T, Ishiguro H, Ohara H, Kamisawa T, Sakagami J, Sata N, Takeyama Y, Hirota M, Miyakawa H, Igarashi H, et al. Evidence-based clinical practice guidelines for chronic pancreatitis 2015. J Gastroenterol. 2016;51:85–92.
39. Ma Y, Zhou W, He S, Xu W, Xiao J. Tyrosine kinase inhibitor sunitinib therapy is effective in the treatment of bone metastasis from cancer of unknown primary: identification of clinical and immunohistochemical biomarkers predicting survival. Int J Cancer. 2016;139:1423–30.
40. Layer P, Yamamoto H, Kalthoff L, Clain JE, Bakken LJ, DiMagno EP. The different courses of early- and late-onset idiopathic and alcoholic chronic pancreatitis. Gastroenterology. 1994;107:1481–7.

19

Prognostic value of progesterone receptor in solid pseudopapillary neoplasm of the pancreas: evaluation of a pooled case series

Feiyang Wang[1,2†], Zibo Meng[2†], Shoukang Li[3], Yushun Zhang[2] and Heshui Wu[2*]

Abstract

Background: The role of progesterone receptor (PR) has been reported in a series of pancreatic cysts. However, the relationship between PR and prognosis of solid pseudopapillary neoplasm of the pancreas (SPNP) has not been elucidated so far. The aim of our study was to evaluate the prognostic value of PR in SPNP.

Methods: A total of 76 patients with SPNP treated in our institution from January 2012 to December 2017 were included. Demographic parameters, laboratory data, pathologic information and clinical outcomes were analyzed by the use of survival analysis. In addition, a pooled case series was performed to evaluate the results.

Results: The institutional data included 76 patients (17 male and 59 female) ranging from 8 to 90 years (median, 30 years) in age. Kaplan-Meier survival analysis confirmed negative PR result was significantly associated with poorer disease-free survival (DFS) and disease-specific survival (DSS) (both $P < 0.001$). In the pooled analysis, a total of 62 studies comprising 214 patients with SPNP were included. After multivariable cox analysis, negative PR result remained an independent prognostic factor for SPNP (DFS HR: 14.50, 95% CI: 1.98–106.05, $P = 0.008$; DSS HR: 9.15, 95% CI: 1.89–44.17, $P = 0.006$).

Conclusion: Our results indicated the role of PR in predicting adverse outcome of patients with SPNP and negative PR result may serve as a potential prognostic factor.

Keywords: Progesterone receptor, Solid pseudopapillary tumor, Pancreas, Prognosis

Background

Solid pseudopapillary neoplasm of the pancreas (SPNP), also called Frantz's tumor, was first described in 1959 [1]. It is a rare pancreatic neoplasm of uncertain lineage, relatively indolent and female predominant, accounting for 1–2% of exocrine pancreatic neoplasms and 5% of cystic pancreatic tumors [2–4]. The World Health Organization currently classifies SPNP as low grade pancreatic malignancy, so excellent survival result is achieved after aggressive surgical resection [5]. The overall survival rate after 5 years surgical resection is about 95–98% [3, 6]. Solid pseudopapillary neoplasm of the pancreas usually show benign in nature, but approximately 10–15% of SPNP demonstrate malignant behavior with adjacent organ invasion, recurrence and metastasis [7, 8]. Albeit with low malignant potential of SPNP, surgical resection is first choice to ensure long term survival even in cases where metastasectomy is required [9, 10].

Owing to the favorable prognosis of SPNP, including the presence of local recurrence and metastasis, predictive factors of survival are difficult to identify. Research have shown the correlation between large tumor size, male sex and younger age with poor prognosis in SPNP [11–14]. While other studies failed to confirm these results [12, 15, 16]. Immunohistochemistry is a common method to diagnosis SPNP in pathology, and some of

* Correspondence: heshuiwu@hust.edu.cn
†Feiyang Wang and Zibo Meng contributed equally to this work.
[2]Department of Pancreatic Surgery, Union Hospital, Tongji Medical College, Huazhong University of Science and Technology, Wuhan 430022, China
Full list of author information is available at the end of the article

these parameters are speculated to be the indicators of poor prognosis in different pancreatic cysts. Report found high Ki-67 immunoreactivity, a proliferative index, was related to the recurrence and metastasis of SPNP [17]. The loss of progesterone receptor (PR) expression was also observed in pancreatic neuroendocrine tumor (PanNET) patients with shorter survival time [18]. The role of sex hormone in the origin of SPNP is still enigma, although SPNP always show a tendency to affect young women and positive PR expression [19, 20]. Whilst, more recent studies have not elaborated the effect of PR expression in SPNP prognosis predicting like in PanNET. The aim of this study was to elucidate the prognostic value of PR in SPNP compared with clinicopathological features and immunohistochemistry index such as Ki-67. We also present a pooled case series of published literature for SPNP.

Methods

Patients and data collection

We retrospectively analyzed the data from 76 patients admitted in Pancreas Surgery Department of Wuhan Union hospital with pathologically confirmed SPNP from January 2012 to December 2017. All these patients received surgical resection in our hospital. Data collected included patient demographic characteristics, imaging and laboratory data, operative method and pathology through patients' electronic medical records and paper charts. Patient outcomes were obtained from outpatient records and telephone interview. Patients status were classified as disease free, alive with disease or died of disease and endpoint of follow up was February 28, 2018.

Pathologic immunohistochemistry for PR

Formalin fixed, paraffin wax embedded tissues were cut into 4 μm sections and mounted on glucose coated slides. Then slides were incubated with mouse anti-human monoclonal PR antibody (1:50, DAKO, Denmark) according to the manufacturer's guidelines. Two pathologists examined the pathologic slides blinded to the clinical data. The interpretation of PR reactivity was performed as either negative or positive according to the criteria of Reiner et al [21].

Review of literature

Literature search of PubMed was performed for all articles in English published from 1998 through 2017, using the following Medical Subject Heading (MeSH): Frantz tumor, Solid pseudopapillary tumor, Solid pseudopapillary neoplasm, Pancreas, Pancreatic, Prognosis, Survival and Outcome.

Inclusion criteria included original articles, case series and case reports of patients with pathologically confirmed SPNP. Exclusion criteria included reviews, abstracts and studies with limited data such as loss of follow up information. As a result, 62 studies and 214 patients were included. Forty of publications were case reports, and the remaining twenty-two were case series. Schematic diagram regarding selection of studies and patient data was in the Fig. 1. Whenever available, patient data containing demographics, pathology, immunohistochemical results and clinical outcome were extracted. If relevant data were lack in studies, additional information were sought from the corresponding authors. However, only 24 patients with PR result had follow up information, which showed that clinicians did not attach attention to this marker in predicting survival for SPNP.

Statistical analysis

Statistical Production and Services Solution 19.0 (SPSS 19.0, SPSS) and GraphPad Prism 7 were used in statistical analysis. Continuous data and categorical variables were presented as mean ± standard derivation (SD) and frequency respectively. Categorical variables comparison was performed using chi-square or Fisher exact test and continuous variables were compared by using of Student's t test. For variables nonparametrically distributed, the Mann Whitney U test was used for comparison. All variables with statistically significant prognostic value in univariable were selected for further multivariable analysis. A COX regression model was used in multivariable analysis. Hazard ratios (HR) and 95% confidence intervals (95% CIs) were presented. Receiver operating characteristic (ROC) curve was performed to determine the optimal discriminator values for continuous variables such as age and tumor size. The optimal cut-off values were determined by Youden index. Evaluation of disease-free survival (DFS) and disease-specific survival (DSS) were obtained by Kaplan-Meier method. P value< 0.05 showed a statistically difference.

Results

Clinicopathological features of SPNP patients in our cohort

A total of 76 patients with surgical resection in Wuhan Union Hospital and confirmed with SPNP in pathology from January 2012 to December 2017 were included in this study. The clinicopathologic characteristics of 76 patients were presented in Table 1. There were 17 male (22.4%) and 59 female (77.6%), with a median age of 30 years (range, 8–90 years). Forty tumors (52.6%) located in head/neck of the pancreas, and thirty-six tumors (47.4%) located in body/tail. The most common symptom was asymptomatic (47.4%), with tumors occasionally found through physical examination, followed by abdominal pain (38.2%) and mass (6.6%). All tumors were resected, including twenty-three pancreaticoduodenectomy (30.7%), seven duodenum preserving pancreatic head resection (9.3%), thirty distal pancreatectomy with

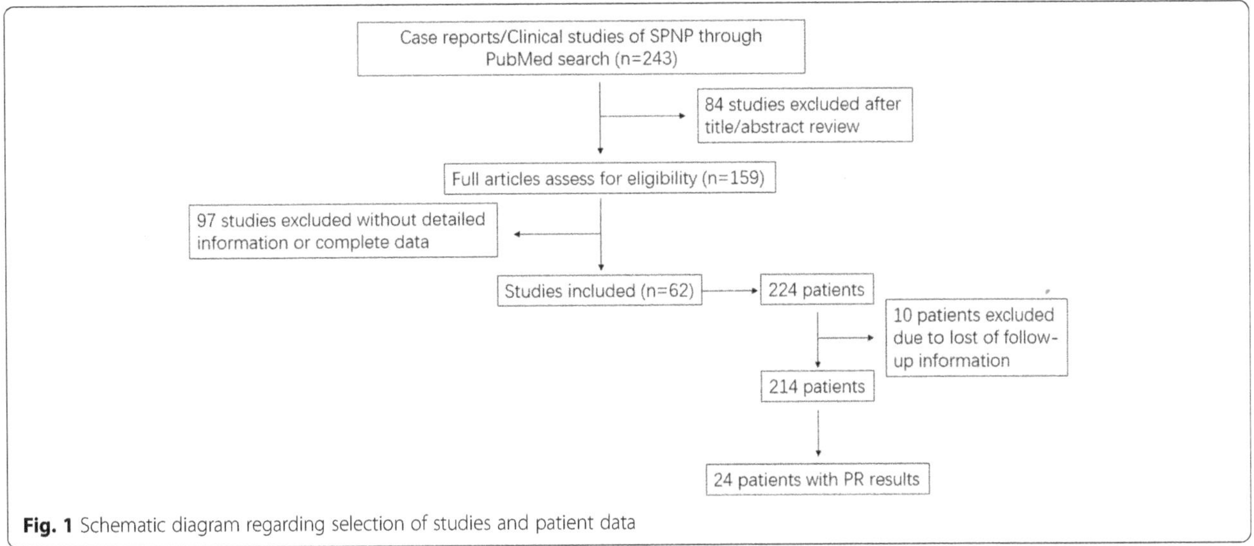

Fig. 1 Schematic diagram regarding selection of studies and patient data

splenectomy (40.0%), five distal pancreatectomy (6.7%), eight central pancreatectomy (10.7%) and two enucleation (2.7%). The tumors ranged from 1.2 to 16 cm in maximum diameter with medium size 5 cm. In immunohistochemistry, all cases showed vimentin (Vim) (71/71, 100%) and β-catenin (73/73, 100%) positive, and most of cases showed PR (68/69, 98.6%), synaptophysin (Syn) (43/70, 61.4%) and CD 10 (68/72, 94.4%) positive. A majority of cases preformed Ki-67 and Chromogranin A (CgA) low proliferation activity (69/71, 97.2%) and negative results (67/71, 94.4%). The mean value of tumor marker in carcinoembryonic antigen (CEA), carbohydrate antigen 19–9 (CA 19–9) and neuron-specific enolase (NSE) were 1.41 ± 0.83, 16.25 ± 31.33 and 21.87 ± 14.64 respectively.

Clinical outcomes and prognostic factors of SPNP patients in our cohort

Survival data of SPNP patients in our institution were summarized in Table 1. Survival data of Sixty-six patients were eventually selected for analysis because of loss of follow up information in other patients. At a median follow up of 23.5 months (range, 4–68 months), six patients (9.1%) occurred recurrence or metastasis and five patients (7.6%) suffered from SPNP related deaths. The 1-, 3- and 5-year DFS was 97.1, 95.0 and 93.2%. And, the 1-, 3- and 5-year DSS was 98.9, 96.4 and 96.4%, respectively.

By the use of ROC analysis, the optimal cut-off value of age and tumor size were 40 years and 7 cm. Kaplan-Meier survival analyses and univariable analysis showed that tumor size (≥7 cm) ($P = 0.003$), high Ki-67 proliferation activity (≥5%) ($P = 0.044$) and negative PR result ($P = 0.001$) were associated with the recurrence and metastasis of SPNP. While, large tumor size (≥7 cm) ($P = 0.006$) and negative PR result ($P < 0.001$) were also significantly related to the death of SPNP patients. To the contrary, factors such as age, sex, presence of symptom, tumor location, tumor markers and other immunohistochemical parameters were not associated with the prognosis of SPNP (Additional file 1: Table S1). The DFS and DSS of SPNP patients in our cohort with different PR result and tumor size (≥7 cm) were shown in Figs. 2, 3 by using Kaplan-Meier survival analyses. Multivariable analysis could not be performed here because of the small number of cases.

PR is an independent prognostic factor for SPNP

According to the literature review, a total of 62 reports and 214 patients with SPNP were included based on our inclusion criteria. The demographic and clinicopathology features of 214 patients were summarized in Additional file 1: Table S2. Combined with 66 SPNP patients in our cohort with follow up information, there were eventually 280 patients in the following prognostic analyses. In the univariable cox regression analysis, we observed age (≥40 years) ($P = 0.03$), high Ki-67 proliferation activity (≥5%) ($P = 0.006$) and negative PR results ($P < 0.001$) were significantly correlated with the incidence of recurrence or metastasis of SPNP. Whilst, tumor size (≥7 cm) ($P = 0.018$) and negative PR result ($P < 0.001$) were related with the death of SPNP. Then, these characteristics showed statistical difference ($P < 0.05$) above were performed in multivariable analysis. The PR result could be an independent prognostic factor of DFS and DSS in SPNP patients (DFS HR: 14.50, 95% CI: 1.98–106.05, $P = 0.008$; DSS HR: 9.15, 95% CI: 1.89–44.17, $P = 0.006$) (Table 2).

Kaplan-Meier curves of DFS and DSS for patients included in the pooled analysis were shown in Fig. 4. The DFS and DSS of SPNP patients according to PR

Table 1 Demographic and clinicopathological characteristics of 76 patients with SPNP in our cohort

Characteristics			Parameters
Age (Σ = 76)		Mean (y, ±SD)	33.03 ± 17.05
		Median (y, range)	30 (8–90)
Gender (Σ = 76)		Male (%)	17 (22.4%)
		Female (%)	59 (77.6%)
Location (Σ = 76)		Head/Neck (%)	40 (52.6%)
		Body/Tail (%)	36 (47.4%)
Tumor size (Σ = 76)		Mean (cm, ±SD)	5.9 ± 3.3
		Median (cm, range)	5.0 (1.2–16.0)
Symptom (Σ = 76)		Abdominal pain (%)	29 (38.2%)
		Asymptomatic (%)	36 (47.4%)
		Mass (%)	5 (6.6%)
		Other (%)	6 (7.9%)
Immunohistochem istry	Σ71	Vim (Pos itive, %)	71 (100 .0%)
	Σ69	PR (Positive, %)	68 (98.6%)
	Σ70	Syn (Positive, %)	43 (61.4%)
	Σ72	CD10 (Positive, %)	68 (94.4%)
	Σ71	Ki67 (Low proliferation activity, %)	69 (97.2%)
	Σ73	β-catenin (Positive, %)	73 (100.0%)
	Σ71	CgA (Negative, %)	67 (94.4%)
Tumor marker	Σ72	CEA (ng/ ml, ±SD)	1.41 ± 0.83
	Σ72	CA199 (U/ml, ±SD)	16.25 ± 31.33
	Σ45	NSE (ug/L, ±SD)	21.87 ± 14.64
Operation Method (Σ = 75)		Pancreaticoduodenectomy (%)	23 (30.7%)
		Duodenum preserving pancreatic head resection (%)	7 (9.3%)
		Enucleation (%)	2 (2.7%)
		Central pancreatectomy (%)	8 (10.7%)
		Distal pancreatectomy (%)	5 (6.7%)
		Distal pancreatectomy with splenectomy (%)	30 (40.0%)
Follow-up (Σ = 66)		Mean (mo, ±SD)	28.65 ± 19.22
		Median (mo, range)	23.5 (4.0–68.0)
Recurrence/metas tasis (Σ = 66)			6 (9.1%)
Disease related mortality (Σ = 66)			5 (7.6%)

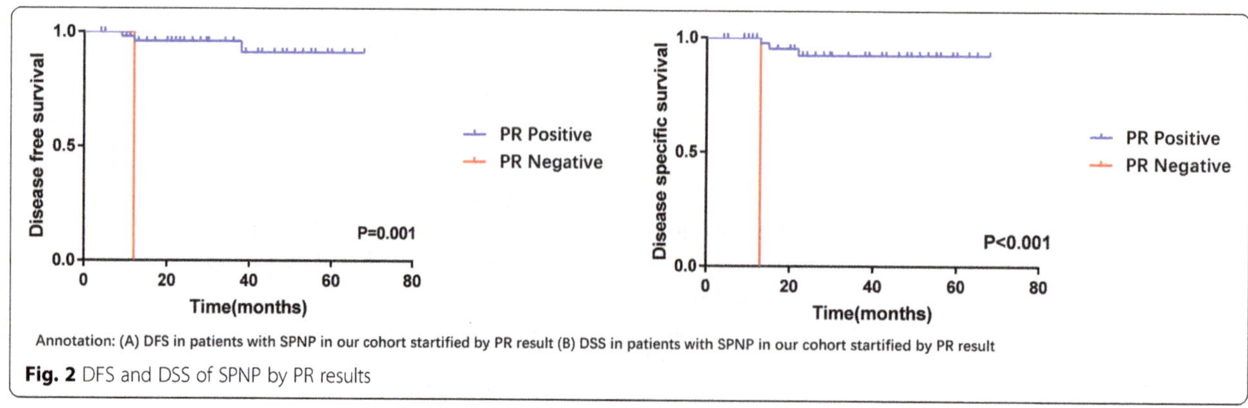

Annotation: (A) DFS in patients with SPNP in our cohort startified by PR result (B) DSS in patients with SPNP in our cohort startified by PR result

Fig. 2 DFS and DSS of SPNP by PR results

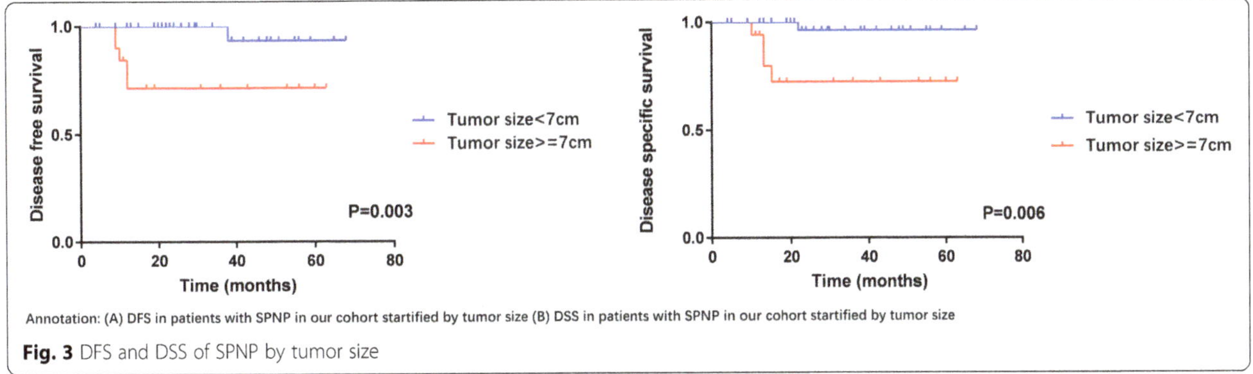

Fig. 3 DFS and DSS of SPNP by tumor size

results were shown in Fig. 5. Negative PR result was associated with poorer DFS and DSS ($P < 0.001$).

Comparison of clinicopathological parameters between SPNP with different PR results

The clinicopathological features of 93 SPNP patients with PR results were compared in the Table 3 according to the different PR results. The results showed that PR results were significantly related to the tumor size ($P = 0.01$) and Ki-67 ($P < 0001$). And the clinical outcomes of SPNP patients with PR negative result were worse than that of PR positive patients ($P < 0.001$). Therefore, negative PR result was a risk factor for prognosis of SPNP patients.

Discussion

With advances in imaging strategies, the number of detected SPNP was obviously increased in the last decades. More and more research about SPNP were also reported. As a neoplasm with low malignant potential, SPNP usually have a good prognosis after aggressive surgical resection, while further observations found some cases showed a short survival time when recurrence or metastasis happened. Therefore, identifying SPNP that have the potential for malignancy seems particularly important. Researchers have tried to find markers to predict the malignant behavior of SPNP for many years, and contradictory results are reported constantly [11–16]. In this study, we retrospectively analyzed the relationship between clinicopathologic features and clinical outcomes in our institution and a pooled case series. Our result showed that DFS and DSS were significantly shorter in patients with negative PR result and PR was classified as an independent prognostic factor for SPNP after multivariable analysis. To the best of our knowledge, this is the first study to evaluate that negative PR result could effectively predict a poorer prognosis of SPNP patients after surgical resection.

Table 2 Prognostic factors for DFS and DSS in patients with SPNP according to cox regression models

	Univariate COX model			Multivariate COX model		
Prognostic factors	β	Hazard ratio (95%CI)	*P* value	β	Hazard ratio (95%CI)	*P* value
DFS (*n* = 280)						
Age (≥40 y)	0.982	2.67 (1.10–6.48)	0.030	0.536	1.71 (0.38–7.79)	0.872
Gender (male)	−0.615	0.54 (0.18–1.59)	0.265			
Location (Head/Neck)	0.399	1.49 (0.64–3.45)	0.351			
Tumor size (≥7 cm)	0.809	2.25 (0.87–5.77)	0.093			
*Ki67 (≥5%)	1.770	5.87 (1.65–20.95)	0.006	0.2 93	1.34 (0.19–9.68)	0.771
*PR negative)	2.962	19.34 (5.08–73.61)	< 0.001	2.674	14.50 (1.98–106.05)	0.008
DSS (*n* = 280)						
Age (≥40 y)	0.454	1.58 (0.41–6.09)	0.511			
Gender (male)	−1.295	0.27 (0.07–1.06)	0.061			
Location (Head/Neck)	−0.067	0.94 (0.27–3.23)	0.916			
Tumor size (≥7 cm)	1.878	6.54 (1.39–30.82)	0.018	1.7 16	5.56 (0.60–51.19)	0.130
*Ki67 (≥5%)	1.214	3.37 (0.65–17.48)	0.149			
*PR (negative)	2.800	16.45 (3.66–73.87)	< 0.001	2.2 13	9.15 (1.89–44.17)	0.006

*Number of SPN patients with Ki67 and PR results are 82 and 83 respectively

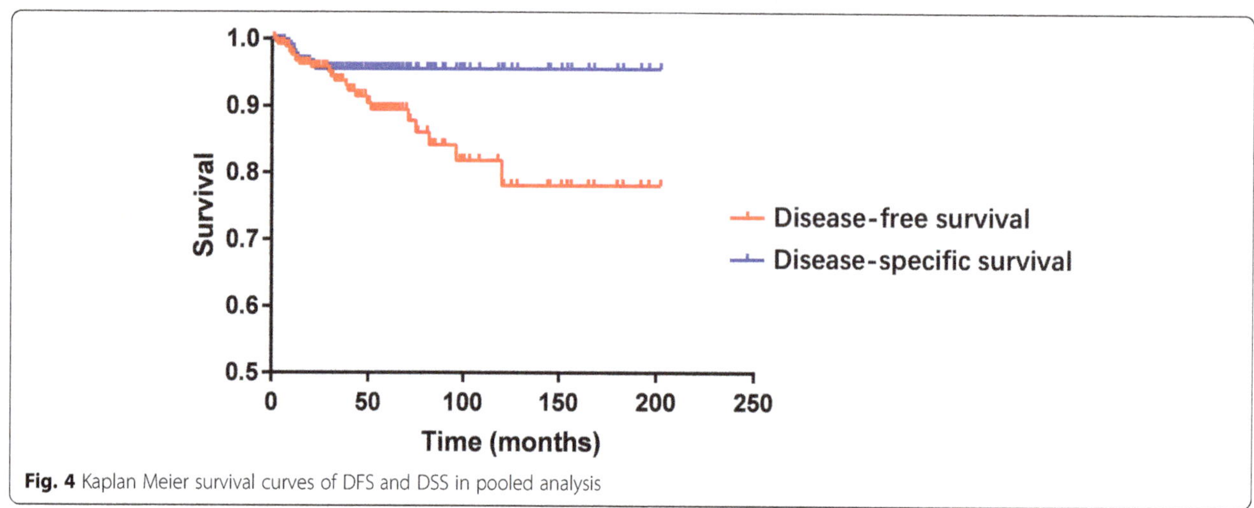

Fig. 4 Kaplan Meier survival curves of DFS and DSS in pooled analysis

Progesterone receptor, the effector of progesterone, is widely distributed in reproductive system, immune tissue, cardiomyocytes, brain, lung and other organs [22–24]. As a neuroendocrine organ, pancreas also show PR expression in normal pancreatic islets suggesting a possible role for progesterone in pancreatic islets function [25, 26]. A hormonal influence on pathogenesis of SPNP has been postulated in view of its high prevalence in young women. Some previous research attempted to study the role of female sex hormone in SPNP, but conflicting results emerged. PR is consistently positive in SPNP irrespective of sex and hormonal changes, while immunolabeling for estrogen receptor is negative [20, 27]. It is still a mystery whether sex hormone participate in the origin of SPNP. Of note, studies have indicated that PR has prognostic value in many other pancreatic malignancies such as PanNET [18, 28]. They found the loss of PR expression can provide information on shorter DFS in PanNET patients. We know that the activation of PR can have an inhibitory effect on cell proliferation, differentiation and tumorigenesis under the change of gene expression, post-translational modification of proteins and intracellular Ca^{2+} level [29–31]. And in the research of Jeannelyn [32], they found PR play a crucial role in advanced PanNET through the regulation of PI3K-AKT pathway. All above may explain how PR could be the prognostic factor of some malignancies, but the mechanism of PR in predicting SPNP prognosis need further research.

Previous studies have suggested that some clinicopathologic features such as tumor size, younger age and male sex could indicate the malignant potential of SPNP [11, 12, 14]. However, we found there were a shorter DFS and DSS when tumor size ≥7 cm in our institution, but only DSS was related to tumor size in the pooled series. Kang [14] et al. considered tumor size larger than 5 cm showed a malignant potential of SPNP. And in immunohistochemistry, high Ki-67 proliferative activity showed a significant correlation with DFS in both of our institution and pooled series, but not with DSS. In Yang's study [17], a Ki-67 index ≥4% remained associated with poorer prognosis of patients with SPNP. We also observed age ≥ 40

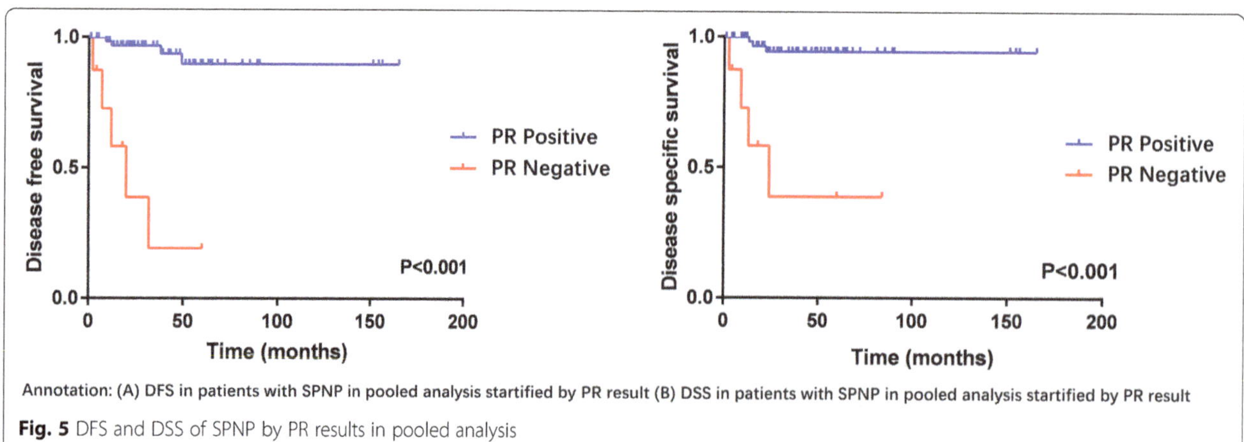

Annotation: (A) DFS in patients with SPNP in pooled analysis startified by PR result (B) DSS in patients with SPNP in pooled analysis startified by PR result

Fig. 5 DFS and DSS of SPNP by PR results in pooled analysis

Table 3 Comparison of clinicopathological parameters between SPN with different PR results

Characteristics		PR (+)	PR (−)	*P* value
Age (Σ = 93)		85	8	0.091
	Mean (y, ±SD)	32.85 ± 16.71	44.13 ± 17.61	
	Median (y, range)	32 (8–90)	43 (20–71)	
Gender (Σ = 93)		85	8	0.194
	Male (%)	15 (17.6%)	0 (0.0%)	
	Female (%)	70 (82.4%)	8 (100.0%)	
Location (Σ = 93)		85	8	0.924
	Head/Neck (%)	44 (51.8%)	4 (50.0%)	
	Body/Tail (%)	41 (48.2%)	4 (50.0%)	
Tumor Size (Σ = 92)		84	8	0.010
	Mean (cm, ±SD)	5.95 ± 3.25	9.99 ± 4.29	
	Median (cm, range)	5.0 (1.2–16.0)	11.0 (2.2–15.5)	
Immunohistochemistry				
	Syn (Positive, %) Σ = 93	47/85 (55.3%)	4/8 (50.0%)	0.774
	CD10 (Positive, %) Σ = 79	68/74 (91.9%)	5/5 (100.0%)	0.508
	Ki67 (Low proliferation activity, %) Σ = 75	65/69 (94.2%)	3/6 (50.0%)	< 0.001
	CgA (Negative, %) Σ = 91	75/84 (89.3%)	7/7 (100.0%)	0.362
Recurrence/metas tasis (Σ = 83)		4/75 (5.3%)	5/8 (62.5%)	< 0.001
Disease related mortality (Σ = 83)		3/75 (4.0%)	4/8 (50.0%)	< 0.001

years was a risk factor of short DFS in univariable analysis. In addition to these parameters, we failed to identify other clinicopathological features in predicting prognosis of SPNP. The reason for different or conflicting results may lie in the fact that some studies used blurred criteria of malignancy or small sample size. Meanwhile, clinicians attach more attention on this kind of tumor in recent decades because of the improvement of imaging and pathology method, so more studies about SPNP were reported.

Due to the recurrence or metastasis of some SPNP after surgical resection, the World Health Organization classified SPNP as low-grade malignant tumor with malignant features of surrounding tissue invasion, perineural invasion, vascular invasion on microscopic pathology and metastasis [33]. Therefore, some studies regarded these malignant performances including muscular vessel invasion, adjacent organ or lymph node invasion and distant metastasis at diagnosis were the prognostic factors of SPNP [34–36]. While, these performances always present late progress of SPNP with poor prognosis, we need a predictive factor on prognosis of SPNP without malignant features at relatively early stage.

Conclusion

This study highlights the potential prognostic value of PR in patients with SPNP, which may help in risk stratification according to the surgical pathologic report. Although SPNP usually has a good clinical outcome, long term follow-up is necessary because of possible recurrence or metastasis. These patients should be scheduled every 1–2 months follow up visits during the first year after surgery and every 3–6 month for years after [17]. And the effect of adjuvant chemotherapy for high risk SPNP need further confirm. There are several limitations in this study. As a retrospective study, the role of PR in SPNP requires to be investigated in a prospective validation study. The small sample size and short length of follow up precluded the difference between all other effective marker. Multicenter prospective studies with large sample size and long follow up are necessary in the future. What's more, we did not notice the effect of adjuvant chemotherapy in this study. Nevertheless, pooled analysis is essential for prediction of prognosis of rare disease. The methodology of our study could be reliable [37, 38].

Abbreviations

CA19–9: Carbohydrate antigen 19–9; CEA: Carcinoembryonic antigen; CgA: Chromogranin A; DFS: Disease-free survival; DSS: Disease-specific survival; MeSH: Medical Subject Heading; NSE: Neuron-specific enolase; PanNET: Pancreatic neuroendocrine tumor; PR: Progesterone receptor; SPNP: Solid pseudopapillary neoplasm of the pancreas; Syn: Synaptophysin; Vim: Vimentin

Acknowledgements
The authors thank the staff from Pancreatic Surgery of Wuhan Union Hospital for their support during the study. We sincerely appreciated the data provided by Pancreas Surgery of Wuhan Union Hospital. At the same time, i would like to appreciate my girlfriend for supporting and accompany during this period time. So, Miss Gu, will you marry with me?

Funding
No funding was obtained for this study.

Authors' contributions
FY and HS designed the study; FY and ZB wrote the main manuscript text; FY and SK did the article search; ZB and YS analyzed the data; all authors have read and approved the manuscript.

Consent for publication
Not applicable.

Competing interests
The authors declare that they have no competing interests.

Author details
[1]Department of General Surgery, Shanghai Jiaotong University Affiliated First People's Hospital, Shanghai 200080, China. [2]Department of Pancreatic Surgery, Union Hospital, Tongji Medical College, Huazhong University of Science and Technology, Wuhan 430022, China. [3]Department of Thoracic Surgery, Union Hospital, Tongji Medical College, Huazhong University of Science and Technology, Wuhan 430022, China.

References
1. Franz VK. Papillary tumors of the pancreas: benign or malignant? In: Tumors of the pancreas. Atlas of tumor pathology; 1959. p. 32–3.
2. Kallichanda N, Tsai S, Stabile BE, et al. Histogenesis of solid pseudopapillary tumor of the pancreas: the case for the centroacinar cell of origin. Exp Mol Pathol. 2006;81:101–7.
3. Papavramidis T, Papavramidis S. Solid pseudopapillary tumors of the pancreas: review of 718 patients reported in English literature. J Am Coll Surg. 2005;200:965–72.
4. De Castro SM, Singhal D, Aronson DC, et al. Management of solid-pseudopapillary neoplasms of the pancreas: a comparison with standard pancreatic neoplasms. World J Surg. 2007;31(5):1130–5.
5. Bosman FT, Carneiro F, Hruban R, Theise ND. WHO classification of tumors of the digestive system, ed 4. Geneva: WHO; 2010.
6. Raffel A, Cupisti K, Krausch M, et al. Therapeutic strategy of papillary cystic and solid neoplasm (PCSN): a rare non-endocrine tumor of the pancreas in children. Surg Oncol. 2004;13(1):1–6.
7. Geers C, Moulin P, Gigot JF, et al. Solid and pseudopapillary tumor of the pancreas review and new insights into pathogenesis. Am J Surg Pathol. 2006;30(10):1243–9.
8. Sperti C, Berselli M, Pasquali C, et al. Aggressive behavior of solid pseudopapillary tumor of the pancreas in adults: a case report and review of the literature. World J Gastroenterol. 2008;14(6):960–5.
9. Martin RC, Klimstra DS, Brennan MF, et al. Solid pseudopapillary tumor of the pancreas: a surgical enigma? Ann Surg Oncol. 2002;9:35–40.
10. Tipton SG, Smyrk TC, Sarr MG, et al. Malignant potential of solid pseudopapillary neoplasm of the pancreas. Br J Surg. 2006;93:733–7.
11. Machado MC, Machado MA, Bacchella T, et al. Solid pseudopapillary neoplasm of the pancreas: distinct patterns of onset, diagnosis, and prognosis for male versus female patients. Surgery. 2008;143:29–34.
12. Lee SE, Jang JY, Hwang DW, et al. Clinical features and outcome of solid pseudopapillary neoplasm: differences between adults and children. Arch Surg. 2008;143:1218–21.
13. Butte JM, Brennan MF, Gonen M, et al. Solid pseudopapillary tumors of the pancreas. Clinical features, surgical outcomes, and long-term survival in 45 consecutive patients from a single center. J Gastrointest Surg. 2011;15:350–7.
14. Kang CM, Kim KS, Choi JS, et al. Solid pseudopapillary tumor of the pancreas suggesting malignant potential. Pancreas. 2006;32:276–80.
15. Goh BK, Tan YM, Cheow PC, et al. Solid pseudopapillary neoplasms of the pancreas: an updated experience. J Surg Oncol. 2007;95:640–4.
16. Yang F, Jin C, Long J, et al. Solid pseudopapillary tumor of the pancreas: a case series of 26 consecutive patients. Am J Surg. 2009;198:210–5.
17. Yang F, Yu X, Bao Y, et al. Prognostic value of Ki-67 in solid pseudopapillary tumor of the pancreas: Huashan experience and systematic review of the literature. Surgery. 2016;159:1023–31.
18. Kim SJ, An S, Lee JH, Kim JY, et al. Loss of progesterone receptor expression is an early tumorigenesis event associated with tumor progression and shorter survival in pancreatic neuroendocrine tumor patients. J Pathol Transl Med. 2017;51:388–95.
19. Pettinato G, Di Vizio D, Manivel JC, et al. Solid-pseudopapillary tumor of the pancreas: a neoplasm with distinct and highly characteristic cytological features. Diagn Cytopathol. 2002;27(6):325–34.
20. Adams AL, Siegal GP, Jhala NC. Solid pseudopapillary tumor of the pancreas: a review of salient clinical and pathologic features. Adv Anat Pathol. 2008;15:39–45.
21. Reiner A, Neumeister B, Spona J, et al. Immunohistochemical localization of estrogen and progesterone receptor and prognosis in human primary breast cancer. Cancer Res. 1990;50:7075–61.
22. Kim JJ, Kurita T, Bulun SE. Progesterone action in endometrial cancer, endometriosis, uterine fibroids, and breast cancer. Endocr Rev. 2013;34:130–62.
23. Lee JH, Lydon JP, Kim CH. Progesterone suppresses the mTOR pathway and promotes generation of induced regulatory T cells with increased stability. Eur J Immunol. 2012;42:2683–96.
24. Thomas P, Pang Y. Protective actions of progesterone in the cardiovascular system: potential role of membrane progesterone receptors (mPRs) in mediating rapid effects. Steroids. 2013;78:583–8.
25. Arnason T, Sapp HL, Barnes PJ, et al. Immunohistochemical expression and prognostic value of ER, PR and HER2/neu in pancreatic and small intestinal neuroendocrine tumors. Neuroendocrinology. 2011;93:249–58.
26. Viale G, Doglioni C, Gambacorta M, et al. Progesterone receptor immunoreactivity in pancreatic endocrine tumors: an immunocytochemical study of 156 neuroendocrine tumors of the pancreas, gastrointestinal and respiratory tracts, and skin. Cancer. 1992;70:2268–77.
27. Lam KY, Lo CY, Fan ST. Pancreatic solid cystic papillary tumor: clinicopathologic features in eight patients from Hong Kong and review of the literature. World J Surg. 1999;23:1045–50.
28. Jang KT, Park SM, Basturk O, et al. Clinicopathologic characteristics of 29 invasive carcinomas arising in 178 pancreatic mucinous cystic neoplasms with ovarian-type stroma: implications for management and prognosis. Am J Surg Pathol. 2015;39:179–87.
29. Shchelkunova TA, Morozov IA. Molecular basis and tissue specificity of the progestins action. Mol Biol. 2015;49:728–48.
30. Goncharov AI, Maslakova AA, Polikarpova AV, et al. Progesterone inhibits proliferation and modulates expression of proliferation-related genes in classical progesterone receptor-negative human BxPC3 pancreatic adenocarcinoma cells. J Steroid Biochem Mol Biol. 2017;165:293–304.
31. Zuo L, Li W, You S. Progesterone reverses the mesenchymal phenotypes of basal phenotype breast cancer cells via a membrane progesterone receptor mediated pathway. Breast Cancer Res. 2010;12:R34.
32. Estrella JS, Broaddus RR, Mathews A, et al. Progesterone receptor and PTEN

expression predict survival in patients with low-and intermediate-grade pancreatic neuroendocrine tumors. Arch Pathol Lab Med. 2014;138:1027–36.
33. Kleihues P, Sobin LH. World Health Organization classification of tumors. Cancer. 2000;88(12):2887.
34. Estrella JS, Li L, Rasid A, et al. Solid Pseudopapillary neoplasm of the pancreas Clinicopathologic and survival analyses of 64 cases from a single institution. Am J Surg Pathol. 2014;38:147–57.
35. Kang CM, Choi SH, Kim SC, et al. Predicting recurrence of pancreatic solid pseudopapillary tumors after surgical resection: a multicenter analysis in Korea. Ann Surg. 2014;260:348–55.
36. Kim CW, Han DJ, Kim J, et al. Solid pseudopapillary tumor of the pancreas: can malignancy be predicted? Surgery. 2011;149:625–34.
37. Howard JE, Dwivedi RC, Masterson L, et al. Langerhans cell sarcoma: a systematic review. Cancer Treat Rev. 2015;41:320–31.
38. De Jong MC, Kors WA, De Graaf P, et al. Trilateral retinoblastoma: a systematic review and meta-analysis. Lancet Oncol. 2014;15:1157–67.

20

Reduced lymphocyte count as an early marker for predicting infected pancreatic necrosis

Xiao Shen[1†], Jing Sun[2†], Lu Ke[1], Lei Zou[1], Baiqiang Li[1], Zhihui Tong[1], Weiqin Li[1*], Ning Li[2] and Jieshou Li[2]

Abstract

Background: Early occurrence of immunosuppression is a risk factor for infected pancreatic necrosis (IPN) in the patients with acute pancreatitis (AP). However, current measures for the immune systems are too cumbersome and not widely available. Significantly decreased lymphocyte count has been shown in patients with severe but not mild type of AP. Whereas, the correlation between the absolute lymphocyte count and IPN is still unknown. We conduct this study to reveal the exact relationship between early lymphocyte count and the development of IPN in the population of AP patients.

Methods: One hundred and fifty-three patients with acute pancreatitis admitted to Jinling Hospital during the period of January 2012 to July 2014 were included in this retrospective study. The absolute lymphocyte count and other relevant parameters were measured on admission. The diagnosis of IPN was based on the definition of the revised Atlanta classification.

Results: Patients were divided into two groups according to the presence of IPN. Thirty patients developed infected necrotizing pancreatitis during the disease course. The absolute lymphocyte count in patients with IPN was significantly lower on admission (0.62×10^9/L, interquartile range [IQR]: $0.46–0.87 \times 10^9$/L vs. 0.91×10^9/L, IQR: $0.72–1.27 \times 10^9$/L, $p < 0.001$) and throughout the whole clinical course than those without IPN. Logistic regression indicated that reduced lymphocyte count was an independent risk factor for IPN. The optimal cut-offs from ROC curve was 0.66×10^9/L giving sensitivity of 83.7 % and specificity of 66.7 %.

Conclusions: Reduced lymphocyte count within 48 h of AP onset is significantly and independently associated with the development of IPN.

Keywords: Acute pancreatitis, Infected pancreatic necrosis, Lymphocyte count, Immunosuppression

Background

Acute pancreatitis (AP) is a sudden inflammation of the pancreas with a mortality rate of 6–10 % [1]. In the past, the Atlanta classification was commonly used to grade the severity of AP, briefly, mild and severe AP. Patients with severe acute pancreatitis (SAP) are usually associated with multiple organ dysfunction (MODS) and poor prognosis. About 5–10 % of the AP patients would develop necrosis of the pancreatic or peripancreatic tissue [2] and the necrotic tissue can remain sterile or be infected, becoming infected pancreatic necrosis (IPN). IPN is known to be an independent risk factor for ultimate mortality [3] and always develops during the second or third week after the onset of the disease [4, 5]. It is recently reported that more than 80 % of the mortality occurs at the late stage as a result of infection [6]. Thus, it is of great importance to distinguish those patients with higher risk for IPN at the initial stage of the disease and make preventive intervention.

Recently, more and more studies have shown that immunosuppression is a key pathogenesis of SAP. Early alterations of the immune system comprising decreased activation of T lymphocyte [7] and down regulation of human leukocyte antigen (HLA) DR [8] may cause IPN, leading to multiple organ failure (MOF) and high mortality. In this way, these immunological indexes might be useful predictors for the prognosis of AP patients.

* Correspondence: njzy_pancrea@163.com
†Equal contributors
[1]Surgical Intensive Care Unit (SICU), Department of General Surgery, Jinling Hospital, Medical School of Nanjing University, No. 305 Zhongshan East Road, Nanjing 210002, Jiangsu Province, China
Full list of author information is available at the end of the article

However, due to the complexity of the measurement methods, the abovementioned indexes are not monitored routinely in the clinical work. Recently, the prognostic value of the neutrophil-lymphocyte ratio (NLR) had also been evaluated, but turned out with controversial results [9]. The absolute lymphocyte count was also assessed as an important part of the immune system. In 1985, Christophi et al. first declared the absolute lymphocyte count had a prognostic significance in the severity of acute pancreatitis [10]. Whereas, no further studies regarding the role of the absolute lymphocyte count as an independent factor for disease severity or mortality in AP patients were carried out after that [11].

Our investigation was the first study to compare the early alteration of the absolute lymphocyte count in the peripheral blood of AP patients with and without IPN. The aim of this study was to determine whether the lymphocyte count was a strong predictor for IPN in patients with acute pancreatitis and how strongly the absolute lymphocyte count was associated with the prognosis.

Methods

Patients

This was a retrospective observational study conducted in the Department of General Surgery, Jinling Hospital, China. The data collection for this study was approved by the Institutional Review Board of our hospital. One hundred fifty-three patients with a diagnosis of acute pancreatitis consecutively treated in our center during January 2012 to July 2014 were included for potential analysis. The diagnostic criteria of AP were according to two of the following three clinical features [2]: upper abdominal pain, significantly increased serum levels of lipase (or amylase) activity and imaging findings consistent with acute pancreatitis. The inclusion criteria were AP patients aged 18 years or older who admitted to our center within 48 h after the onset of the disease and received systemic laboratory evaluations on admission. Patients during pregnancy, with a history of cancer or bone marrow diseases or a medical history of immunosuppressive agents were excluded from this study.

Data collection

All the patients with AP were evaluated for blood routine and biochemical tests at arrival in the central laboratory of our hospital. Hemoglobin, hematocrit, platelet, C-reactive protein (CRP), white blood cells as well as the absolute neutrophil and lymphocyte counts were obtained from an automatic blood cell analyzer (CELL-DYN3700, Chicago, Abbott). NLR was calculated using the values of the absolute neutrophil and lymphocyte counts. Serum levels of albumin, amylase and lipase were detected using an Aeroset (Hitachi 7060 Automatic Biochemical Analyzer, Tokyo, Japan). HLA-DR and T lymphocyte subsets were also assayed in our central laboratory in 30 patients (24 in non-IPN group and 6 in IPN group) by the direct fluorescence method for the whole blood using flow cytometer in a flow cytometer (FACS-Calibur, Becton Dickinson, San Jose, Calif., USA) and double straining (FITC/PE) monoclonal antibodies (Marseilles, France). HLA-DR expression was measured in the monocyte population and T lymphocyte subsets were measured in the lymphocytes population. Analysis of the data was performed by CellQuest software. Demographic variables, possible etiology of acute pancreatitis were reviewed and recorded by two independent physicians.

Baseline characteristics, including age, gender, body mass index, Acute Physiology and Chronic Health Enquiry II (APACHE II) score and computed tomography (CT) severity index, were also collected and recorded.

Definition

The diagnosis of IPN was according to the imaging findings and/or bacterial culture result: either the presence of extraluminal gas in the pancreatic and/or peripancreatic tissues on contrast-enhanced computed tomography (CECT) or positive bacterial culture of aspiration and drainage content of pancreatic and/or peripancreatic tissues could confirm the diagnosis [2]. Lymphocytopenia was defined as the absolute lymphocyte count below 0.8×10^9/L. Organ dysfunction was evaluated in three organ systems (respiratory, renal and cardiovascular) within 24 h after admission and the definition of organ dysfunction was based on the modified Marshall scoring system, defining as a score of 2 or more [12]. The definition of local complications, including portal vein thrombosis, intra-abdominal hypertension and hemorrhage, deep vein thrombosis (DVT) and gastrointestinal fistula, judged by two independent physicians, was according to the recently revised Atlanta criteria [2]. Disease severity of AP was assessed based on the presence of sterile/infected pancreatic necrosis and transient/persistent organ failure, namely, mild, moderate, severe and critical AP [13].

Statistic analysis

Continuous variables in the data were presented as medians plus interquartile range (IQR) and categorical variables were presented as absolute numbers and percentage. Mann–Whitney *U* test was used in continuous variables and Chi-square test was used to analyze categorical variables for group comparisons. Logistic regression was constructed to evaluate the relationship between the relevant parameters and secondary infection. Multivariate logistic regression only involved in the variables that showed statistic significance in univariate analysis. Further receiver operating characteristic (ROC) curve was displayed for accuracy assessment. Statistical analyses were performed using SPSS (version 22.0) statistical software (IBM Analytics, Armonk, NY). A probability (p value) of <0.05 was considered statistically significant.

Results

1096 patients were initially screened for the study and eventually 153 patients were enrolled for analysis (Fig. 1). Patients were divided into two groups according to the presence of IPN, namely, IPN ($n = 30$) and non-IPN ($n = 123$) group. Except for the acute physiology and chronic health enquiry II (APACHE II) score, the baseline characteristics showed no significant differences between the two groups (Table 1). Also, no significant difference was seen in the distribution of etiology. Lymphocytopenia developed in 42 (34.1 %) patients in non-IPN group and 19 (63.3 %) patients in IPN group ($p = 0.006$). The median absolute lymphocyte count in peripheral blood of the patients with IPN was significantly lower than those patients without IPN on admission (0.62×10^9/L, interquartile range [IQR]: 0.46–0.87 × 10^9/L vs. 0.91 × 10^9/L, IQR: 0.72–1.27 × 10^9/L, p < 0.001) and also in the following days (Fig. 2). Consistent with the previous studies, the median value of NLR was significantly higher in the patients with IPN compared to those without (15.5, IQR: 12.0–23.8 vs. 10.9, IQR: 7.7–18.2, $p = 0.002$), indicating immunosuppression occurred at the very onset of AP in the patients with IPN. As for other immunological indexes, we also measured the expression of HLA-DR on peripheral monocytes and T lymphocyte subsets on peripheral lymphocytes. Down-regulated expression of HLA-DR (15.5 %, IQR: 12.9–31.7 % vs. 30.3 %, IQR: 22.4–51.9 %, $p = 0.026$) and decreased proportion of mature T lymphocytes (44.8 %, IQR: 31.4–51.5 % vs. 51.5 %, IQR: 40.4–63.9 %, $p = 0.203$) in the patients with IPN also confirmed the presence of immunosuppression (Fig. 3). As a result of immunosuppression, patients who developed IPN suffered higher mortality and longer hospital durations.

Table 2 represented the comparison of complications and outcome between the two groups. The incidence of organ dysfunction was 30.9 % (38/123) in the patients of non-IPN group and 86.7 % (26/30) in those of IPN group ($p < 0.001$). Acute respiratory distress syndrome (ARDS) and acute kidney injury (AKI) were two most common organ dysfunctions in both groups, followed by shock, mainly septic shock. Higher percentage of organ dysfunctions in the patients with IPN led to increased need for mechanical ventilation and continuous renal replacement therapy (CRRT). Intra-abdominal hemorrhage and hypertension were the most common complications in both two groups, followed by fistula. Four patients in the non-IPN group died during hospitalization: MOF for two patients, pulmonary embolism and unexplained cardiac arrest for the remaining two patients, respectively. The hospital mortality was much higher in the patients with IPN, above 40 %. All patients but one died of MOF.

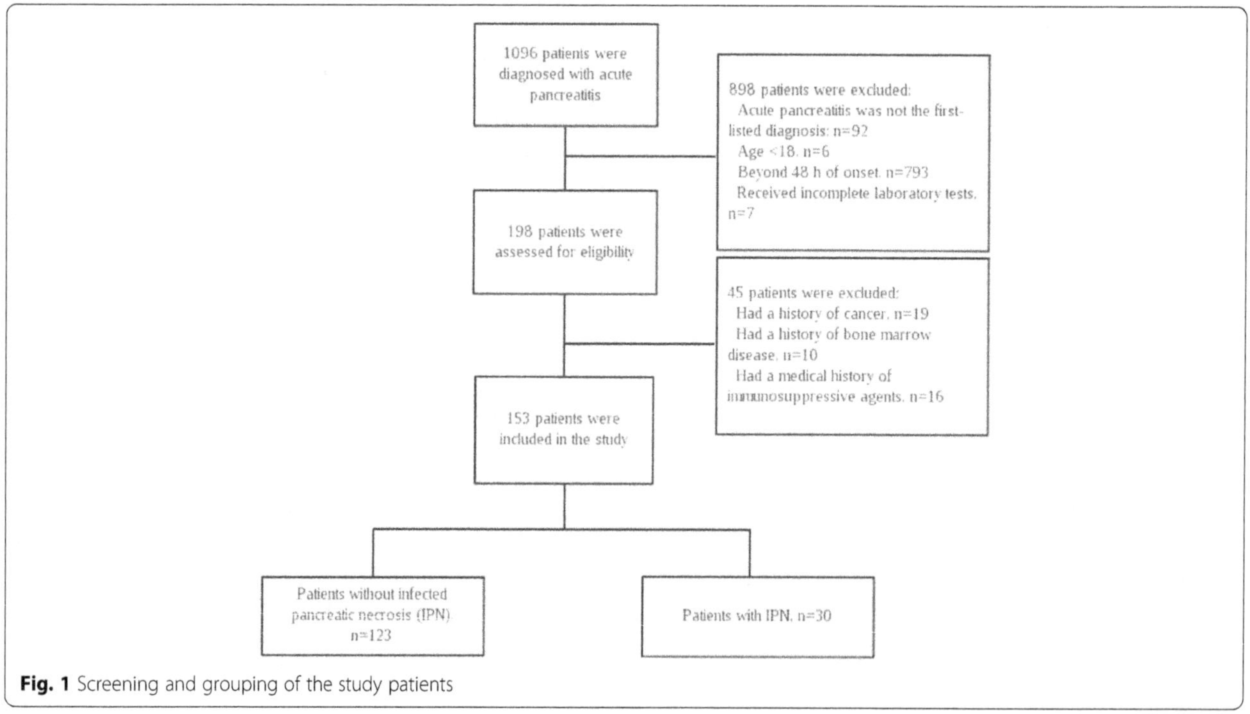

Fig. 1 Screening and grouping of the study patients

Table 1 Baseline characteristics and clinical features of the AP patients with or without IPN

Variable	Non-IPN group ($n = 123$)	IPN group ($n = 30$)	p Value
Age, years	45 (36, 56)	47 (38, 57)	0.529
Gender, male/female	79/44	21/9	0.068
BMI	26.1 (23.3, 28.8)	27.3 (23.0, 28.4)	0.155
APACHE II score	13 (12, 15)	20 (14, 29)	<0.001
CT severity index	3 (3, 6)	8 (6, 8.5)	<0.001
Laboratory data			
Hemoglobin, g/L	135 (116, 150)	126 (101, 149)	0.247
Hematocrit	0.40 (0.34, 0.45)	0.36 (0.29, 0.44)	0.211
Platelet, $\times 10^9$/L	158 (117, 204)	116 (81, 166)	0.002
CRP, mg/L	161.0 (71.8, 208.8)	202.7 (158.7, 251.5)	0.001
WBC, $\times 10^9$/L	13.0 (9.6, 17.3)	11.8 (8.7, 14.6)	0.152
Lymphocyte count, $\times 10^9$/L	0.91 (0.72, 1.27)	0.62 (0.46, 0.87)	<0.001
NLR	10.9 (7.7, 18.2)	15.5 (12.0, 23.8)	0.002
Albumin, g/L	35.6 (34.0, 38.2)	34.4 (31.6, 36.2)	0.010
Amylase, U/L	276 (138, 544)	270 (183, 934)	0.129
Lipase, U/L	1095 (457, 1916)	972 (579, 1814)	0.963
Aetiology of acute pancreatitis, no. (%)			
Gallstone	59 (48.0)	14 (46.7)	1.000
Hypertriglyceridemia	49 (39.8)	15 (50.0)	0.409
Alcohol	11 (8.9)	1 (3.3)	0.462
Post-ERCP	2 (1.6)	0 (0)	1.000
Other	2 (1.6)	0 (0)	1.000

AP acute pancreatitis, *IPN* infected pancreatic necrosis, *BMI* Body Mass Index, *APACHE II score* Acute Physiology and Chronic Health Enquiry II score, *CT* computed tomography, *CRP* C-reactive protein, *WBC* white blood cells, *NLR* Neutrophil-lymphocyte ratio, *ERCP* Endoscopic Retrograde Cholangiopancreatography

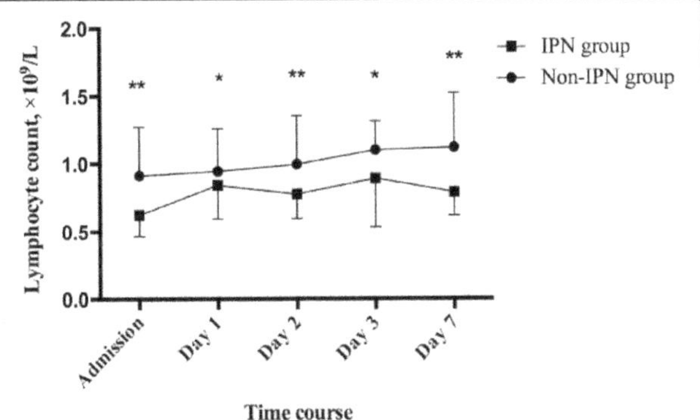

Fig. 2 Change of the absolute lymphocyte count during the disease course of acute pancreatitis in the patients of different groups. Values were presented with median ± interquartile range (IQR); IPN: infected pancreatic necrosis. $*p < 0.05$ for IPN vs. non-IPN group, $**p < 0.001$ for IPN vs. non-IPN group

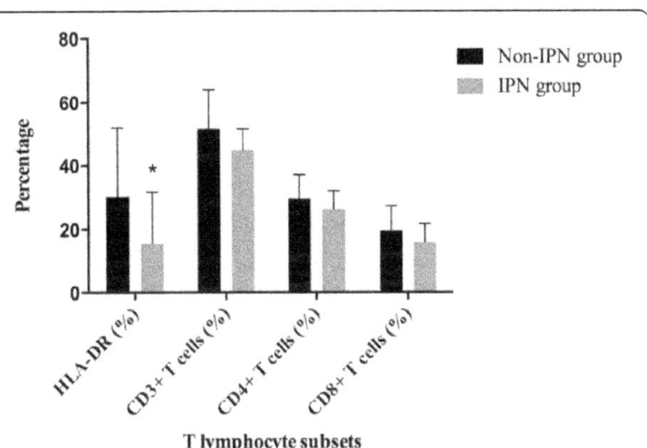

Fig. 3 Change of Human leukocyte antigen (HLA)-DR and T lymphocyte subsets in patients of different groups. Values were presented with median ± IQR; IPN: infected pancreatic necrosis. $*p < 0.05$ for IPN vs. non-IPN group, $**p < 0.001$ for IPN vs. non-IPN group

Table 2 Complications and outcomes of the AP patients with or without IPN

	Non-IPN group ($n = 123$)	IPN group ($n = 30$)	p Value
Severity of AP, no. (%)			<0.001
Mild	59 (48.0)	0 (0)	
Moderate	26 (21.1)	0 (0)	
Severe	38 (30.9)	4 (13.3)	
Critical	0 (0)	26 (86.7)	
Organ dysfunction, no. (%)			
Respiratory	34 (27.6)	19 (63.3)	<0.001
Renal	20 (16.3)	22 (73.3)	<0.001
Cardiovascular	5 (4.1)	12 (40.0)	<0.001
Mechanical ventilation, no. (%)	21 (17.1)	18 (60.0)	<0.001
CRRT, no. (%)	20 (16.3)	19 (63.3)	<0.001
Complication, no. (%)			
Pancreatic pseudocyst	8 (6.5)	1 (3.3)	1.000
Invasive fungal infection	0 (0)	2 (6.7)	0.037
Intra-abdominal hemorrhage	1 (0.8)	9 (30.0)	<0.001
Deep vein thrombosis	5 (4.1)	2 (6.7)	0.624
Portal thrombosis	1 (0.8)	1 (3.3)	0.355
IAH	6 (4.9)	8 (26.7)	0.001
Encephalopathy	1 (0.8)	0 (0)	1.000
Fistula	0 (0)	5 (16.7)	<0.001
Hospital stay, days	10 (6, 14)	30 (18, 54)	<0.001
ICU stay, days	6 (3, 9)	17 (9, 48)	<0.001
Mortality rate, no. (%)	4 (3.3)	13 (43.3)	<0.001

IPN infected pancreatic necrosis, *AP* acute pancreatitis, *CRRT* continuous renal replacement therapy, *IAH* intra-abdominal hypertension, *ICU* intensive care unit

Univariate logistic regression analysis (Table 3) was performed to evaluate the predictive power of the absolute lymphocyte count, NLR and other related parameters for IPN. Results indicated significant correlations between IPN and APACHEII score, platelet, CRP, lymphocyte count, NLR, albumin as well as amylase. Further stepwise multivariate logistic regression was constructed and displayed in Table 4. The final model suggested that APACHEII score (Odds Ratio: 1.299, 95 % confidence interval [CI]: 1.153–1.464, $p < 0.001$) and reduced lymphocyte count (Odds Ratio: 0.006, 95 % CI: 1.153–1.464, $p < 0.001$) were strongly and independently associated with IPN. The area under the ROC curve (Fig. 4) showed the reduced absolute lymphocyte count (0.842, 95 % CI: 0.769–0.914, $p < 0.001$) had a moderate to high accuracy in predicting IPN, higher than APACHEII score (0.819, 95 % CI: 0.722–0.917, $p < 0.001$). The optimal cut-offs from ROC curve was 0.66×10^9/L giving sensitivity of 83.7 % and specificity of 66.7 %.

Discussion

About one third of the patients with necrotizing pancreatitis would develop IPN progressively [14]. IPN would prolong the hospital stay and increase the incidence of complications as well as mortality. Briefly, the development of IPN determines the management of acute pancreatitis and has a great influence on the prognosis. In accordance with previous studies, the incidence of complications and mortality were much higher in the patients with IPN than those without. Also, MOF caused by pancreatic infection or sepsis was the major death cause in both two groups. Hence, it is urgent to find a simple and early marker that could predict IPN at the very onset of the disease. In the literature, several biochemical parameters such as procalcitonin, CRP and NLR have been investigated but turned out with unsatisfying results. Our study first assessed the predictive power of the absolute lymphocyte count for IPN in the patients with acute pancreatitis and demonstrated that the absolute lymphocyte count was a strong predictor for IPN in AP patients with a moderate to high accuracy. Patients who developed IPN in the late course of AP had significantly lower lymphocyte count in the peripheral blood at the initial stage (within 48 h of AP onset) than those without IPN. Contrast to the study

Table 3 Univariate logistic regression analysis for IPN

Elements	Odds ratio	95 % Confidence Interval	*p* Value
Age	1.005	0.977–1.034	0.734
Gender	0.447	0.199–1.006	0.052
BMI	1.105	0.942–1.296	0.218
APACHE II score	1.288	1.168–1.421	<0.001
Hemoglobin	0.991	0.976–1.006	0.221
Hematocrit	0.025	0.000–5.185	0.175
Platelet	0.988	0.981–0.996	0.002
CRP	1.010	1.004–1.017	0.001
WBC	0.941	0.865–1.023	0.153
Lymphocyte count	0.020	0.003–0.123	<0.001
NLR	1.059	1.015–1.104	0.008
Albumin	0.858	0.762–0.967	0.012
Amylase	1.001	1.000–1.001	0.034
Lipase	1.000	1.000–1.000	0.750
HLA-DR	0.909	0.806–1.025	0.120
CD3+ T cell	0.945	0.872–1.025	0.173
CD4+ T cell	0.944	0.844–1.055	0.310
CD8+ T cell	0.930	0.807–1.071	0.312
CD4+/CD8+ T cell	0.953	0.254–3.580	0.944

IPN infected pancreatic necrosis, *BMI* Body Mass Index, *APACHE II score* Acute Physiology and Chronic Health Enquiry II score, *CRP* C-reactive protein, *WBC* white blood cells, *NLR* Neutrophil-lymphocyte ratio, *ERCP* Endoscopic Retrograde Cholangiopancreatography, *HLA-DR* human leukocyte antigen-DR

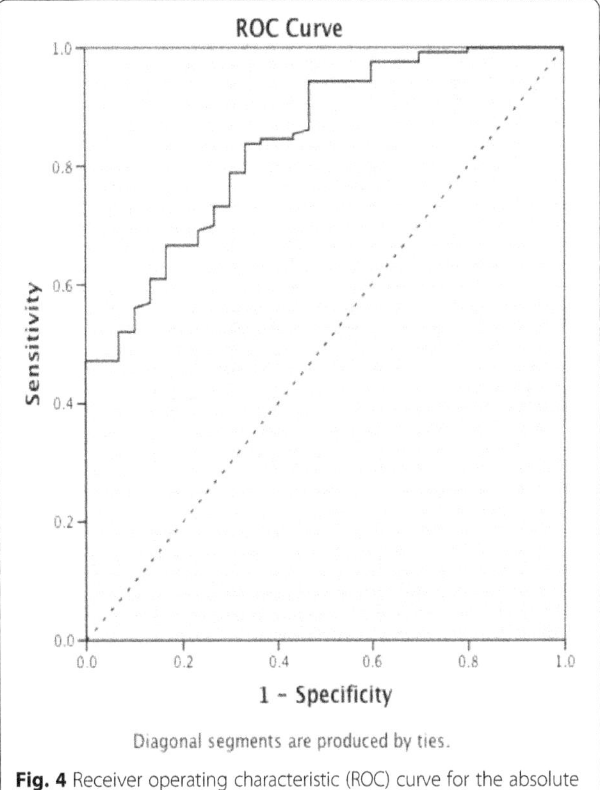

Fig. 4 Receiver operating characteristic (ROC) curve for the absolute lymphocyte count in predicting infected pancreatic necrosis (IPN)

of Azab et al., our study indicated that NLR did not show good prognostic value when compared with lymphocyte count [15]. However, in Azab et al.'s study, the primary outcome was severity instead of secondary infection, which might contribute to the difference of the results in the two studies.

Currently, immunosuppression is well accepted as an important risk factor for IPN in AP patients [8]. HLA-DR is a crucial immunological index and shows close relationship with sepsis and late mortality in SAP patients in many studies [16–18]. Early alteration of T lymphocyte subsets is also proved to have significant influence on the prognosis of AP patients [19]. Nonetheless, those immunological indexes need to be examined by flow cytometry, which are not routinely performed in every hospital due to its high cost and complexity. Furthermore, the accuracy of flow cytometer largely depends on the laboratory technician who carried out the experiment.

The absolute lymphocyte count, as a simple immunological index, can roughly and rapidly reflect the general change of the immune system. More importantly, the lymphocyte count can be easily assessed and is available in every hospital. Christophi et al. first evaluated the prognostic value of the absolute lymphocyte count in 104 male patients and 50 female patients with acute pancreatitis. They classified the patients according to their severities, mild and severe group. They found that the mean absolute lymphocyte count in the patients with SAP was significantly lower than those with mild AP and concluded that the absolute lymphocyte count had an accurate predictive power for AP severity. However, major flaws in that study were as follows: First, the patients included in that study were not restricted to those in the acute phase. Second, the results of the statistic analysis were not powerful enough to get such a solid conclusion. More recently, a study performed by Conlledo et al. confirmed that early lymphocyte count was

Table 4 Multivariate stepwise logistical regression and receiver operator characteristic (ROC) curve to predict IPN

Element	Odds Ratio (95 % CI)	*p* Value	AUROC (95 % CI)	*p* Value
Lymphocyte count	0.006 (0.000–0.100)	<0.001	0.842 (0.769–0.914)	<0.001
APACHE II score	1.299 (1.153–1.464)	<0.001	0.819 (0.722–0.917)	<0.001

ROC receiver operator characteristic, *IPN* infected pancreatic necrosis, *AUROC* area under receiver operating characteristic curve, *CI* confidence interval, *APACHE II score* Acute Physiology and Chronic Health Enquiry II score

independently associated with increased mortality in patients with sepsis or septic shock [20]. Besides, the study also indicated that the absolute lymphocyte count was closely associated with late infection.

One latest retrospective study by Zeng et al. identified the independent risk factors for pancreatic infection in 163 patients with acute pancreatitis [11]. They performed multiple logistic analyses and concluded that increased lactate dehydrogenase (LDH), high CT severity index, delayed fluid resuscitation and hypoxemia were independent risk factors for predicting IPN in patients with SAP. Nonetheless, they did not integrate the absolute lymphocyte count into their analysis.

Circulating lymphocyte subsets in acute pancreatitis have also been studied for a long time in the literature [21]. Many studies suggested that dysregulation of T lymphocytes played a vital role in the process of acute pancreatitis [22, 23] and down regulation of HLA-DR indicated IPN development and poor prognosis [16, 24]. In our patients, significantly down-regulated HLA-DR was also seen in those AP patients with IPN. However, the relationship between HLA-DR and IPN was not strong enough, probably attributing to the limited sample size. Similar to previous studies [19], the percentage of mature T lymphocyte was also a bit lower in the patients with IPN, as well as the percentages of CD 4+ and CD8+ T lymphocytes. These results demonstrated that the occurrence of immunosuppression at the early stage of acute pancreatitis might be a strong independent risk factor for IPN development in the late stage. To verify this hypothesis, further larger studies might be needed.

Several limitations of our study were listed as follows: Firstly, because of the small number of the IPN patients, the predictive power might be slightly influenced. Secondly, the retrospective nature of the study limited the extension of the study. Lastly, there were some data missing in the respect of HLA-DR and T lymphocyte subsets, which may also have some influence over the results. However, the majority of the abovementioned limitations were not thought to have too much influence on the results as they were equally existed in the two groups.

Conclusion

In summary, early immunosuppression always occurs in AP patients who might develop IPN in the late stage of the disease. Reduced lymphocyte count at the initial stage of the disease (within 48 h of AP onset), which simply and generally reflects the dysfunction of the immune system, might be an early and powerful predictor for IPN in AP patients.

Competing interests

The authors declare that they have no competing interests.

Authors' contributions

XS and JS carried out the studies and drafted the manuscript. LK and LZ carried out the data collection and performed statistical analysis. BQL and ZHT participated in the participated in the design of the study and performed the statistical analysis. WQL, NL and JSL conceived of the study, and participated in its design and coordination and helped to draft the manuscript. All authors read and approved the final manuscript.

Acknowledgements

This research was supported by the National Science Foundation of China (81170438 and 81200334). The authors gratefully acknowledge this support.

Author details

[1]Surgical Intensive Care Unit (SICU), Department of General Surgery, Jinling Hospital, Medical School of Nanjing University, No. 305 Zhongshan East Road, Nanjing 210002, Jiangsu Province, China. [2]Department of General Surgery, Jinling Hospital, Medical School of Nanjing University, No. 305 Zhongshan East Road, Nanjing 210002, Jiangsu Province, China.

References

1. Neoptolemos JP, Raraty M, Finch M, Sutton R. Acute pancreatitis: the substantial human and financial costs. Gut. 1998;42(6):886–91.
2. Banks PA, Bollen TL, Dervenis C, Gooszen HG, Johnson CD, Sarr MG, et al. Classification of acute pancreatitis—2012: revision of the Atlanta classification and definitions by international consensus. Gut. 2013;62(1):102–11.
3. Petrov MS, Shanbhag S, Chakraborty M, Phillips AR, Windsor JA. Organ failure and infection of pancreatic necrosis as determinants of mortality in patients with acute pancreatitis. Gastroenterology. 2010;139(3):813–20.
4. Besselink MG, van Santvoort HC, Boermeester MA, Nieuwenhuijs VB, van Goor H, Dejong CH, et al. Timing and impact of infections in acute pancreatitis. Br J Surg. 2009;96(3):267–73.
5. van Santvoort HC, Besselink MG, Bakker OJ, Hofker HS, Boermeester MA, Dejong CH, et al. A step-up approach or open necrosectomy for necrotizing pancreatitis. N Engl J Med. 2010;362(16):1491–502.
6. Gloor B, Muller CA, Worni M, Martignoni ME, Uhl W, Buchler MW. Late mortality in patients with severe acute pancreatitis. Br J Surg. 2001;88(7):975–9.
7. Rau BM, Kruger CM, Hasel C, Oliveira V, Rubie C, Beger HG, et al. Effects of immunosuppressive and immunostimulative treatment on pancreatic injury and mortality in severe acute experimental pancreatitis. Pancreas. 2006;33(2):174–83.
8. Qin Y, Pinhu L, You Y, Sooranna S, Huang Z, Zhou X, et al. The role of Fas expression on the occurrence of immunosuppression in severe acute pancreatitis. Dig Dis Sci. 2013;58(11):3300–7.
9. Binnetoglu E, Akbal E, Gunes F, Sen H. The prognostic value of neutrophil-lymphocyte ratio in acute pancreatitis is controversial. J Gastrointest Surg. 2014;18(4):885.
10. Christophi C, McDermott F, Hughes ES. Prognostic significance of the absolute lymphocyte count in acute pancreatitis. Am J Surg. 1985;150(3):295–6.
11. Zeng YB, Zhan XB, Guo XR, Zhang HG, Chen Y, Cai QC, et al. Risk factors for pancreatic infection in patients with severe acute pancreatitis: an analysis of 163 cases. J Dig Dis. 2014;15(7):377–85.
12. Marshall JC, Cook DJ, Christou NV, Bernard GR, Sprung CL, Sibbald WJ. Multiple organ dysfunction score: a reliable descriptor of a complex clinical outcome. Crit Care Med. 1995;23(10):1638–52.
13. Dellinger EP, Forsmark CE, Layer P, Levy P, Maravi-Poma E, Petrov MS, et al. Determinant-based classification of acute pancreatitis severity: an international multidisciplinary consultation. Ann Surg. 2012;256(6):875–80.
14. Isenmann R, Beger HG. Natural history of acute pancreatitis and the role of infection. Bailliere's Best Prac Res Clin Gastroenterol. 1999;13(2):291–301.
15. Azab B, Jaglall N, Atallah JP, Lamet A, Raja-Surya V, Farah B, et al. Neutrophil-lymphocyte ratio as a predictor of adverse outcomes of acute pancreatitis. Pancreatology. 2011;11(4):445–52.
16. Ho YP, Sheen IS, Chiu CT, Wu CS, Lin CY. A strong association between down-regulation of HLA-DR expression and the late mortality in patients with severe acute pancreatitis. Am J Gastroenterol. 2006;101(5):1117–24.

17. Yu WK, Li WQ, Li N, Li JS. Mononuclear histocompatibility leukocyte antigen-DR expression in the early phase of acute pancreatitis. Pancreatology. 2004;4(3–4):233–43.
18. Satoh A, Miura T, Satoh K, Masamune A, Yamagiwa T, Sakai Y, et al. Human leukocyte antigen-DR expression on peripheral monocytes as a predictive marker of sepsis during acute pancreatitis. Pancreas. 2002;25(3):245–50.
19. Pietruczuk M, Dabrowska MI, Wereszczynska-Siemiatkowska U, Dabrowski A. Alteration of peripheral blood lymphocyte subsets in acute pancreatitis. World J Gastroenterol. 2006;12(33):5344–51.
20. Conlledo R, Rodriguez A, Godoy J, Merino C, Martinez F. Total globulins and lymphocyte count as markers of mortality in sepsis and septic shock. Rev Chilena Infectol. 2012;29(2):192–9.
21. Pezzilli R, Billi P, Beltrandi E, Maldini M, Mancini R, Morselli Labate AM, et al. Circulating lymphocyte subsets in human acute pancreatitis. Pancreas. 1995;11(1):95–100.
22. Chaloner C, Laing I, Heath DI, Imrie CW, Braganza JM. Dysregulation of T cell-macrophage network in severe acute pancreatitis. Biochem Soc Trans. 1993;21(4):451S.
23. Qin Y, Liao P, He S, Yin Y, Song S, Hu J, et al. Detection of FasL mRNA, sFasL and their regulatory effect on T lymphocyte subsets in patients with severe acute pancreatitis. Xi bao yu fen zi mian yi xue za zhi = Chinese journal of cellular and molecular immunology. 2013;29(11):1189–92.
24. Lin ZQ, Guo J, Xia Q, Yang XN, Huang W, Huang ZW, et al. Human leukocyte antigen-DR expression on peripheral monocytes may be an early marker for secondary infection in severe acute pancreatitis. Hepatogastroenterology. 2013.

An indeterminate mucin-producing cystic neoplasm containing an undifferentiated carcinoma with osteoclast-like giant cells: a case report of a rare association of pancreatic tumors

Marco Chiarelli[1], Angelo Guttadauro[2], Martino Gerosa[1], Alessandro Marando[3], Francesco Gabrielli[2], Matilde De Simone[4] and Ugo Cioffi[4*]

Abstract

Background: Only few case reports of mucinous cystic pancreatic neoplasm containing an undifferentiated carcinoma with osteoclast-like giant cells have been described in the literature. In the majority of cases this unusual association of tumors seems related to a favorable outcome. We present the second case of an indeterminate mucin-producting cystic neoplasm containing an area of carcinoma with osteoclast-like giant cells. The specific features of the two histotypes and the rapid course of the disease make our clinical case remarkable.

Case presentation: A 68 year old female came to our attention for a pancreatic macrocystic mass detected with ultrasonography. Her past medical history was silent. The patient reported upper abdominal discomfort for two months; nausea, vomiting or weight loss were not reported. Physical examination revealed a palpable mass in the epigastrium; scleral icterus was absent. Cross-sectional imaging showed a complex mass of the neck and body of the pancreas, characterized by multiple large cystic spaces separated by thick septa and an area of solid tissue located in the caudal portion of the lesion. The patient underwent total pancreatectomy with splenectomy. Pathological examination revealed a mucinous cystic neoplasm with a component of an undifferentiated carcinoma with osteoclast-like giant cells. Because of the absence of ovarian-type stroma, the lesion was classified as an indeterminate mucin-producing cystic neoplasm of the pancreas. The immunohistochemical studies evidenced no reactivity of osteclast-like giant cells to epithelial markers but showed a positive reactivity to histiocytic markers. Numerous pleomorphic giant cells with an immunohistochemical sarcomatoid profile were present in the undifferentiated carcinoma with osteoclast-like giant cells. A rapid tumor progression was observed: liver metastases were detected after 4 months. The patient received adjuvant chemotherapy (Gemcitabine) but expired 10 months after surgery.

Conclusion: Our case confirms that the presence of a solid area in a cystic pancreatic tumor at cross-sectional imaging should raise a suspicion of malignant transformation. The lack of ovarian-type stroma in a pancreatic mucinous cystic neoplasm and the presence of pleomorphic giant cells in an undifferentiated carcinoma with osteoclast-like giant cells could be a marker of a poor prognosis.

Keywords: Mucinous cystic neoplasm, Intraductal papillary mucinous neoplasm, Osteoclast-like giant cells carcinoma, Pleomorphic giant cell carcinoma, Pancreas

* Correspondence: ugocioffi5@gmail.com
[4]Department of Surgery, University of Milan, Milan, Italy
Full list of author information is available at the end of the article

Background

The World Health Organization (WHO) classifies pancreatic mucin-producing cystic tumors into two different pathological entities: mucinous cystic neoplasm (MCN) and intraductal papillary mucinous neoplasm (IPMN) [1]. MCNs are thick-walled macrocystic tumors characterized by the absence of communication with ductal system. The distinctive histological feature of an MCN is a columnar mucin-producing epithelium supported by an ovarian-type stroma; this neoplasm occurs typically in premenopausal women [1–3]. IPMNs are intraductal tumors characterized by epithelial papillary proliferation and mucin hypersecretion causing a typical cystic dilatation of the pancreatic ductal system. IPMNs occur frequently in the head of the gland and are characterized by the communication between the tumor and the pancreatic ducts [1, 3]. IPMN has an equal gender distribution and occurs frequently in the seventh decade of life [1]. On the basis of epithelial atypia and invasiveness, cystic neoplasms are classified as adenoma, non-invasive carcinoma and invasive carcinoma [1, 3].

The undifferentiated carcinoma is a rare and aggressive form of pancreatic neoplasm. The WHO classification describes two distinct histological types: osteoclast-like giant cell carcinoma (OGCC) and pleomorphic giant cell carcinoma (PGCC) [1]. PGCC shows a sarcomatoid growth pattern, characterized by the presence of pleomorphic mononucleated and multinucleated bizarre giant cells [1, 4]. OGCC is composed of spindle-shaped or ovoidal mononuclear cells and scattered giant cells with multiple small regular nuclei [1, 4].

In 1981, Posen described for the first time the association of a giant cell tumor of the osteoclastic type with a mucous secreting cystic pancreatic neoplasm and since then only 12 cases have been reported [5, 6]. In a recent review Wada et al. analyzing all the cases in the literature, reported a favourable prognosis for this particular tumor association [6]. We present the second case in the literature of a patient with an indeterminate mucin-producing cystic neoplasm containing a single area of undifferentiated carcinoma with osteoclast- like giant cells, characterized by a rapid disease progression.

Case presentation

Clincal history and treatment

A 68 year old caucasian female with a pancreatic cystic neoplasm diagnosed on ultrasonography (US) presented at our Institute in December 2013. Her past medical history was silent. No abuse of ethanol or smoking was reported. The patient reported upper abdominal discomfort for 2 months; nausea, vomiting or weight loss were not referred. The physical examination revealed a palpable mass in the epigastrium; scleral icterus was absent. No other clinical abnormalities were detected.

The US showed a 5 × 6 cm pancreatic macrocystic lesion localized in the body of the gland. Laboratory tests showed that blood cell counts and C-reactive protein were normal. Levels of serum glucose, creatinine, albumin, aminotransferase, gamma-glutamyl transferase, alkaline phosphatase and lipase were all within normal limits. The serum levels of the following tumor markers were elevated: carcino-embryonic antigen (CEA) was 196 ng/ml (normal range <5 ng/ml) and carbohydrate antigen 19-9 (CA 19-9) was 66 U/ml (normal range <33 U/ml).

The patient underwent a triphasic multidetector computed tomography (CT) scan and a T1, T2-weighted and DWI contrast enhanced magnetic resonance imaging (MRI) with intravenous Gadolinium administration.

The CT scan showed a large complex cystic and solid mass measuring 5 × 3 × 6 cm involving the neck and the body of the pancreas (Fig. 1a). The tumor had a predominant central component characterized by multiple large cystic spaces (up to 3 cm in diameter) separated by thick septa. A 2 cm area of low attenuation solid tissue was located between cyst walls in the caudal portion of the lesion. The main pancreatic duct was enlarged in its entirity (diameter 12 mm) with a more marked dilatation in the body and tail region. Irregular calcifications were evident in the peripheral portion of the tumor. There was compression of superior mesenteric vein by the mass with a minimal infiltration of the splenic vein. The CT scan of the chest and abdomen did not show any lymphadenopathy, hepatic and pulmonary metastasis.

MRI confirmed the complex pancreatic lesion featured by a large cystic portion with inner irregular septa and a peripheral solid area measuring 2 cm in the lower portion of the tumor (Fig. 1b). Cholangiopancreatographic images did not demonstrate a communication between the enlarged main pancreatic duct and the cystic mass; ectatic branch ducts were present in the body and tail region.

At laparotomy a large cystic mass involving the body and the neck of pancreas was confirmed. Further exploration showed an infiltration of the head of the gland but ruled out neoplastic spreading to adjacent organs and lymph nodes; the splenic vein was infiltrated by the mass at superior mesenteric veinous junction. Patient underwent total pancreatectomy with splenectomy and lymph node dissection. A US performed on 7th post-operative day ruled out any intra-abdominal fluid collection. Patient developed post-pancreaectomy diabetes which was difficult to control by insulin therapy. The patient was discharged 14 days after the operation.

Histopathological findings

Macroscopically the pancreas was involved by a 6 cm well-circumscribed round mass localized in the neck and the body with infiltration of the head; stomach, duodenum, common bile duct and spleen were not infiltrated.

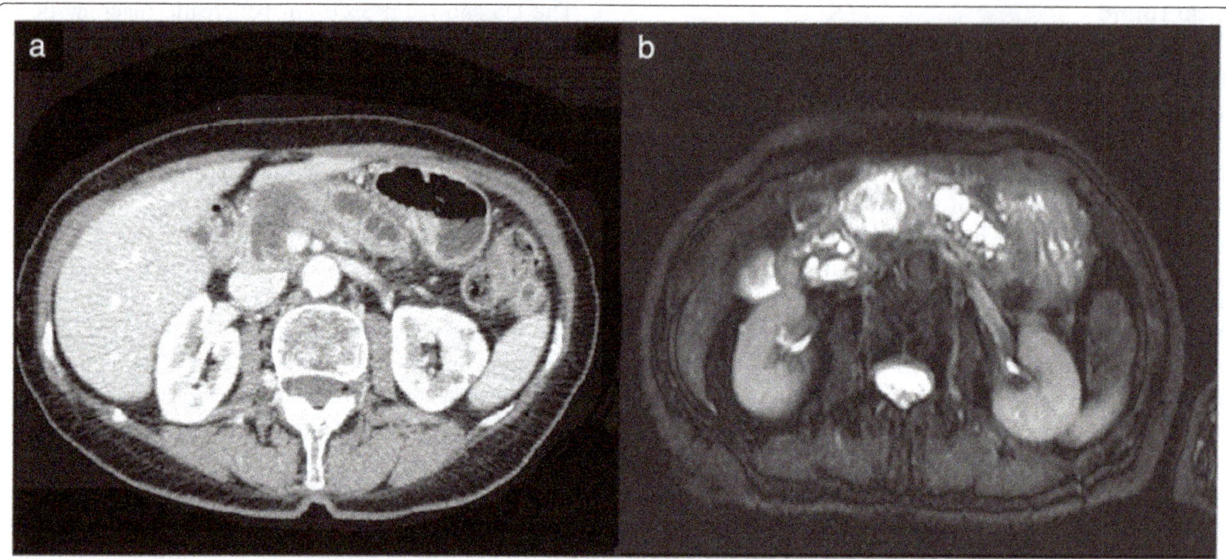

Fig. 1 a Contrast enhanced CT scan demonstrates a complex pancreatic macrocystic mass involving the neck and the body of the pancreas with a peripheral solid portion. **b** Axial T2-weighted MRI shows the high-intensity central cystic portion of the mass with inner irregular septa and the peripheral less intense solid tissue determining main duct dilatation

Externally the tumor presented a smooth reddish surface and the pancreatic parenchyma not involved by the lesion appeared fibrotic. On cut-section the lesion showed multilocular macrocystic spaces separated by fibrous septa and filled by a clear viscous mucoid fluid. The main pancreatic duct was ectatic but it was not possible to recognize a communication with the cystic lesion. A 2 cm single yellow solid area was located in the caudal portion of the mass.

Microscopically the tumor was principally composed of a cystic mucinous part characterized by a columnar mucinous epithelium with atypical nuclei, copious mitoses and stromal invasion. It was not possible to find an ovarian-like stroma (Fig. 2a). In the caudal part of the neoplasm there was a solid area containing mononuclear spindle cells, associated with pleomorphic giant cells (PGCs) and scattered multinucleated osteoclast-like giant cells (OGCs) (Fig. 2b).

The surgical margins were negative for neoplastic infiltration. No lymph node metastases were shown. There was no evidence of perineural or vascular infiltration.

The mononuclear spindle cells and pleomorphic giant cells were immunoreactive for epithelial markers including CK8/18 and CK19, and for vimentin and expressed a weak immunoreactivity for CD68 and a focal immunoreactivity for actin and CD10. The proliferative index (Ki-67) of the mononuclear spindle cells and pleomorphic giant cells was high (approximately 30 %) (Fig. 3a). Multinucleated

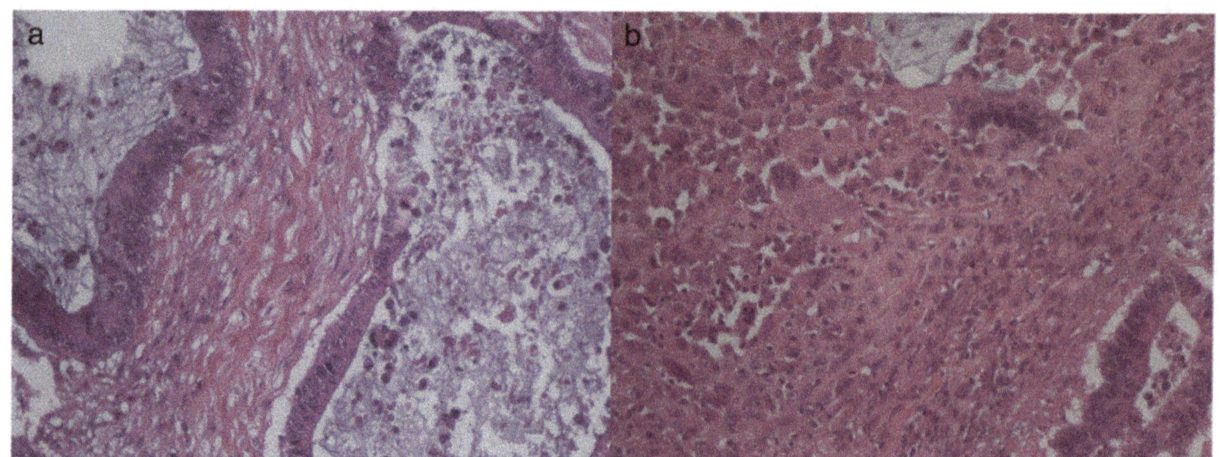

Fig. 2 a Microscopically the tumor is characterized by a predominant cystic lesion composed of a columnar mucinous epithelium with atypical nuclei, numerous mitoses and stromal invasion. An ovarian-type stroma is absent (hematoxylin/eosin staining, 20x). **b** The solid area contains mononuclear spindle-shaped cells, pleomorphic giant cells and scattered multinucleated osteoclast-like giant cells (hematoxylin/eosin staining, 20x)

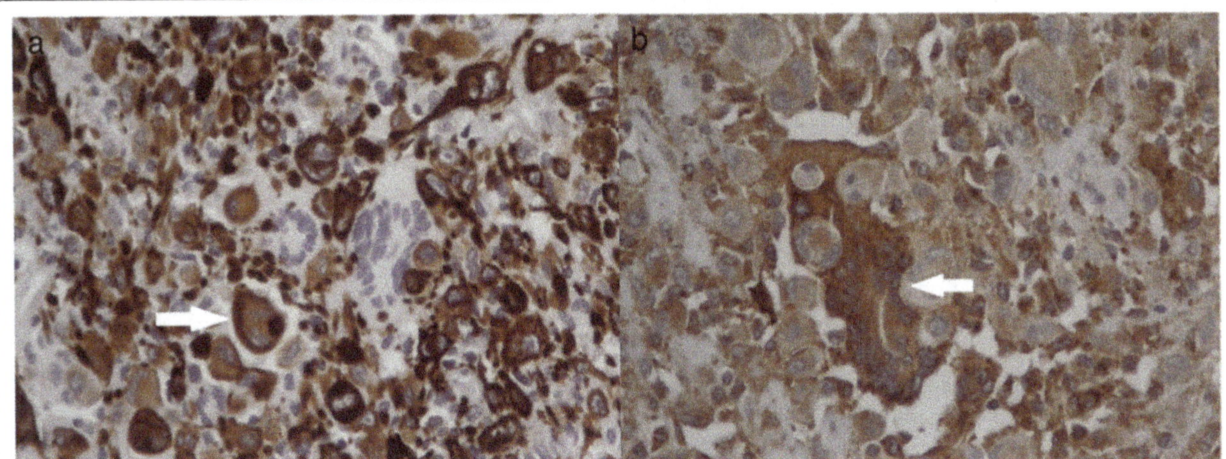

Fig. 3 a Mononuclear spindle-shaped cells and pleomorphic giant cells (*arrow*) are immunoreactive for epithelial markers (CK8/18), while multinucleated osteoclast-like giant cells are negative (40x). **b** Mononuclear spindle-shaped cells and pleomorphic giant cells stain weakly for histiocytic marker CD68; in contrast, multinucleated osteoclast-like giant cells show an intense immunoreactivity for CD68 (*arrow*) (40x)

osteoclast-like giant cells intensely expressed histiocytic marker (CD68) and vimentin but they were negative for epithelial markers (CK8/18 and CK19) and actin. In these cells Ki-67 immunoreaction was negative (Fig. 3b).

The histopathological findings supported the diagnosis of indeterminate mucin-producing cystic neoplasm with a component of osteoclast-like giant cell carcinoma.

Follow-up

Two months after surgery serum CEA and CA 19-9 decreased to 83 ng/ml and 31 U/ml, respectively. Nevertheless after 4 months serum CEA increased to 144 ng/ml and hepatic metastases were founded at follow-up CT scan. Gemcitabine single agent chemotherapy was started (1,00 mg/m^2 weekly × 7, then weekly × 3 every 4 weeks). CT scan performed 8 months after surgery showed the progression of liver metastases and appearance of lung metastases. The patient expired 10 months after surgery.

Discussion

International Consensus Guidelines have established how to diagnose and manage pancreatic cystic tumors [7]. Although their clinical, radiological and pathological features have been defined, in some cases the differential diagnosis between mucinous forms is difficult [8].

In our case the assessment of a correct preoperative diagnosis was difficult due to the clinical and radiological findings. Patient's age and main duct dilatation were elements in favor of IPMN, while female gender and the involvement of the body of the gland leaned towards MCN. However the diagnosis of IPMN was excluded as there was no communication between the cystic mass and the main pancreatic duct.

Tumor size, peripheral calcifications, irregular septa, and the presence of an intramural nodule pointed towards malignant transformation and led to surgical resection. Indeed all these radiological findings are very frequently associated with malignant histology [9].

On the basis of microscopic criteria (nuclear atypia, number of mitoses, and invasion into the stroma), the lesion should be categorized as a mucinous cystoadenocarcinoma. Nevertheless the absence of ovarian-type stroma made us to classify it as an indeterminate mucin-producing cystic neoplasm of the pancreas [7]. In the literature the lack of ovarian-type stroma is more frequent in postmenopausal women and MCNs that do no express ovarian-type stroma have a worse prognosis compared to those which have ovarian-type stroma [2, 10].

OGCC is rare pancreatic neoplasm: a US population study based on Surveillance, Epidemiology and End Result (SERR) database evidenced that its incidence is 11 % of all undifferentiated carcinomas of the pancreas [11].

In the past decades the histogenesis of OGCC was debated, but the more recent immunohistochemical studies demonstrate that OGCs present no reactivity to epithelial markers and show a positive reactivity to histiocytic marker CD68; by contrast, spindle-shaped mononuclear cells express epithelial markers [12, 13]. The immunoreactivity for Ki-67 reveals a low proliferative activity of OGCs and a high proliferative activity for mononuclear cells [13]. These data, as our findings, confirm the hypothesis that spindle-shaped mononuclear cells are neoplastic elements, while OGCs are not neoplastic and may have a histiocytic lineage [12, 13].

In our case numerous PGCs were detected in the solid area of the neoplasm. These cells are frequently characterized by immunoreactivity for epithelial markers like cytokeratins and CEA and by a high proliferative index; in some cases, PGCs express mesenchymal markers like vimentin [14]. These data support the hypothesis that PGCs are undifferentiated neoplastic cells derived from epithelial elements with a sarcomatoid profile. These histological changes are typical of the epithelial-mesenchimal transition which is a marker of tumor de-differentiation and invasiveness [15].

The simultaneous presence of PGCs and OGCs within the same tumor indicates a possible overlap between the two histological types: some authors propose to classify the mixed giant cell carcinoma as a different histopathological entity containing both osteoclastic and pleomorphic giant cells in significant proportion [4, 14, 16].

Incongruous data is there in the literature about OGCC prognosis. Early reports based on single case suggested that it might have a better outcome than ordinary ductal carcinoma [17]. However in a series of nine cases all patients but one died within 1 year from diagnosis [12]. In a retrospective analysis of 15 patients with anaplastic carcinoma of the pancreas, all long-term survivors presented a neoplasm containing OGCs and the median survival was significantly better in this histological type [18]. In two small series, OGCCs with a high proportion of PGCs were associated with a shorter survival [13, 19] and in an overall analysis of the few reported cases, the presence of a cell population expressing epithelial markers seemed to predict a worse prognosis [20].

Ours is the second case described in the english literature of an indeterminate mucin-producting cystic neoplasm containing an area of undifferentiated carcinoma with osteoclast-like giant cells. In a review that analyzed all cases of MCN associated with OGCC, 10 of 12 patients were alive at follow-up [6]. By contrast our report was remarkable for the rapid progression of the tumor. It is interesting to note that both cystic and solid components of the neoplasm presented histological features of malignancy. Only further studies based on large series with longer follow-up will clarify if the absence of ovarian-type stroma and the presence of PGCs could be related with the outcome of these tumors.

Conclusions

There are only few case reports in literature of an MCN with a component of OGCC. Due to limited data it is difficult to establish accurately radiological presentation and clinical outcome of these patients. Our case confirms that the presence of solid area in a cystic tumor at cross-sectional imaging should raise a suspicion of malignant transformation. In conclusion, the peculiar histological features of the two neoplasms and the rapid course of the disease make our case remarkable.

Consent

Written informed consent was obtained from the patient for publication of this Case report and any accompanying images. A copy of the written consent is available for review by the Editor of this journal.

Abbreviations

WHO: World Health Organization; SEER: Surveillance, Epidemiology and End Result; MCN: Mucinous cystic neoplasm; IPMN: Intraductal papillary mucinous neoplasm; OGCC: Osteoclast-like giant cell carcinoma; PGCC: Pleomorphic giant cell carcinoma; OGCs: Osteoclast-like giant cells; PGCs: Pleomorphic giant cells; CEA: Carcino-embryonic antigen; CA 19-9: Carbohydrate antigen 19-9; US: Ultrasonography; CT: Computed tomography; MRI: Magnetic resonance imaging; CK8/18: Cytokeratin 8/18; CK19: Cytokeratin 19; CD68: Cluster of differentiation 68; CD10: Cluster of differentiation 10.

Competing interest

None of the contributing authors have any conflict of interest, including specific financial interests or relationships and affiliations relevant to the subject matter or materials discussed in the manuscript.

Authors' contributions

MC: carried out the study, drafted the manuscript and revised it. AG: collected information of patient and revised the contents of discussion and conclusions of the manuscript. MG: collected information of patient and wrote the contents of clinical history, treatment and follow-up of the manuscript. AM: checked the histopathology and wrote the contents of histopatological findings of the manuscript. FG: revised the contents of the discussion and conclusions of the manuscript. MDS: revised the manuscript. UC: carried out the concept and the design of the study and revised the manuscript. All authors read and approve the final manuscript.

Acknowledgements

We thank Dr. Gerardo Cioffi, native speaker, for reviewing the English language.

Author details

[1]Department of Surgery, Ospedale Alessandro Manzoni, Lecco, Via dell'Eremo 9/11, 23900 Lecco, LC, Italy. [2]Department of Surgery, University of Milan-Bicocca, Istituti Clinici Zucchi, Via Zucchi, 24, 20900 Monza, MB, Italy. [3]Department of Pathology, Ospedale Alessandro Manzoni, Lecco, Via dell'Eremo 9/11, 23900, Lecco LC, Italy. [4]Department of Surgery, University of Milan, Milan, Italy.

References

1. Bosman FT, Carniero F, Hruban RH, Theise ND, editors. WHO classification of tumours of the digestive system. 4th ed. Lyon: IARC; 2010.
2. Thompson LDR, Becker RC, Przygodzki RM, Adair CF, Heffess CS. Mucinous cystic neoplasm (mucinous cystoadenocarcinoma of low-grade malignant potential) of the pancreas. A clinicopathologic study of 130 cases. Am J Surg Pathol. 1999;23:1–16.
3. Campbell F, Azadeh B. Cystic neoplasm of the exocrine pancreas. Histopathology. 2008;52:539–51.
4. Moore JC, Bentz JS, Hilden K, Adler DG. Osteoclastic and pleomorphic giant cell tumors of the pancreas: a review of clinical, endoscopic, and pathologic features. World J Gastrointest Endosc. 2010;2:15–9.
5. Posen JA. Giant cell tumor of the pancreas of the osteoclastic type associated with a mucous secreting cystadenocarcinoma. Hum Pathol. 1981;12:944–7.
6. Wada T, Itano O, Oshima G, Chiba N, Ishikawa H, Koyama Y, et al. A male case of an undifferentiated carcinoma with osteoclast-like giant cells originating in an indeterminate mucin-producing cystic neoplasm of the pancreas. A case report and review of the literature. World J Surg Oncol. 2011;9:100.
7. Tanaka M, Chari S, Adsay V, Fernandez-del Castillo C, Falconi M, Shimizu M, et al. International consensus guidelines for management of intraductal papillary mucinous neoplasm and mucinous cystic neoplasm of the pancreas. Pancreatology. 2006;6:17–32.

8. Sarr MG, Murr M, Smyrk TC, Yeo CJ, del-Castillo Fernandez C, Hawes RH, et al. Primary cystic neoplasm of the pancreas: neoplastic disorders of emerging importance – current state-of-the-art and unanswered questions. J Gastrointest Surg. 2003;7:417–28.
9. Sarr MG, Carpenter HA, Prabhakar LP, Orchard TF, Hughes S, van Heerden JA, et al. Clinical and pathologic correlation of 84 mucinous cystic neoplasm of the pancreas. Ann Surg. 2000;231:205–12.
10. Zamboni G, Scarpa A, Bogina G, Iacono C, Bassi C, Talamini G, et al. Mucinous cystic tumors of the pancreas: clinicopathological features, prognosis, and relationship to other mucinous cystic tumors. Am J Surg Pathol. 1999;23:410–22.
11. Clark CJ, Graham RP, Arun JS, Harmsen WS, Reid-Lombardo KM. Clinical outcomes for anaplastic pancreatic cancer: a population-based study. J Am Coll Surg. 2012;215:627–34.
12. Molberg KH, Heffess C, Delgado R, Albores-Saavedra J. Undifferentiated carcinoma with osteoclast-like giant cells of the pancreas and periampullary region. Cancer. 1998;82:1279–87.
13. Deckard-Janatpour K, Kragel S, Teplitz RL, Min BH, Gumerlock PH, Frey CF, et al. Tumors of the pancreas with osteoclast-like and pleomorphic giant cells. An immunohistochemical and ploidy study. Arch Pathol Lab Med. 1998;122: 266–72.
14. Watanabe M, Miura H, Inoue H, Uzuki M, Noda Y, Fujita N, et al. Mixed osteoclastic/pleomorphic – type giant cell tumor of the pancreas with ductal adenocarcinoma: histochemical and immunohistochemical study with review of the literature. Pancreas. 1997;15:201–8.
15. Lewandrowski KB, Weston L, Dickersin GR, Rattner DW, Compton CC. Giant cell tumor of the pancreas of mixed osteoclastic and pleomorphic cell type: evidence for a histogenetic relationship and mesenchymal differentiation. Hum Pathol. 1990;21:1184–7.
16. Ezenekwe AM, Collins BT, Ponder TB. Mixed osteoclastic/pleomorphic giant cell tumor of the pancreas. Acta Cytol. 2005;49:549–53.
17. Jeffrey I, Crow J, Ellis BW. Osteoclast-type giant cell tumor of the pancreas. J Clin Pathol. 1983;36:1165–70.
18. Strobel O, Hartwig W, Bergmann F, Hinz U, Hackert T, Grenacher L, et al. Anaplastic pancreatic cancer: presentation, surgical management, and outcome. Surgery. 2011;149:200–8.
19. Moore JC, Hilden K, Bentz JS, Pearson RK, Adler DG. Osteoclastic and pleomorphic giant cell tumors of the pancreas diagnosed via EUS-guided FNA: unique clinical, endoscopic, and pathologic findings in a series of 5 patients. Gastrointest Endosc. 2009;69:162–6.
20. Machado MA, Herman P, Montagnini AL, Jukemura J, Leite KR, Machado MC. Benign variant of osteoclast-type giant cell tumor of the pancreas. Importance of the lack of epithelial differentiation. Pancreas. 2001;22:105–7.

Prevalence of Non-Alcoholic Fatty Pancreas Disease (NAFPD) and its risk factors among adult medical check-up patients in a private hospital

Cosmas Rinaldi A. Lesmana[1,2*], Levina S. Pakasi[1], Sri Inggriani[3], Maria L. Aidawati[3] and Laurentius A. Lesmana[1]

Abstract

Background: The clinical significance of non-alcoholic fatty pancreatic disease (NAFPD) or fatty pancreas is largely unknown. It is often an incidental finding on abdominal ultrasound, which is not explored further, especially its association with metabolic condition and the risk of pancreatic malignancy. The aim of this study is to evaluate the presence of NAFPD and its associated risk factors among adult medical check-up patients.

Method: A large cross-sectional study was done among adult medical check-up patients underwent abdominal ultrasound between January and December 2013 in Medistra Hospital, Jakarta. Data was obtained from the patients' medical record and include demographic data, blood pressures, fasting blood glucose level, and lipid profile. The presence of fatty pancreas was diagnosed by ultrasound. Bivariate and multivariate analyses were done to find associated risk factors for NAFPD. Statistical analysis was done using SPSS version 17.

Results: A total of 1054 cases were included in this study; pancreas cannot be visualized in 153 cases and were excluded from the analysis. Fatty pancreas was present in 315 (35.0 %) patients. Bivariate analyses found associations among fatty pancreas and several risk factors such as gender, age, systolic and diastolic blood pressures, body mass index (BMI), fasting plasma glucose (FPG), triglycerides (TG) and cholesterol levels.

Conclusion: Fatty pancreas is a common finding during medical check-up with a prevalence of 35 %. Fatty pancreas has significant association with metabolic factors and it might have an important role in risk of malignancy.

Keywords: Fatty pancreas, Metabolic syndrome, Non-alcoholic fatty pancreas disease, Risk factors

Background

High energy intake in human may lead to excessive fat which could be accumulated in visceral organs that are unusual for adipose tissue storage, the so-called ectopic fat [1]. Fatty pancreas or nonalcoholic fatty pancreatic disease (NAFPD) is an excessive fat infiltration of the pancreas due to obesity in the absence of significant alcohol intake [2]. Fatty pancreas is a common ultrasound finding which has increased echogenicity when compared to the normal pancreas [3].

On the contrary to the nonalcoholic fatty liver disease (NAFLD), the potential systemic and local consequences of excessive fat accumulation in the pancreas have not been well established. Fatty infiltration in the pancreas has been showed to correlate with the metabolic risk factors and may represent a meaningful manifestation of metabolic syndrome., [4, 5] Epidemiology study also suggests that obesity is a risk factor for pancreatic cancer [6]. Based on a recent study, fatty infiltration in the pancreas may increase the risk of pancreatic ductal adenocarcinoma beyond the effect of obesity alone [7]. The problem with

* Correspondence: medicaldr2001id@yahoo.com
[1]Digestive Disease & GI Oncology Center, Medistra Hospital, Jakarta, Indonesia
[2]Department of Internal Medicine, Hepatobiliary Division, Cipto Mangunkusumo Hospital, University of Indonesia, Jakarta, Indonesia
Full list of author information is available at the end of the article

the organ location needs the more accurate imaging diagnostic procedures, such as abdominal MRI or even Endoscopic Ultrasound (EUS). The fat content of the pancreas also can be estimated by 3D two point Dixon techniques. However, in population or medical checkup settings, it would be unpractical and also costly to examine the pancreas [8–10].

Since the clinical implication of fatty pancreas is still a mater of debate, especially in countries where alcohol consumption is not an issue, therefore, this study was aimed to evaluate the presence of fatty pancreas and estabslihed its associated risk factors.

Method

Study design and subject

The study design was an analytical cross-sectional study among medical check-up patients in Medistra Hospital which has been approved from the Medistra hospital's local ethics committee between January and December 2013. Inclusion criteria was adult patients aged more than 18 years, no serious illness at the time of examination, having routine laboratory check-up for liver function test, fasting plasma glucose (FPG) levels, and lipid profile, and underwent abdominal ultrasound assessment. None of the patients had a history of significant alcohol drinking (<20 g/day). Patients were excluded from analyses if the pancreas was not visualized on ultrasound or laboratory data was incomplete. Risk factors of NAFPD tested were gender, age group, history of diabetes, body mass index (BMI), systolic and diastolic blood pressures (BP), FPG, triglycerides, total cholesterol, low-density lipoprotein (LDL)-cholesterol, and high-density lipoprotein (HDL)-cholesterol levels. Diabetes mellitus (DM) is diagnosed based on clear history from patient's interview and the blood glucose database. The metabolic data parameters were collected as the parameters which become our hospital medical check-up standard examination. The minimum sample size for estimating one population proportion at an anticipated proportion of 50 %, 99 % level of confidence and 5 % margin of error was 664 patients.

Diagnosis of fatty pancreas

Fatty pancreas or pancreas lipomatosis was diagnosed using abdominal ultrasound technique performed by one experienced radiologist in the hospital using a high-resolution ultrasound machine equipped with a 3.5 MHz convex-array probe (LOGIC S7, GE System, US). The radiologist who performed the ultrasound examinations was blinded to the laboratory data; the results were evaluated by another experienced radiologist to ensure unbiased evaluation. Pancreatic echogenicity was compared to the liver echogenicity at the same depth on a longitudinal scan taken near the abdominal midline [11]. If the liver also showed increased echogenicity, comparison was also made with the renal cortex. Diagnosis of pancreas lipomatosis was established if there is increased echogenicity of the pancreas over the liver or renal cortex.

Laboratory tests

All subjects underwent laboratory tests for standard medical check-up consisting of complete peripheral blood test, liver function test, fasting plasma glucose and lipid profiling. These tests were performed after an overnight fast for a minimum of 10 h.

Statistical analyses

Characteristics of the study subjects were presented descriptively. Bivariate analyses between the presence of NAFPD and risk factors were performed using the Chi-square test. A p value of less than 0.05 was considered significant. Multivariate logistic regression was used to find independent risk factors for NAFPD. Statistical analysis was done using SPSS version 17.0.

Results

Characteristics of the study subjects

There were 1054 cases enrolled in the analysis; 720 (68.3 %) of them were men. The mean age was 43.1 ± 12.19 years old. Other characteristics were summarized in Table 1. Pancreas was non-visualized in 153 (14.5 %) cases. In the remaining 901 cases, fatty pancreas was found in 315 (35 %) patients.

Associations among metabolic risk factors and fatty liver

The presence of fatty pancreas were significantly associated with male gender, age >35 years, higher systolic and diastolic blood pressures, fasting blood glucose >100 mg/

Table 1 Characteristics of the study subject ($N = 1054$)

Characteristic	Mean (SD)	N	%
Male gender		720	68.3
Age (years)	43.1 ± 12.19		
Age >35 years old		723	68.6
Body mass index (kg/m^2)	24.9 ± 3.96		
Systolic blood pressure (mmHg)	120 ± 37.2		
Diastolic blood pressure (mmHg)	75 ± 9.9		
Fasting plasma glucose (mg/dL)	96.7 ± 24.69		
Triglyceride levels (mg/dL)	127.1 ± 89.15		
Total cholesterol levels (mg/dL)	205.4 ± 59.0		
LDL-cholesterol	133.2 ± 35.29		
HDL-cholesterol	51.1 ± 12.87		
NAFLD			
No		516	49.0
Yes		538	51.0

dL, triglycerides, total and LDL-cholesterol, and lower HDL cholesterol levels (Table 2).

Association between fatty pancreas and fatty liver

Fatty liver was present in 538 (51.0 %) of the total study subjects. Among 901 patients with visualized pancreas, fatty pancreas coexisted with fatty liver in 232 (25.7 %) patients; both were absent in 381 (42.3 %) patients. In addition, fatty pancreas with normal liver was found in 83 patients (16.0 %) and fatty liver with normal pancreas was seen in 205 (39.4 %) patients. There was a significant association between fatty pancreas and fatty liver (OR: 5.195; 95 %CI: 3.838-7.032; $p < 0.001$).

When the 381 patients with neither fatty liver nor fatty pancreas were excluded, fatty pancreas coexisted with fatty liver in 232 patients (44.6 %). This number can be brokendown further, revealing that fatty pancreas was found in 53.1 % of patients with fatty liver whereas fatty liver can be found in 73.7 % of patients with fatty pancreas (Fig. 1).

Association between fatty pancreas and diabetes mellitus

Type 2 diabetes mellitus was present in 62 (6.9 %) of the study subects and fatty pancreas was detected in 31 (50 %) of them. Statistically, diabetes has significant associated with fatty pancreas (OR 1.953; 95 % CI: 1.164–3.280; $p < 0.001$). However, when entered into the multivariate analyses; diabetes failed to show a significant association, suggesting that it was a confounding factor rather than an independent risk factor.

Discussion

Characteristics of the study subjects

With a detection rate of 35 %, our study showed that the prevalence of nonalcoholic fatty pancreas is high among adult patients underwent routine medical check-up. A recent study involving 8097 subjects underwent health check-up in Taiwan found only 16 % prevalence of fatty pancreas detected by abdominal ultrasound [12]. On the contrary, a Korean study found that 67.9 % of 293 subjects visiting an obesity clinic had fatty pancreas detected by abdominal ultrasound. Larger sample size allows more valid generalization into the general population; therefore, the estimated prevalence of fatty pancreas in the real community may be best represented by the Taiwanese study. The subjects of our study might give an over-estimate result because most of our hospital's medical check-up subjects came from high social economic groups. Our study may also not represent the true Indonesian population since the patients were recruited from a referral private hospital. However, the high prevalence of NAFPD has given a new insight in patient's follow up and screening as the risk of malignancy might also be increasing. A more accurate estimation might be shown by a recent study among 685 Hong Kong Chinese healthy volunteers; the prevalence of fatty pancreas detected by fat-water magnetic resonance imaging was 16.1 % [13].

Association between fatty pancreeas and metabolic risk factors

Our results showed significant association between fatty pancreas and metabolic risk factors (Table 2). Table 3 showed independent risk factors to predict fatty pancreas. These results were consistent with previous epidemiological report in Hong Kong Chinese population [10]. The OR of DM and other variables mostly around the value of 2.0; therefore although systolic BP have higher OR, the difference with DM or triglycerides can be considered not too wide. However, the number of subjects with DM is relatively small compared to other variables. It could affect the statistical calculation of OR and may explain the slight difference with systolic BP.

Table 2 Associations among risk factors and the presence of fatty pancreas ($n = 901$)

Risk Factor	Fatty pancreas		Odds ratio	p value
	Yes ($n = 315$)	No ($n = 586$)	(95 % CI)	(χ^2)
Male sex ($n = 574$)	228 (72.4 %)	346 (59.0 %)	1.818 (1.351–2.446)	<0.001
Age > 35 years ($n = 612$)	268 (85.1 %)	344 (58.7 %)	4.011 (2.824–5.697)	<0.001
Systolic BP ≥ 130 mmHg ($n = 201$)	99 (31.4 %)	102 (17.4 %)	2.175 (1.580–2.994)	<0.001
Diastolic BP ≥ 85 mmHg ($n = 111$)	54 (17.1 %)	57 (9.7 %)	1.920 (1.286–2.866)	0.001
Body mass index ≥ 25 kg/m^2 ($n = 390$)	206 (65.4 %)	184 (31.4 %)	4.129 (3.088–5.520)	<0.001
Type 2 diabetes mellitus ($n = 62$)	31 (9.8 %)	31 (5.3 %)	1.954 (1.164–3.280)	0.010
FPG ≥ 100 mg/dL ($n = 187$)	99 (31.4 %)	88 (15.0 %)	2.594 (1.867–3.603)	<0.001
Triglycerides ≥ 150 mg/dL ($n = 226$)	105 (33.3 %)	121 (20.6 %)	1.921 (1.412–2.615)	<0.001
Total cholesterol ≥ 200 mg/dL ($n = 491$)	203 (64.4 %)	288 (49.1 %)	1.875 (1.415–2.486)	<0.001
LDL-C ≥ 100 mg/dL ($n = 742$)	275 (87.3 %)	467 (79.7 %)	1.752 (1.189–2.582)	0.004
HDL-C < 40 (M) or < 50 (F) mg/dL ($n = 194$)	86 (27.3 %)	108 (18.4 %)	1.662 (1.202–2.298)	0.002

BMI body mass index, ***FPG* fasting plasma glucose**, *LDL-C* low-density lipoprotein cholesterol, *HDL-C* high-density lipoprotein cholesterol

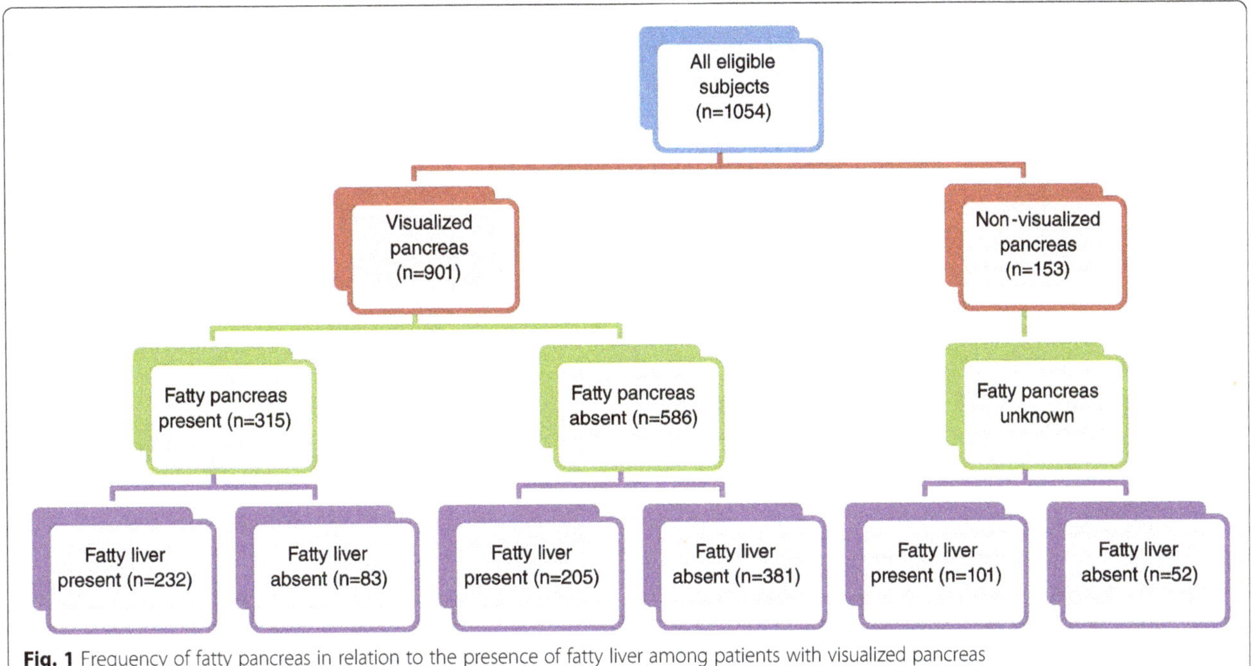

Fig. 1 Frequency of fatty pancreas in relation to the presence of fatty liver among patients with visualized pancreas

From the statistical point of view, clinical value of an OR occurs when it is more than 1.5. Compared to age or BMI (which have OR >4.0), the ORs of DM and systolic BP are much weaker, it's also the same with other variables with OR value less than 2.0. From the metabolic point of view, DM is considered as part of metabolic syndrome with could confound other variables within the metabolic markers group (such as cholesterol or TG). On the other hand, blood pressure is a hemodynamic marker. High blood pressure in metabolic syndrome is a consequence of insulin resistance with various underlying mechanisms [14]. Therefore, higher OR of systolic BP might reflect that is more important as risk factor than DM or other lipid parameters.

Association between fatty pancreas and fatty liver

Fatty liver was reported as a predictor of "hyperechogenic pancreas" seen during endoscopic ultrasound [15]. A postmortem study collected from 80 cadavers found that total pancreatic fat was a significant predictor of NAFLD, but no correlation was found between pancreatic fat and NAFLD activity score after corrected for body mass index [16]. Our study showed significant correlation between fatty pancreas and fatty liver, however whether with these two entities might doubling the risk of malignancy is still unknown.

Despite the presence of statistical association, the pathophysiology underlying both conditions might be coincidence rather than causative. Both fatty pancreas and fatty liver are significantly associated with metabolic risk factors due to excessive energy intake.

Association between fatty pancreas and diabetes mellitus

Based on our study, even though there is a significant association between the presence of fatty pancreas and diabetes mellitus, however the association was not observed in the multivariate analysis. Different result was reported among 7464 subjects underwent physical check-up in Taiwan. This might be due to the smaller size effect in the subgroup analysis. The investigators did found an independent association between fatty pancreas and diabetes (OR: 1.379; 95 %CI: 1-047-1.816) [17]. However, this study

Table 3 Independent risk factors to predict fatty pancreas ($N = 901$)

Risk factor	β	SE (β)	β/SE	OR_{adj}	95 % CI	*p* value
Age > 35 years	1.077	0.191	5.639	2.936	2.020–4.267	<0.001
BMI ≥ 25 kg/m²	1.261	0.154	8.188	3.529	2.607–4.775	<0.001
FPG ≥ 100 mg/dL	0.531	0.183	2.902	1.701	1.189–2.434	0.004
Total cholesterol ≥ 200 mg/dL	0.491	0.157	3.127	1.634	1.201–2.223	<0.001
Constant	−2.423					

BMI body mass index, ***FPG*** **fasting plasma glucose**

was not designed to establish a direct causal relationship between diabetes mellitus and fatty pancreas or *vice versa* and should be interpreted as such. The complex factor in insulin resistance pathway might play an important factor. High free fatty acid (FFA) will induce the accumulation of pancreatic fat and the fat deposition will disrupt the beta cell function. The beta cell dysfunction results in unmet relative insulin need to maintain optimal glycemic control and in combination with insulin resistance at the periphery synergistically contributes to the long-term hyperglycemia. This is an important pathway for the development of diabetes mellitus. In return, the insulin resistance condition where induced by FFA source in the pancreas might induce the chronic inflammation stage where this can become a malignancy risk [18]. With these findings, we might also need to screen our diabetes patients for pancreatic malignancy risk.

This study has several limitations. First, the study was designed as a cross-sectional study which cannot prove causal link between fatty pancreas and the associated factors. However, the large sample size in this study could provide generalization to the larger population of interest. Body mass index (BMI) as a risk for pancreatic lipomatosis might be a confounding factor to detect the presence of fatty pancreas. Second, the data about diabetes medication not being reported based on our MCU standard examination record. But this study has given the importance of metabolic factors associated with the presence of NAFPD. Third, the need to differentiate between simple steatosis and steatosis with inflammation in the pancreas has not been elucidated. The transabdominal ultrasound study might not be the best of choice, but ultrasound is still a qualified technique in an experienced hand, and also cheaper when compared to MRI in the community setting. Further study with ethical consideration will be needed to perform pancreas biopsy using EUS study.

Conclusion

The prevalence of NAFPD in Indonesia is high and it is strongly correlated with other metabolic conditions. The clinical significance of routine fatty pancreas screening needs to be included in our clinical practice. However, it would need further investigation about the long standing condition of fatty pancreas and the usefulness of pancreatic biopsy to see the possibility of disease progression.

Abbreviations

NAFPD: Non-alcoholic Fatty Pancreas Disease; NAFLD: Non-alcoholic Fatty Liver Disease; EUS: Endoscopic Ultrasound; BMI: Body Mass Index; FPG: Fasting Plasma Glucose; TG: Triglyceride; LDL: Low Density Lipoprotein; HDL: High Density Lipoprotein; BP: Blood Pressure.

Competing interests

The authors declare that they have no competing interests.

Author contribution

CRAL and LSP designed and conducted the study; LSP performed statistical analysis and drafted the manuscript. SR, MLA performed abdominal ultrasound, interpreted the data and contributed to the discussion. LAL supervised the study and contributed to the discussion, edited and approved the manuscript. All authors read and approved the manuscript.

Author details

[1]Digestive Disease & GI Oncology Center, Medistra Hospital, Jakarta, Indonesia. [2]Department of Internal Medicine, Hepatobiliary Division, Cipto Mangunkusumo Hospital, University of Indonesia, Jakarta, Indonesia. [3]Department of Radiology, Medistra Hospital, Jakarta, Indonesia.

References

1. Britton KA, Fox CS. Ectopic fat depots and cardiovascular disease. Circulation. 2011;124:e837–41.
2. Mathur A, Marine M, Lu D, Swartz-Basile DA, Saxena R, Zyromski NJ, et al. Nonalcoholic fatty pancreas disease. HPB (Oxford). 2007;9:312–8.
3. Marks WM, Filly RA, Callen PW. Ultrasonic evaluation of normal pancreatic echogenicity and its relationship to fat deposition. Radiology. 1980;137:475–9.
4. Lee JS, Kim SH, Jun DW, Han JH, Jang EC, Park JY, et al. Clinical implications of fatty pancreas: correlations between fatty pancreas and metabolic syndrome. World J Gastroenterol. 2009;15:1869–75.
5. Wu WC, Wang CY. Association between non-alcoholic fatty pancreatic disease (NAFPD) and the metabolic syndrome: case–control retrospective study. Cardiovasc Diabetol. 2013;12:77 (6 pages).
6. Patel AV, Rodriguez C, Bernstein L, Chao A, Thun MJ, Calle EE. Obesity, recreational physical activity, and risk of pancreatic cancer in a large U.S. Cohort. Cancer Epidemiol Biomarkers Prev. 2005;14:459–66.
7. Hori M, Takahashi M, Hiraoka N, Yamaji T, Mutoh M, Ishigamori R, et al. Association of pancreatic fatty infiltration with pancreatic ductal adenocarcinoma. Clin Translat Gastroenterol. 2014;5:e53. doi:10.1038/ctg.2014.5.
8. Sandrasegaran K, Lin C, Akisik FM, Tann M. State of the art pancreatic MRI. Am J Rad. 2010;195:42–53.
9. Sijens PE, Edens MA, Bakker SJ, Stolk RP. MRI determined fat content of human liver, pancreas and kidney. World J Gastroenterol. 2010;16(16):1993–8.
10. Powis ME, Chang KJ. Endoscopic ultrasound in the clinical staging and management of pancreatic cancer: Its impact on cost of treatment. Cancer Control. 2000;7(5):413–20.
11. Worthen NJ, Beabeu D. Normal pancreatic echogenicity: relatin to age and body fat. AJR. 1982;139:1095–8.
12. Wang C-Y, Ou H-Y, Chen M-F, Chang T-C, Chang C-J. Enigmatic ectopic fat: prevalence of nonalcoholic fatty pancreas disease and its associated factors in a Chinese population. J Am Heart Assoc. 2014;3:e000297.
13. Wong VW, Wong GL, Yeung DK, Abrigo JM, Kong AP, Chan RS, et al. Fatty pancreas insulin resistance, and β-cell function: a population study using fat-water resonance imaging. Am J Gastroenterol. 2014;109:589–97.
14. Yanai H, Tomono Y, Ito K, Furutani N, Yoshida H, Tada N. The underlying mechanisms for development of hypertension in the metabolic syndrome. Nutr J. 2008;7:10.
15. Al-Haddad M, Khashab M, Zyromski N, Pungpapong S, Wallace MB, Scolapio J, et al. Risk factors for hyperechogenic pancreas on endoscopic ultrasoundL a case–control study. Pancreas. 2009;38:672–5.
16. van Geenen EJ, Smits MM, Schreuder TC, van der Peet DL, Bloemena E, Mulder CJ. Nonalcoholic fatty liver disease is related to nonalcoholic fatty pancreas disease. Pancreas. 2010;39:1185–90.
17. Ou H-Y, Wang C-Y, Yang Y-C, Chen M-F, Chang C-J. The association between nonalcoholic fatty pancreas disease and diabetes. PLoS ONE. 2013;8:e62561.
18. Cerf ME. Beta cell dysfunction and insulin resistance. Front Endocrinol. 2013; 4(37):1–7.

LDP vs ODP for pancreatic adenocarcinoma: a case matched study from a single-institution

Miaozun Zhang[1], Ren Fang[1], Yiping Mou[2*], Ronggao Chen[1], Xiaowu Xu[2], Renchao Zhang[2], Jiafei Yan[1], Weiwei Jin[1] and Harsha Ajoodhea[1]

Abstract

Background: Laparoscopic distal pancreatectomy (LDP) showed advantage of perioperation outcomes for benign and low-grade tumor of the pancreas. The application of LDP for pancreatic ductal adenocarcinoma (PDAC) didn't gain popular acceptance and the number of LDP for PDAC remains low. We designed a case-matched study to analysis the short- and long-term outcomes of the patients undergoing either Laparoscopic distal pancreatectomy or open distal pancreatectomy for PDAC.

Method: From 2003 to 2013, 17 patients were underwent LDP and 34 patients were underwent ODP for PDAC were matched by tumor size, age and body mass index (BMI). The two groups' demographic information, perioperative outcomes and survival data were compared.

Results: Baseline characteristics were comparable between the LDP and ODP groups. The intraoperative blood loss, first flatus, first oral intake and postoperative hospital stay were significantly less in LDP group than ODP group (50 ml vs400ml, $P = 0.000$; 3d vs 4d, $P = 0.001$; 3d vs 4d, $P = 0.003$; 13d vs 15.5d, $P = 0.022$). The mean operation time, overall postoperative morbidity and postoperative pancreatic fistula rates were similar in the two groups. 5 patients (29.4 %) in LDP group and 7 patients (20.6 %) in ODP group underwent extended resections. There were no significant differences in tumor sizes (3.5 cm vs 3.9 cm, $P = 0.664$) and number of harvested lymph nodes (9 vs8 $P = 0.534$). The median overall survival for both groups was 14.0 months. Cox proportional hazards analysis showed extended resections, R1 resection, perineural invasion and tumor differentiation were associated with worse survival.

Conclusion: LDP is technically feasible and safe for PDAC in selected patients and the short-term oncologic outcomes were not inferior to ODP in this small sample study. However the long-term oncologic safety of LDP for PDAC has to be further evaluated by multicenter or randomized controlled trials.

Keywords: Pancreatic ductal adenocarcinoma, Laparoscopic surgery, Open surgery, Distal pancreatectomy, Case matched study

Background

In the last few decades, with the development of laparoscopic instruments and skills, Laparoscopic distal pancreatectomy (LDP) has become widely accepted by surgeons for benign and low-grade tumors of the pancreas. Recent reviews and meta-analysis showed that LDP has the advantage of less blood loss and fewer hospital stay days as well as fewer postoperative complications compared with open distal pancreatectomy [1–3]. However, application of laparoscopic approach has been restricted for malignant pancreatic lesions due to concerns over oncologic safety [4]. Unlike other gastrointestinal regions, such as stomach and colon, until now, only a few pioneer studies reported direct comparisons of oncologic outcomes between LDP and open distal pancreatectomy (ODP) for pancreatic ductal adenocarcinoma (PDAC) [5–9]. In this study, we designed a 1:2 case-matched retrospective study from a single institution and analysed the short-term and long-

* Correspondence: yipingmou@126.com
[2]Department of General Surgery, Zhejiang Provincial People's Hospital, Wenzhou Medical University, 158 Shangtang Road, Hangzhou 310014, Zhejiang Province, China
Full list of author information is available at the end of the article

term outcomes of the patients undergoing either LDP or ODP for PDAC.

Methods

Patient sample and data collection

From April 2003 to December 2013, 68 distal pancreatectomies were performed for PDAC. All the patients were given detailed information about LDP and OPD for PDAC, four experienced surgeons decided the type of operation according to patient's condition with informed consent. An informed consent was signed by every patient before the study. The exclusion criterias for LDPwere: (1) borderline resectable according to NCCN guidelines [10]; (2) intra-abdominal dissemination; (3) tumor size > 5 cm (located in pancreatic body) or >10 cm (located in pancreatic tail). Invasion of adjacent organs were not considered as contraindications. Cases who underwent laparoscopic exploration before definitive open surgery were not included in either LDP or ODP groups. Finally 17 LDP cases were enrolled in this study and were matched with 34 ODP cases in a 1:2 case-matched design. The patients were matched by three parameters: tumor size (±0.5 cm), age (±5 years), BMI (±1.0). The study was approved by the Institutional Review Board of Sir Run Run Shaw Hosptial of Zhejiang University. All patient data were retrospectively reviewed from cohort database including demographic information, perioperative outcomes and survival data. The following data were collected: gender, age, American Society of Anesthesiologists (ASA), body mass index (BMI), comorbidity, operation time, intraoperative blood loss (EBL), resection margin status, length of hospital stay, postoperative pancreatic fistulae (POPF), postoperative complications, mortality, adjuvant therapy, recurrence, tumor size, tumor differentitation, tumor stage, number of harvested lymph nodes and ration of N1.

Operative technique

Laparoscopic pancreatic surgery has been carried at our institution since 2003. The first LDP for PDAC was performed in 2004. The standardized technique for LDP at our institution has been previously described [11, 12]. The first 10-mm trocar was inserted below the umbilicus, then the main working trocar (12 mm) and another three assistant trocars (5 mm) were inserted into the right upper flank, left upper flank, left flank, and right flank quadrants respectively; these five trocars were arranged in a V-shape. Briefly, the gastrocolic ligament was divided by a harmonic scalpel (Harmonic Ace; Ethicon Endo-Surgery, Cincinnati, OH, United States) and the lesser sac was entered. Then, the superior border of the pancreas was mobilized and the proximal splenic artery was freed. After mobilization of the inferior border of the pancreas, a retropancreatic tunnel was created under the neck of the pancreas and the pancreas was transected using an endoscopic linear stapler (Endocutter 60 stapler, white or blue cartridge; Ethicon Endo-Surgery, Cincinnati, OH, United States). The splenic artery and the splenic vein were divided at the root. The soft tissue around the common hepatic artery and the celiac trunk were dissected. Then dissection was performed in a "medial – to - lateral" fashion and the distal pancreas along with the spleen were removed. In cases of invasion to adjacent organs such as stomach, left adrenal gland and even left lobe of liver, en bloc resection was performed by laparoscopic approach. The resected specimen was removed using an endoscopic bag by enlarging the incision at the periumbilical port. ODP was performed in a traditional manner or same method as LDP depending on the habit of the surgeon. Frozen section biopsy was applied to ascertain the resection margin.

Postoperative management Oral intake was started after the first flatus passed. The gastric tube was removed immediately after surgery and the urethral catheter was removed on the following day. Patient were discharged if they could tolerate semifluid diet without obvious discomfort and they felt sufficiently recovered without any major complications. Postoperative complications were recorded using the modified Clavien-Dindo classification [13]. Mortality was defined as death occurring during hospitalization or within 30 days. Postoperative pancreatic fistulae were defined as any measurable volume of fluid output (amylase level three times greater than the normal serum level) from drainage tube on or after postoperative day 3 according to the International Study Group on (ISGPF) [14]. R1 resection was considered as tumor extension within 1 mm of margin [15]. TMN stage was applied by the American Joint Committee on Cancer (7th edition). Adjuvant therapy refers to use of motherapy or radiation therapy perioperative or postoperative.

Patient follow-up

All patients were regularly followed up through outpatient service at the 1, 3, 6, 12 months and 6-month intervals thereafter by telephone call. Recurrences or metastasis were recorded by evidence of imaging examination, laboratory tests or pathologic results from biopsy, cytology or surgical resection. The last follow-up was conducted in Feburary 2015.

Statistical analysis

Continuous variables were presented as median and range and analyzed using the Student t test (parametric distribution) or Mann–Whitney test (nonparametric distribution). Categorical variables were analyzed using Chi Squared and or Fisher's exact test. Kaplan-Meier method with log rank testing was applied for estimating the survival analysis. Cox proportional hazards analysis was applied to investigate the prognostic factor for overall survival following distal pancreatectomy and variables were entered into the multivariate regression analysis when P value was less than 0.2. $P < 0.05$ was considered statistically significant.

Results

Baseline characteristics

The baseline characteristics of patients undergoing distal pancreatectomy for PDAC are summarized at Table 1. Seventeen patients underwent LDP while 34 patients underwent ODP. Of the 17 patients in LDP group 2 cases (11.8 %) were converted to open procedure because of local invasion of superior mesenteric artery. The baseline characteristics such as age, gender, BMI, ASA score, comorbidity and ration of extended resection were comparable between LDP and ODP. The most common comorbidity was hypertension and diabetes mellitus (DM).

Comparison of surgical outcomes for PDAC

Comparison of surgical outcomes of distal pancreatectomy for PDAC is summarized in Table 2. The mean operation time in LDP group and ODP group was similar (190 min vs 245 min, $P = 0.064$). The intraoperative blood loss was significantly lower in LDP group than in ODP group (50 ml vs 400 ml, $P = 0.000$). The first flatus time and diet start time were shorter in LDP group (3d vs 4d, $P = 0.001$; 3d vs 4d, $P = 0.003$). The postoperative length of hospital stay was shorter in LDP group (13d vs 15.5d, $P = 0.022$).

In LDP group 5 patients underwent extended distal pancreatectomy, including resection of stomach in 1 patient, left hepatic lobe in 2 patients and left adrenal gland in 3 patients (in 1 patient both left hepatic lobe and left adrenal gland were resected); while in ODP group, 7 patients had simultaneous resections, including stomach in 1 patient, colon in 1 patient, partial resection portal vein in 1 patient, left hepatic lobe in 2 patients, left adrenal gland in 3 patients (in 1 patient both left hepatic lobe and left adrenal gland were resected). There was one R1 resection in LDP group and five R1 resection in ODP group and showed no significant differences between the two groups ($P = 0.650$).

There were no significant differences in overall postoperative morbidity rate between the two groups ($P = 0.750$). Postoperative pancreatic fistula rates were similar in the two groups ($P = 0.484$) and no C-grade record in LDP group. Only one patient needed reoperation because of intestinal obstruction in ODP group. One death occurred 35 days post-operation during the hospitalization in ODP group. ODP group had 2 (5.9 %) 30 day re-admission because of abdominal infection while LDP group had none ($P = 0.547$).

Table 1 Baseline characteristics of patients undergoing distal pancreatectomy for PDAC

Characteristics	LDP ($n = 17$)	ODP ($n = 34$)	P value
Age	60 (44–75)	64 (40–76)	0.164
Gender (F)	6 (35.3)	15 (44.1)	0.763
BMI	23.4 (18.7–27.6)	23.7 (19.0–28.7)	0.313
ASA score			0.569
1	9 (52.9)	15 (44.1)	
2	8 (47.1)	19 (55.9)	
Comorbidity	7 (41.2)	17 (48.6)	0.769
Extended resection	5 (29.4)	7 (20.6)	0.792
Liver	2 (11.8)	2 (5.9)	
Left adrenal gland	3 (17.6)	3 (8.8)	
Stomach	1 (5.9)	1 (2.9)	
Colon	0 (0)	1 (2.9)	
Portal vein	0 (0)	1 (2.9)	

Table 2 Comparison of surgical outcomes of distal pancreatectomy for PDAC

Variables	LDP ($n = 17$)	ODP ($n = 34$)	P value
Operation time (min)	190 (100–390)	245 (155–420)	0.064
Intraoperative blood loss (mL)	50 (30–500)	400 (100–3900)	0.000
First flatus time (d)	3 (1–4)	4 (2–6)	0.001
First oral intake (d)	3 (1–6)	4 (2–9)	0.003
Pancreatic fistula			0.484
Grade A	6 (35.3)	6 (17.6)	
Grade B	3 (17.6)	9 (26.5)	
Grade C	0 (0)	1 (2.9)	
Clavien-Dindo grade			0.754
Grade I	3 (17.6)	4 (11.8)	
Grade II	3 (17.6)	7 (20.6)	
Grade III	0 (0)	2 (5.9)	
Grade IV	0 (0)	0 (0)	
grade V	0 (0)	1 (2.9)	
Resection margin			0.650
R0	16 (94.1)	29 (85.3)	
R1	1 (5.9)	5 (14.7)	
Postoperative hospital stay (d)	13 (4–23)	15.5 (6–40)	0.022
30 day re-admission	0 (0)	2 (5.9)	0.547

Comparison of clinicopathologic characteristics

Comparison of clinicopathologic characteristics of LDP and ODP for PDAC is shown in Table 3. There were no significant differences in tumor sizes (3.5 cm vs 3.9 cm, $P = 0.664$), number of harvested lymph nodes (9 vs 8 $P = 0.534$), ration of N1 ($P = 0.382$),

Table 3 Comparison of Clinicopathologic Characteristics of distal pancreatectomy for PDAC

Variables	LDP (*n* = 17)	ODP (*n* = 34)	*P* value
Tumor size (cm)	3.5 (2.3–5.5)	3.9 (1.8–5.5)	0.664
Tumor stage			0.090
T1	0 (0)	0 (0)	
T2	3 (17.6)	4 (11.8)	
T3	12 (70.6)	30 (88.2)	
T4	2 (3.9)	0 (0)	
Total LN	9 (5–15)	8 (2–22)	0.534
N1 (positive)	7 (41.2)	19 (55.9)	0.382
Tumor differentitation			0.145
Well	3 (17.6)	7 (23.5)	
Moderate	6 (35.3)	19 (55.9)	
Poor	8 (47.1)	8 (20.6)	
Perineural invasion	12 (70.6)	25 (29.4)	1.000
Adjuvant treatment	13 (76.5)	26 (76.5)	1.000
Recurrences	11 (64.7)	16 (47.1)	0.372

perineural invasion ($P = 1.000$), recurrences ($P = 1.000$). Most patients in both groups had T3 disease. LDP group had 2 (3.9 %) T4 cases. There was no significant difference between the two groups in terms of tumor stage ($P = 0.090$) as well as tumor differentiation ($P = 0.145$). The ration of accepting adjuvant chemotherapy was similar in two groups ($P = 1.000$).

Survival

The mean and median overall survival for the LDP group was 19.9 months and 14.0 months and for ODP group was 22.3 months and 14.0 months. There was no difference in overall survival between the two groups ($P = 0.802$) (Fig. 1). In Cox proportional hazards analysis, tumor size, comorbidity, POPF, tumor stage and adjuvant treatment were not significant for overall survival. Extended resections, R1 resection, perineural invasion and tumor differentitation (Moderate) were associated with worse survival following distal pancreatectomy and the choice of surgical procedure was not associated with the overall survival (Table 4). The mean and median overall survival for group with adjuvant treatment was 27.8 months and 15.0 months while the group without adjuvant treatment was 16.6 months and 13.0 months ($P = 0.363$). The median survival for extended resection group was 8.0 months and for no extended resection group was 15.0 months ($P = 0.004$) (Fig. 2).

Discussion

In recent years, LDP has been gradually accepted as standard approach to treat benign or low grade lesions located in the body or tail of the pancreas. The technical feasibility, safety and clinical benefit has been well confirmed by various matched studies compared with open distal pancreatectomies [16–18]. However, application of Laparoscopic distal pancreatectomies for PDAC was still limited due to the concern of oncologic outcome and surgical quality [4]. But reports emerging from some experienced centers are encouraging. Compared with conventional open approach, they demonstrated the advantages of less blood loss, shorter hospital stay and early return to normal activity with a similar morbidity, POPF, short oncology outcome (R0 resection rate, the number of harvested lymph nodes) and the overall survival rate [5–9, 19, 20]. In this case-matched study we compared the short-term and long-term outcomes of patients undergoing distal pancreatectomy and the results were consistent with these reports.

Surgery remains the only opportunity for long-term survival for patients with resectable PDAC [21]. R0 resection is the most crucial prognostic factor [22]. In a multicenter analysis Kooby et al. [5] reported that the R0 resection rate of LDP and ODP for PDAC was 73.9 % (17/23) and 65.7 % (46/70). A multivariate analysis was conducted in the whole cohort and only blood >500 ml was associated with R1 resection while the method of resection (LDP or ODP) wasn't correlated. Shin et al. [20] reported the largest single-institution study of LDP for PDAC ($n = 70$), the R0 resection rate was 75.7 % (53/70) for LDP while 83.8 % (67/80) for ODP. Lee et al. and Hu et al. [8, 9] reported in their series that patients included in LDP group were relatively in early stage and the R0 resection rate was 100 %. These case–control retrospective studies showed no significant difference of R0 resection between the LDP and ODP groups. In the present study, the R0 resections for LDP and ODP were 94.1 % and 85.3 % ($P = 0.650$) which was in accordance with those former studies. Recently, Sharpe et al. [19] reported outcomes for 769 patients of which 144 in the LDP group for PDAC through the National Cancer Data Base. In this retrospective survey, the LDP group had a decrease in margin positivity rate but the tumor size was smaller compared with the ODP group and LDP was more likely to be performed at academic/research institutions. The results were satisfactory for laparoscopic procedure although the heterogeneity might exist due to the type of study design or selection bias. Besides the essentiality of frozen section, extended resections were required in some cases in order for a definitive margin-negative surgery because of the aggressive nature of the disease [23]. Extended resections are feasible procedures with increased postoperative morbidity and better survival compared with palliative bypass procedures [24]. Although laparoscopic extended resection of the pancreas is technically demanding, its application is increasing in specialized centers. Croome et al. [25]

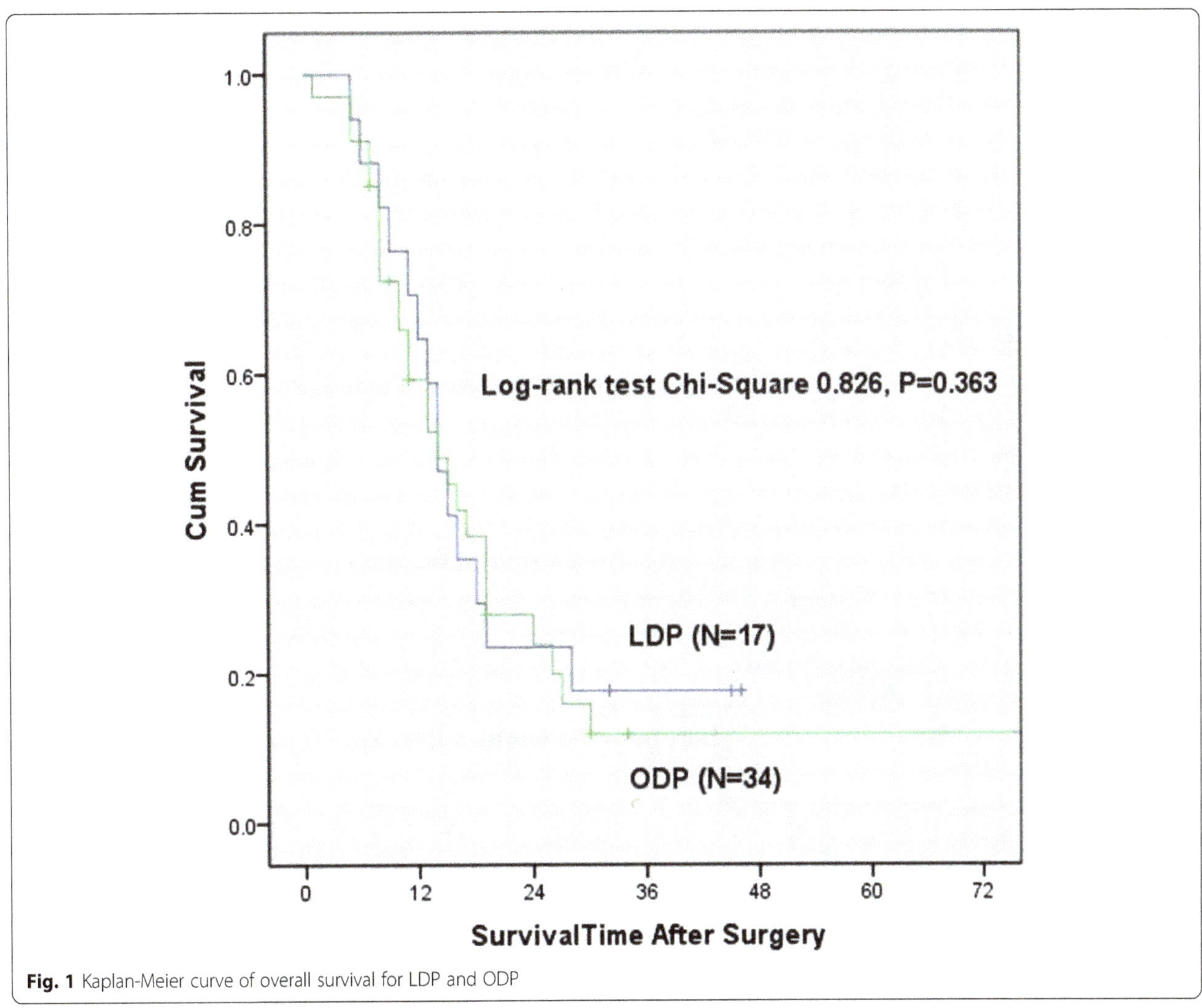

Fig. 1 Kaplan-Meier curve of overall survival for LDP and ODP

Table 4 Cox proportional hazards analysis for overall survival

Viables	Hazard ration	95 % CI	*P* value
Adjuvant treatment (no/yes)	0.407	0.207–1.020	0.056
R 1 (negative/positive)		1.260–15.468	0.020
Extended resection (no/yes)		1.105–5.945	0.028
Operation (LDP/ODP)		0.420–1.863	0.885
N1 (negative/positive)		0.745–4.147	0.198
Perineural invasion (negative/positive)		1.240–6.746	0.014
Tumor stage T2	1.000		
Tumor stage T3	0.776	0.292–2.060	0.611
Tumor stage T4	1.174	0.433–3.180	0.753
Tumor differentitation Well	1.000		
Tumor differentitation Moderate	3.432	1.012–11.645	0.048
Tumor differentitation Poor	6.316	0.980–40.700	0.053

HR hazard ratio
95 % CI, 95 % confidence interval

reported data from Mayo clinic of 31 patients undergoing total laparoscopic pancreaticoduodenectomy with major vascular resection, there was no significant difference of the total complications comparable with open group and with less mean operative blood, less hospital stay. We previously reported the first laparoscopic hepatopancreatoduodenectomy case with favorable perioperative outcome and showed no sign of recurrence over a year [26]. The data of LDP combined with extended resections is rare. Shin et al. [20] reported 6 (8.6 %) cases of concurrent resections for PDAC by laparoscopic procedure including 5 left colectomies and 1 gastrectomy. After propensity score-matched (including age, BMI, tumor size, concurrent resection) analysis, the overall survival was similar between the LDP group and ODP group while concurrent resection ration were balanced between the two groups. Ricci et al. [27] reported 6 (18.7 %) extended resections including resection of liver wedge, stomach, left adrenal gland and colon among 32 LDP. In our study, we had 5 cases (29.4 %) of extended resections in LDP group with 1

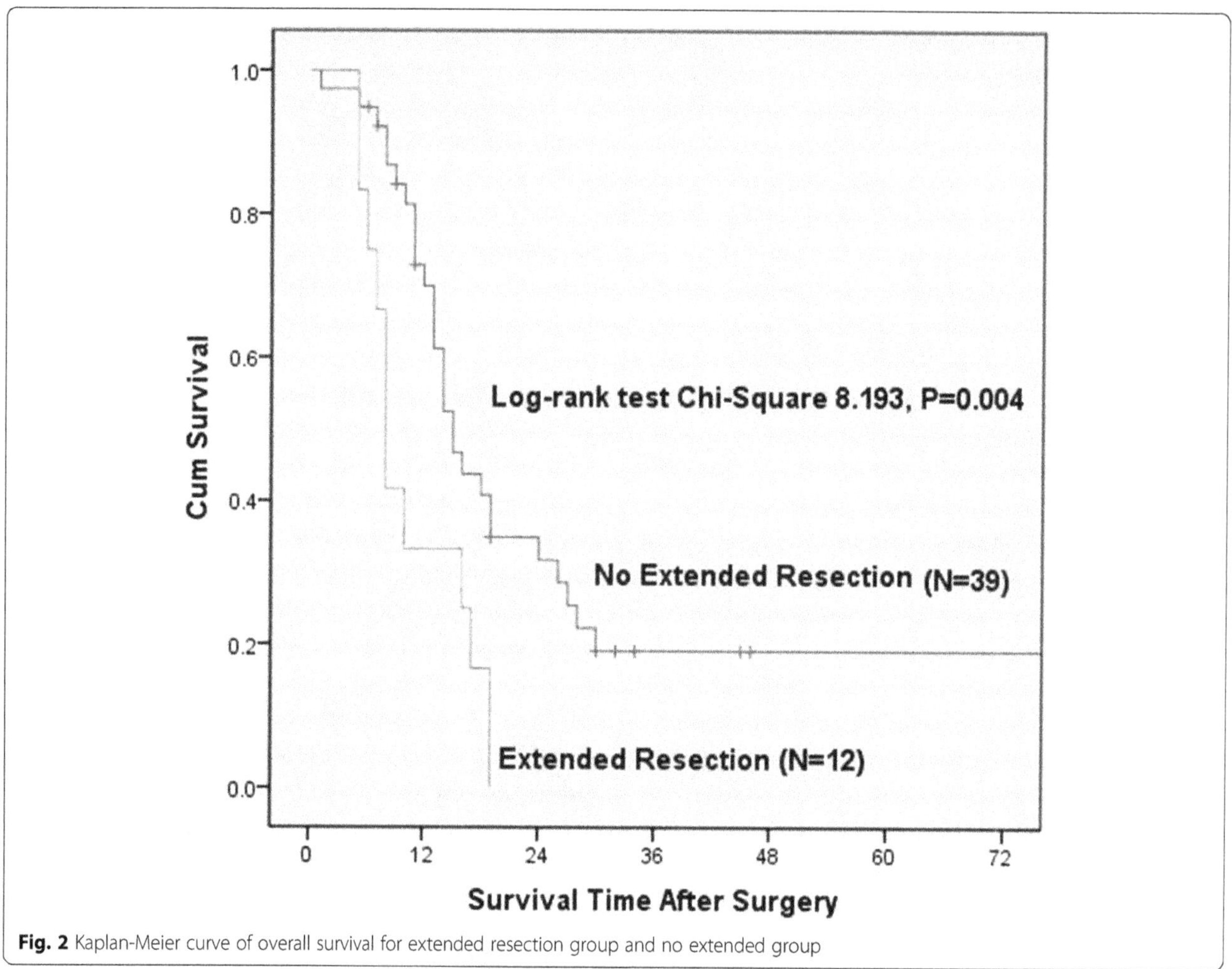

Fig. 2 Kaplan-Meier curve of overall survival for extended resection group and no extended group

R1 resection while 7 cases (20.6 %) in ODP group with 5 R1 resections. We abolished the laparoscopic procedure of two cases because of invasion to superior mesenteric artery (SMA). Despite the sample data was too small to make any persuasive conclusion, it may achieve R0 resection of locally advanced PDAC in selected patients through laparoscopic procedure by skilled surgeons. Completion of the learning curve, a fixed surgical group and suitable selection criteria were efficacious to carry out these complex goals [27, 28] and we insist on using 5 trocars strategy in order for the cooperation of the main surgeon and the first assistant. Until now, there is no standard indication of LDP for PDAC. As reported from previous studies and meta-analysis, surgeons are mostly inclined to conduct LDP for smaller tumor size [2, 6–8]. Although Kooby et al. [5] reported tumor size (>4 cm) was not associated with positive resection margin, a huge tumor would be an obvious obstacle for exposure of the operation field. So, patients forwith tumor size >5 cm in body and >10 cm in tail of the pancreas were reserved for open procedure and were exluded in this study. The median survival was both 14 months in LDP and ODP groups in this series. Kooby et al. [5] reported median survival 16 months both for LDP and ODP groups and Magge et al. [6] reported 19 months for the entire cohort. Lee et al. [8] reported a median follow-up 39 months for the minimally invasive surgery group (including 4 robotic cases) using their inclusion criteria (Yonsei criteria) which mainly consisted of early stage pancreatic cancer. Compared with previous studies, the survival data in this study was not fulfilling. In Cox proportional hazards analysis extended resection, perineural invasion were strong factors for worse survival. The high ration of extended resection (23.5 %) and perineural invasion (72.5 %) of the whole cohort indicated the cases enrolled in this study were relatively in advanced stage due to lack of early diagnosis of the disease probably. The median survival for no extended resection group was 15.0 months and was consistent with the previous case-matched studies.

This study has several critical limitations, including the retrospective design and low number of patients enrolled in the study. Adjuvant treatment is believed to prolong overall survival [29], but in this study the Cox proportional hazards analysis showed no association with overall survival ($P = 0.380$). The poor differentiation was not associated with overall survival but the moderate differentiation showed association. The small sample of this study might be the reason and didn't have sufficient statistical power to evaluate the outcome. The study span lasted 11 years and only 1.3 LDP cases per year were performed. The surgical technique was not standardized between the laparoscopic and open approach. Also the follow-up time was short especially for the LDP group and it was difficult to calculate the 5-year survival. Until now, the oncologic safety and long-term survival were not tested by any randomized controlled study between LDP and ODP for PDAC, so it is not sufficient enough to make a conclusion that LDP is oncologic equivalence to ODP [3, 4]. As Kooby and Kang commented it was difficult to conduct an RCT because of the infrequence of diagnosis and opportunity for operation of PDAC in the pancreatic body and tail [4, 5]. The result of this study could provide valuable evidence to support use of LDP for PDAC even in relatively advanced stage.

Conclusion

In conclusion, the results in our study validated that LDP was technically feasible and safe for PDAC in selected patients and the short-term oncologic outcomes were not inferior to ODP in this small sample study However the long-term oncologic safety of LDP for PDAC has to be further evaluated by multicenter or randomized controlled trials.LDP with extended resection for PDAC is better performed in highly specialized centers and with suitable selection criteria.

Abbreviations

ASA: American Society of Anesthesiologists; BMI: body mass index; DM: diabetes mellitus; LDP: laparoscopic distal pancreatectomy; ODP: open distal pancreatectomy; PDAC: pancreatic ductal adenocarcinoma; POPF: postoperative pancreatic fistulae; SMA: superior mesenteric artery.

Competing interests

The authors declare that they have no competing interests.

Authors' contributions

ZMZ and MYP conceived and designed the study; MYP, XXW, ZMZ and ZRC performed the operation; AH, RF, CRG, YJF, and JWW collected case data; ZMZ wrote the manuscript; MYP proofread and revised the manuscript. All authors read and approved the version to be published.

Acknowledgments

This work was supported by Key Subject of Medical Science Foundation of Zhejiang Province, China (grant No. 11-CX-21).

Author details

[1]Department of General Surgery, Sir Run Run Shaw Hospital, School of Medicine, Zhejiang University, 3 East Qingchun Road, Hangzhou 310016, Zhejiang Province, China. [2]Department of General Surgery, Zhejiang Provincial People's Hospital, Wenzhou Medical University, 158 Shangtang Road, Hangzhou 310014, Zhejiang Province, China.

References

1. Xie K, Zhu YP, Xu XW, Chen K, Yan JF, Mou YP. Laparoscopic distal pancreatectomy is as safe and feasible as open procedure: a meta-analysis. World J Gastroenterol. 2012;18(16):1959–67.
2. Ricci C, Casadei R, Taffurelli G, Toscano F, Pacilio CA, Bogoni S, et al. Laparoscopic versus open distal pancreatectomy for ductal adenocarcinoma: a systematic review and meta-analysis. J Gastrointest Surg. 2015;19(4):770–81.
3. Mehrabi A, Hafezi M, Arvin J, Esmaeilzadeh M, Garoussi C, Emami G, et al. A systematic review and meta-analysis of laparoscopic versus open distal pancreatectomy for benign and malignant lesions of the pancreas: it's time to randomize. Surgery. 2015;157(1):45–55.
4. Kang CM, Lee SH, Lee WJ. Minimally invasive radical pancreatectomy for left-sided pancreatic cancer: current status and future perspectives. World J Gastroenterol. 2014;20(9):2343–51.
5. Kooby DA, Hawkins WG, Schmidt CM, Weber SM, Bentrem DJ, Gillespie TW, et al. A multicenter analysis of distal pancreatectomy for adenocarcinoma: is laparoscopic resection appropriate? J Am Coll Surg. 2010;210(5):779–85. 786–777.
6. Magge D, Gooding W, Choudry H, Steve J, Steel J, Zureikat A, et al. Comparative effectiveness of minimally invasive and open distal pancreatectomy for ductal adenocarcinoma. JAMA Surgery. 2013;148(6):525–31.
7. Rehman S, John SK, Lochan R, Jaques BC, Manas DM, Charnley RM, et al. Oncological feasibility of laparoscopic distal pancreatectomy for adenocarcinoma: a single-institution comparative study. World J Surg. 2014;38(2):476–83.
8. Lee SH, Kang CM, Hwang HK, Choi SH, Lee WJ, Chi HS. Minimally invasive RAMPS in well-selected left-sided pancreatic cancer within Yonsei criteria: long-term (>median 3 years) oncologic outcomes. Surg Endosc. 2014;28(10): 2848–55.
9. Hu M, Zhao G, Wang F, Zhao Z, Li C, Liu R. Laparoscopic versus open distal splenopancreatectomy for the treatment of pancreatic body and tail cancer: a retrospective, mid-term follow-up study at a single academic tertiary care institution. Surg Endosc. 2014;28(9):2584–91.
10. Tempero MA, Malafa MP, Behrman SW, Benson AB 3rd, Casper ES, Chiorean EG, et al. Pancreatic adenocarcinoma, version 2.2014: featured updates to the NCCN guidelines. J Natl Compr Canc Netw. 2014;12(8):1083–93.
11. Zhang RC, Yan JF, Xu XW, Chen K, Ajoodhea H, Mou YP. Laparoscopic vs open distal pancreatectomy for solid pseudopapillary tumor of the pancreas. World J Gastroenterol. 2013;19(37):6272–7.
12. Yan JF, Xu XW, Jin WW, Huang CJ, Chen K, Zhang RC, et al. Laparoscopic spleen-preserving distal pancreatectomy for pancreatic neoplasms: a retrospective study. World J Gastroenterol. 2014;20(38):13966–72.
13. Clavien PA, Barkun J, de Oliveira ML, Vauthey JN, Dindo D, Schulick RD, et al. The Clavien-Dindo classification of surgical complications: five-year experience. Ann Surg. 2009;250(2):187–96.
14. Bassi C, Dervenis C, Butturini G, Fingerhut A, Yeo C, Izbicki J, et al. Postoperative pancreatic fistula: an international study group (ISGPF) definition. Surgery. 2005;138(1):8–13.
15. Hartwig W, Vollmer CM, Fingerhut A, Yeo CJ, Neoptolemos JP, Adham M, et al. Extended pancreatectomy in pancreatic ductal adenocarcinoma: definition and consensus of the International Study Group for Pancreatic Surgery (ISGPS). Surgery. 2014;156(1):1–14.
16. Eom BW, Jang JY, Lee SE, Han HS, Yoon YS, Kim SW. Clinical outcomes compared between laparoscopic and open distal pancreatectomy. Surg Endosc. 2008;22(5):1334–8.
17. Soh YF, Kow AW, Wong KY, Wang B, Chan CY, Liau KH, et al. Perioperative outcomes of laparoscopic and open distal pancreatectomy: our institution's 5-year experience. Asian J Surgery/Asian Surgical Association. 2012;35(1):29–36.
18. Lee SY, Allen PJ, Sadot E, D'Angelica MI, DeMatteo RP, Fong Y, et al. Distal pancreatectomy: a single institution's experience in open, laparoscopic, and robotic approaches. J Am Coll Surg. 2015;220(1):18–27.
19. Sharpe SM, Talamonti MS, Wang E, Bentrem DJ, Roggin KK, Prinz RA, et al. The laparoscopic approach to distal pancreatectomy for ductal adenocarcinoma results in shorter lengths of stay without compromising oncologic outcomes. Am J Surg. 2015;209(3):557–63.
20. Shin SH, Kim SC, Song KB, Hwang DW, Lee JH, Lee D, et al. A comparative study of laparoscopic vs. open distal pancreatectomy for left-sided ductal adenocarcinoma: a propensity score-matched analysis. J Am Coll Surg. 2015; 220(2):177–85.
21. Valle JW, Palmer D, Jackson R, Cox T, Neoptolemos JP, Ghaneh P, et al. Optimal duration and timing of adjuvant chemotherapy after definitive surgery for ductal adenocarcinoma of the pancreas: ongoing lessons from the ESPAC-3 study. J Clin Oncol. 2014;32(6):504–12.

22. Wagner M, Redaelli C, Lietz M, Seiler CA, Friess H, Buchler MW. Curative resection is the single most important factor determining outcome in patients with pancreatic adenocarcinoma. Br J Surg. 2004;91(5):586–94.
23. Hartwig W, Hackert T, Hinz U, Hassenpflug M, Strobel O, Buchler MW, et al. Multivisceral resection for pancreatic malignancies: risk-analysis and long-term outcome. Ann Surg. 2009;250(1):81–7.
24. Konstantinidis IT, Warshaw AL, Allen JN, Blaszkowsky LS, Castillo CF, Deshpande V, et al. Pancreatic ductal adenocarcinoma: is there a survival difference for R1 resections versus locally advanced unresectable tumors? What is a "true" R0 resection? Ann Surg. 2013;257(4):731–6.
25. Croome KP, Farnell MB, Que FG, Reid-Lombardo KM, Truty MJ, Nagorney DM, et al. Pancreaticoduodenectomy with major vascular resection: a comparison of laparoscopic versus open approaches. J Gastrointest Surg. 2015;19(1):189–94. discussion 194.
26. Zhang MZ, Xu XW, Mou YP, Yan JF, Zhu YP, Zhang RC, et al. Resection of a cholangiocarcinoma via laparoscopic hepatopancreato- duodenectomy: a case report. World J Gastroenterol. 2014;20(45):17260–4.
27. Ricci C, Casadei R, Buscemi S, Taffurelli G, D'Ambra M, Pacilio CA, et al. Laparoscopic distal pancreatectomy: what factors are related to the learning curve? Surg Today. 2015;45(1):50–6.
28. Braga M, Ridolfi C, Balzano G, Castoldi R, Pecorelli N, Di Carlo V. Learning curve for laparoscopic distal pancreatectomy in a high-volume hospital. Updates Surg. 2012;64(3):179–83.
29. Oettle H, Neuhaus P, Hochhaus A, Hartmann JT, Gellert K, Ridwelski K, et al. Adjuvant chemotherapy with gemcitabine and long-term outcomes among patients with resected pancreatic cancer: the CONKO-001 randomized trial. JAMA. 2013;310(14):1473–81.

24

Pancreatic hamartoma: a case report and literature review

Daisuke Matsushita[1*], Hiroshi Kurahara[1], Yuko Mataki[1], Kosei Maemura[1], Michiyo Higashi[2], Satoshi Iino[1], Masahiko Sakoda[1], Hiroyuki Shinchi[3], Shinichi Ueno[1] and Shoji Natsugoe[1]

Abstract

Background: Pancreatic hamartoma is an extremely rare benign disease of the pancreas. Only 30 cases have been reported to date.

Case presentation: A 68-year-old man presented with an asymptomatic solid and multi-cystic lesion in the uncus of the pancreas, incidentally detected on abdominal enhanced computed tomography. The tumor was found to be a well-demarcated solid and multi-cystic lesion without any enhancement, measuring 4 cm in diameter. After 28 months of follow-up, the tumor enlarged. At 31 months after initial diagnosis, the patient underwent surgical resection because it was difficult to clinically determine whether the tumor was malignant or not. Macroscopically, the solid tumor consisted of yellow adipose tissue with a smooth thin capsule confined to the pancreatic uncus. The inner structure of the tumor consisted of multiple cysts with a white nodule between the cysts. Histologically, the solid part and the multi-cystic portion consisted of mature adipose tissue and colonization of dilated pancreatic ducts with mild fibrosis, respectively. Immunohistochemical findings revealed cytokeratin 7 and 19 positive staining in the epithelial cells of the ducts. Adipose tissue showed positive staining for S-100 protein and there were only a few MIB-1 positive cells. The tumor was then diagnosed as a pancreatic hamartoma.

Conclusion: Beside on the above findings, we suggest that the term "well-demarcated solid and cystic lesion with chronological morphological changes" could be a clinical keyword to describe pancreatic hamartomas.

Keywords: Pancreas, Hamartoma, Cystic lesion, Pseudotumor, Cytokeratin, S-100

Background

Pancreatic tumor-like cystic lesions are significantly less common than solid lesions, and they account for less than 1 % of all pancreatic tumors [1]. Cystic tumors of the pancreas are categorized as pseudocysts and true lined cysts (e.g., intraductal papillary mucinous neoplasm [IPMN], mucinous cystic neoplasm [MCN], and serous cystic neoplasm [SCN]). Rare pancreatic cysts such as squamous-lined cysts (e.g., lymphoepithelial cyst, epidermoid cyst, dermoid cyst, and squamoid cyst) and solid-pseudopapillary neoplasms (SPNs) have also been reported. In addition, extremely rare non-neoplastic pancreatic tumors such as hamartomas have been reported. The differential clinical diagnosis of these pancreatic benign tumors from malignant disease using abdominal ultrasound (AUS), computed tomography (CT), magnetic resonance imaging (MRI), endoscopic retrograde cholangiopancreatography (ERCP), and endoscopic ultrasound (EUS) remains difficult despite advances in diagnostic imaging equipment [2]. Therefore, histological diagnosis with surgical resection is often needed to diagnose these rare tumors. Here, we report a case of pancreatic hamartoma and review the English literature on this extremely rare pancreatic tumor.

Case presentation

A 68-year-old man presented with an asymptomatic solid and multi-cystic mass in the uncus of the pancreas, incidentally detected on abdominal enhanced CT during a health examination. The patient had no relevant medical history, including chronic pancreatitis. The tumor was demonstrated to be a well demarcated solid and cystic lesion, measuring 4.2 × 3.9 cm in diameter by enhanced CT (Fig. 1a). The tumor consisted of a cystic lesion with

* Correspondence: m7762@m2.kufm.kagoshima-u.ac.jp
[1]Department of Digestive Surgery and Breast and Thyroid Surgery, Graduate School of Medical and Dental Sciences, Kagoshima University, 8-35-1 Sakuragaoka, Kagoshima 890-8520, Japan
Full list of author information is available at the end of the article

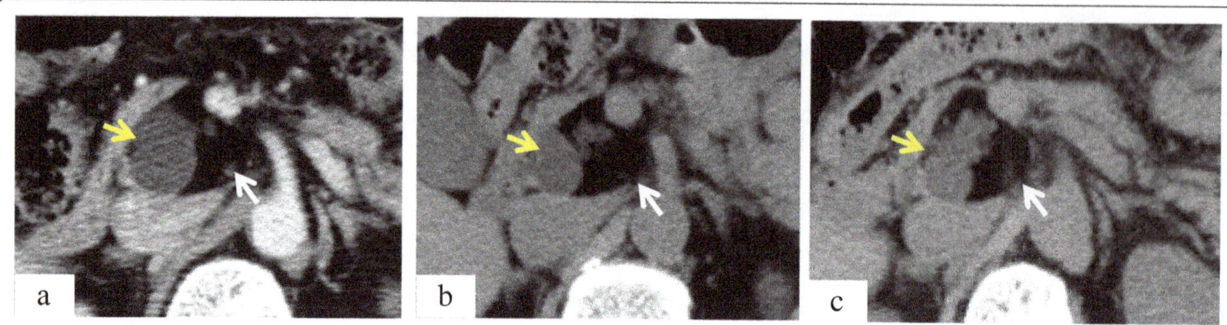

Fig. 1 Chronological changes seen on CT. **a**: First examination. The hypo-enhanced mass was 4.2 × 3.9 cm in size with solid and cystic lesions located in the uncus of the pancreas. **b**: At 21 months after first examination. The tumor shown is 3.9 × 3.6 cm in size. The cystic lesion (*yellow arrow*) had become smaller and the solid lesion (*white arrow*) had become larger. **c**: At 28 months after first examination. The tumor was 4.2 × 3.3 cm in size. The cystic lesion changed and displayed irregular margins

iso- to low-density surrounded by an extremely low-density area similar in density to adipose tissue. MRI and magnetic resonance cholangiopancreatography (MRCP) showed multilocular cysts ranging in size from one to several millimeters in the pancreas uncus. The main pancreatic duct (MPD) showed no dilation and the evidence of communications between the tumor and MPD was not found (Fig. 2a). The morphological feature of the tumor was completely different from pancreatic adenocarcinoma and the tumor was initially diagnosed benign tumor such as lipoma, dermoid cyst or the other rare benign tumor (Table 1). During the first enhanced CT examination, the patient developed an allergic reaction to contrast medium so that the patient was followed-up regularly with plain CT and MRI.

The patient visited for re-examination 21 months after the initial visit because he had no symptoms. The size of the pancreatic tumor had become smaller, measuring 3.9 cm in maximum diameter, and the internal structure showed morphological changes with smaller cysts and a larger solid lesion by plain CT (Fig. 1b) and MRI/MRCP (Fig. 2b). The tumor displayed a honeycomb-like appearance by EUS. At 28 months after the initial visit, the tumor showed an increase in size by plain CT. MRCP showed an increase in the size and number of the cysts, with no infiltration into the pancreatic ducts (Figs. 1c

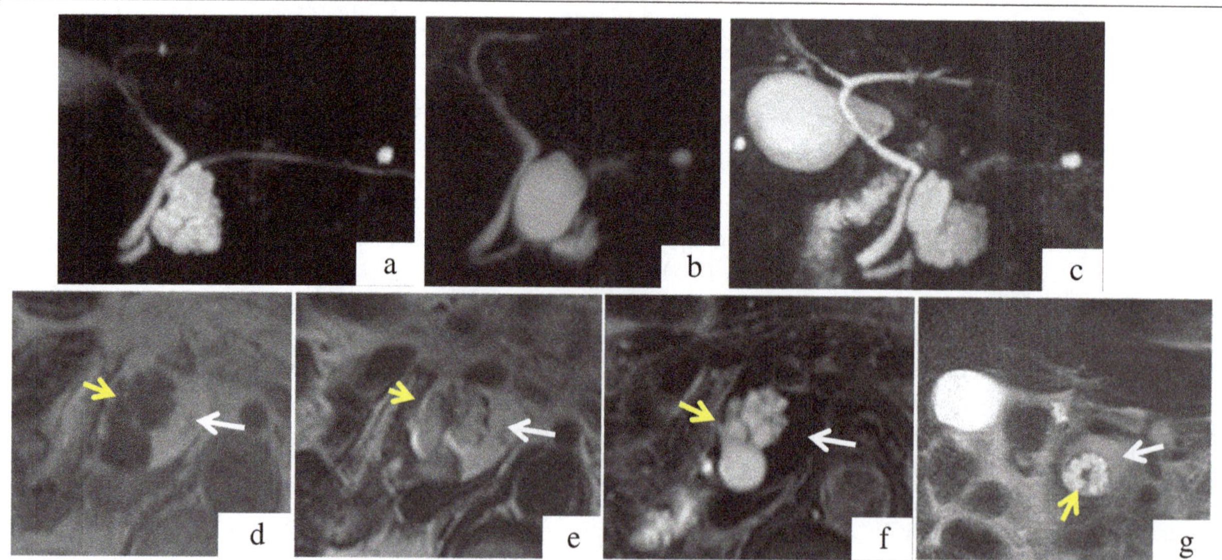

Fig. 2 a, **b**, **c**. Chronological changes seen on MRCP. **a**: At the first examination. The tumor was observed as multiple cystic lesions. **b**: At 21 months after first examination. **c**: At 28 months after first examination. Figure 2-**d**, **e**, **f**, **g**. MRI appearance at 28 months after first examination. **d**: T1WI. A multi-cystic lesion with low intensity was surrounded by a mass with iso-intensity. **e**: T2WI. A multi-cystic lesion displays low- to iso-intensity. The surrounding tissue shows iso- to high intensity. **f**: T2-FAT-SAT. A multi-cystic high intensity lesion is shown. The surrounding tissue shows complete fat suppression. **g**: T2WI (coronal image). A ringed multi-cystic lesion with high intensity is surrounded by a smooth superficial mass. A small nodule is seen inside of the cyst ring

Table 1 Differential diagnosis of the rare cystic lesion of the pancreas

	Age	Gender	Region	Morphology	Contents of the cyst	Histological feature
Lymphoepithelial cyst 1)20)21)	50s-60s	Male		Uni- or multilocular Cyst wall and trabeculae are usually thin.	Serous to cheesy/caseous-appearing depending on the degree of keratin formation.	Lined by well-differentiated stratified squamous epithelium. Surrounding dense lymphoid tissue.
Epidermoid cyst 1)22)	20s-30s	Female	Tail	Uni- or multilocular	Serous to cheesy/casseous-appearing depending on the degree of keratin formation. High levels of CA 19-9 and/or CEA in the serum and in the cystic fluid.	Lined by attenuated squamous cells. Exist with accessory spleens.
Dermoid cyst 1)23)24)	20s-30s	Unknown		Similar to the teratoma	Cheesy or caseous, with keratinaceous and sebaceous secretions.	Skin appendages and sebaceous glands, hair follicles, etc.
Squamoid cyst 1)25)26)	Unknown	Unknown		Unilocular	Acidophilic acinar	Cystically dilated ducts lined by a squamous/transitional epithelium. Basal are positive for p63. Superficial cells are positive for MUC1, MUC6 and involucrin.
Serous cystadenoma 1)27)	60s	M:F=1: 3	Body and tail	Multi-cystic large mass (mean size: 6 cm)	Serous fluid Sponge-like appearance	Cuboidal glycogen-rich epithelial cells positive for GLUT-1. Clear cytoplasm and well-defined cytoplasmic borders. Small, round nuclei with dense homogeneous chromatin. Von Hippel-Lindau gene is detected in 40% cases.
Lipoma 28)29)30)	Unknown	Unknown		Hypodensity (-30 to -120 HU) and homogeneity in enhanced CT	Mature adipose tissue, capsuled by thin collagen layer	No evidence of typical pancreatic tissue.
Hamartoma 1),3)-19)	50s- 60s	M:F=1.4:1	Head	Solid and cystic mass	Mature acini, ducts with architectural disarrangement surrounded by stromal fibrosis. Lack or decrease of islet cells.	C34, CD117 or bcr-2 expression for the stromal fibrosis. S-100 protein expression for the ductal component.

CA19-9; Carbohydrate antigen 19-9, CEA: Carcinoembryonic antigen, GLUT-1: Glucose transporter -1

and 2c). The multi-cystic lesion displayed low intensity on T1-weighted imaging (T1WI), iso-intensity on T2-weighted imaging (T2WI) and high intensity on T2-fat saturation (FAT-SAT) by MRI. The solid lesion surrounding the multi cystic lesion displayed iso-intensity on T1WI, iso- to high intensity on T2WI and low intensity with complete fat-tissue suppression using T2-FATSAT conditions (Fig. 2d-f). These findings demonstrated that the cystic lesion consisted with pancreatic juice and the solid lesion was a fat tissue.

On coronal T2WI imaging, ringed-multilocular cysts with high intensity were surrounded by a smooth superficial mass, and a small nodule was observed inside of the cyst ring (Fig. 2g). These images suggested the possibility of IPMN malignant transformation. At 31 months after the initial diagnosis, the patient underwent surgical resection. There were no symptoms or abnormal levels of tumor markers (carcinoembryonic antigen [CEA], carbohydrate antigen 19-9 [CA19-9]) during follow-up.

Operative findings

A soft and elastic tumor was confirmed in the uncus of the pancreas. The tumor was not exposed and there were no inflammatory changes around the pancreas. Intraoperative ultrasound showed a well demarcated honeycomb-like cystic lesion in the pancreatic uncus, and there was no evidence of venous or ductal invasion (Fig. 3). Pylorus preserving pancreaticoduodenectomy was performed. The operation was completed without any complications.

Macroscopic findings

A solid tumor consisting of yellow adipose tissue with a smooth thin capsule measuring 40 × 40 × 28 mm in size was confirmed in the pancreatic uncus. The inner structure

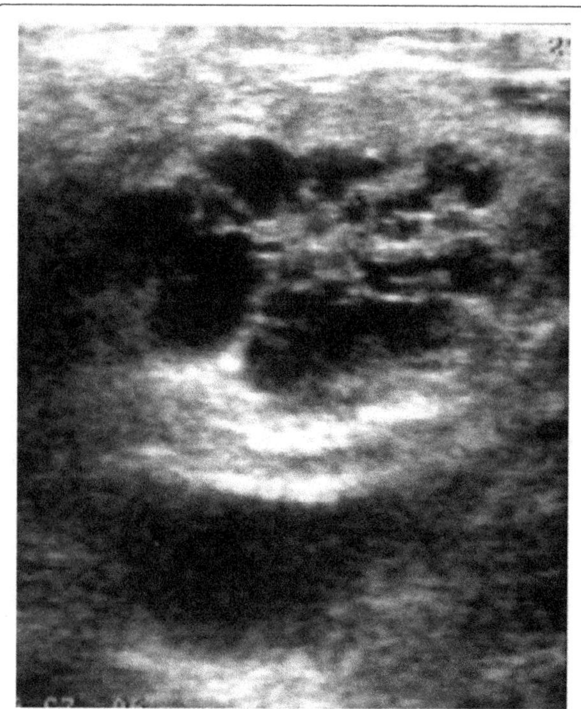

Fig. 3 Intraoperative ultrasound examination. A well-demarcated honeycomb-like cystic lesion in the pancreatic uncus was found. There was no evidence of venous or ductal invasion

of the tumor consisted of multiple cysts, and a white nodule was found between the cysts (Fig. 4a).

Hematoxylin-eosin staining (HE)

The solid part of the mass consisted of mature adipose tissue, and the cystic lesion consisted of colonization of the dilated pancreatic ducts with mild fibrosis and infiltration of monocytes in the circumference. There was no evidence of mucinous products in the cysts, and no evidence of malignancy in the epithelial cells of the cysts. A few normal scattered acini were observed in the solid portion of the lesion, and the nodule located between the cysts consisted of stromal fibrosis without atypical cells (Fig. 4b).

Immunohistochemical staining (IHC)

The epithelial cells of the ducts expressed cytokeratin 7 and cytokeratin 19, but were negative for cytokeratin 20. The adipose tissue was positive for S-100 protein, and mostly negative for MIB-1 (Ki-67). These results suggest that the tumor was non-proliferative (Fig. 5). Based on these findings, the tumor was determined to be composed of a mixture of differentiated cell types that are normally present in the pancreas. It was therefore regarded as a malformation rather than a neoplasm. Giving these findings, the tumor was diagnosed as a pancreatic hamartoma.

After surgical resection, the patient received follow-up examination with plain CT every three to six months and there was no recurrence for 50 months.

Discussion

Pancreatic hamartoma is an extremely rare benign disease of the pancreas. With the improvements in diagnostic imaging equipment over the last decade, it has become increasingly common to discover rare pancreatic tumors such as those listed above. Although these tumors are usually not aggressive, they typically require surgical resection because of the difficulty in prospective clinical diagnosis [2]. Accurate knowledge about these rare pancreatic tumors is therefore necessary. Table 1 shows the clinical features of the rare pancreatic tumors for which differential diagnosis was carried out in the present case [1, 3–31]. The information in Table 1 provides the clinical and histological characteristics of each disease. However, this information alone is not sufficient to be used as decisive diagnostic evidence.

Albrecht [32] first introduced the term "hamartoma" to describe "tumor-like malformations" of the liver, spleen, kidney, and breast that show an abnormal admixture of normal components typical of the organ involved. A hamartoma may be regarded as a malformation rather than a neoplasm. A pancreatic hamartoma is an extremely rare pancreatic tumor, accounting for < 1 % of occurrences of tumor-like cystic lesions of the pancreas [15]. There are only 30 cases of pancreatic hamartoma reported in the English literature to date [3–20], including the first case reported by Anthony et al. in 1977 [3]. All of these reports have described the difficulty in imaging diagnosis, and almost all patients underwent surgical resection because of the possibility of malignant disease.

Table 2 (Additional file 1 shows detailed data) shows the clinical and pathological features of 31 cases of pancreatic hamartoma, including the present case. The median age of the patients was 50.4 years (range, 34 weeks to 78 years), and there were no significant differences in the male-to-female ratio (1.4/1.0). Thirteen of the patients had no clinical symptoms, and the other patients had non-typical symptoms such as abdominal pain and weight loss. Noltenius et al. [33] suggested a relationship between the pancreatic hamartoma-like appearance and chronic pancreatitis in a case study of Wernicke's encephalopathy with alcoholic pancreatitis. In this study, only 4 cases were complicated by pancreatitis. On the other hand, many authors, including Pauser et al. [10], suggested that hamartoma should be distinguished from pancreatitis because chronic pancreatitis may just mimic hamartoma lesions, while lacking acinar cells.

Regarding the morphological features of these cases, 15 cases showed a solid pattern, and 14 cases showed

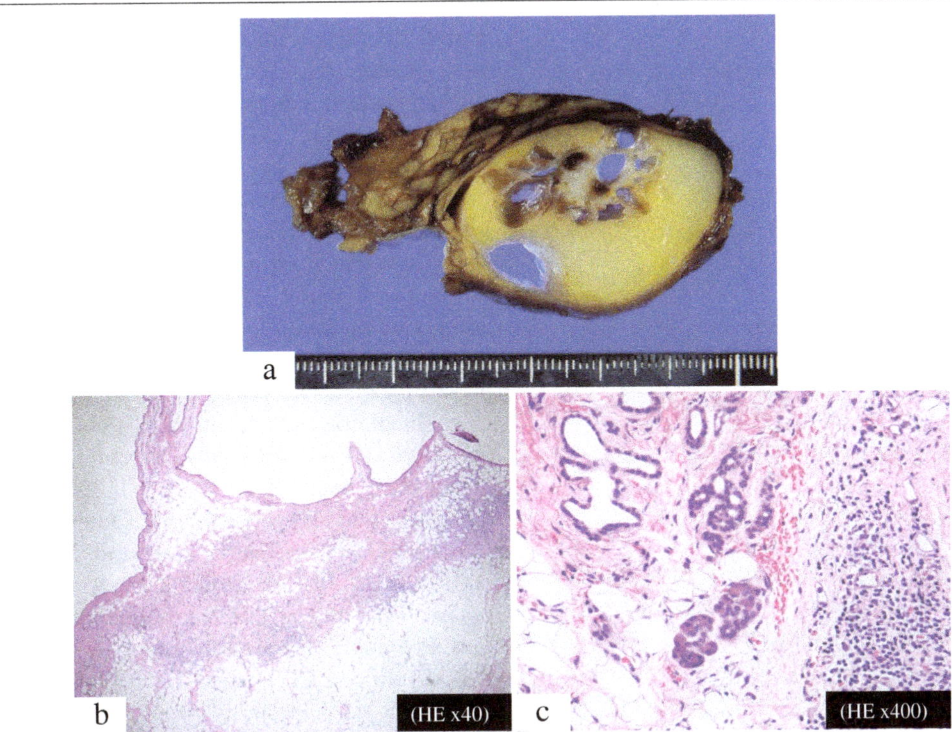

Fig. 4 Macroscopic and pathological findings of the pancreatic hamartoma. **a**: Solid and cystic tumor in the pancreatic uncus with a smooth, thin capsule. Cysts were surrounded by yellow adipose tissue and a white nodule was found between the cysts. **b**: The solid lesion filled with mature adipose tissue. There was no evidence of mucinous products in the cysts and no evidence of malignancy in the epithelial cells of the cysts. **c**: The cystic lesion consisted of dilated ducts. Fibrosis and infiltration of monocytes were observed around the cysts. There were a few normal acini in the solid lesion, and the nodule located between the cysts consisted of stromal fibrosis without atypical cells

both a solid and cystic pattern (this was unknown in two cases). A solitary tumor was observed in 22 patients, and multiple tumors were found in 6 cases (this was unknown in three cases). All cases showed a well-demarcated line and non-invasive growth. The median size of the main tumor was 4.4 cm (range, 0.9–19 cm). Twenty-one of the reported hamartomas were located in the head, four were located in the body, and 4 in the tail of the pancreas. Two cases were identified as diffuse tumors.

There were only a few patients who could be followed for a long period of time. In the present case, we were able to follow the patient over 2 years, during which we

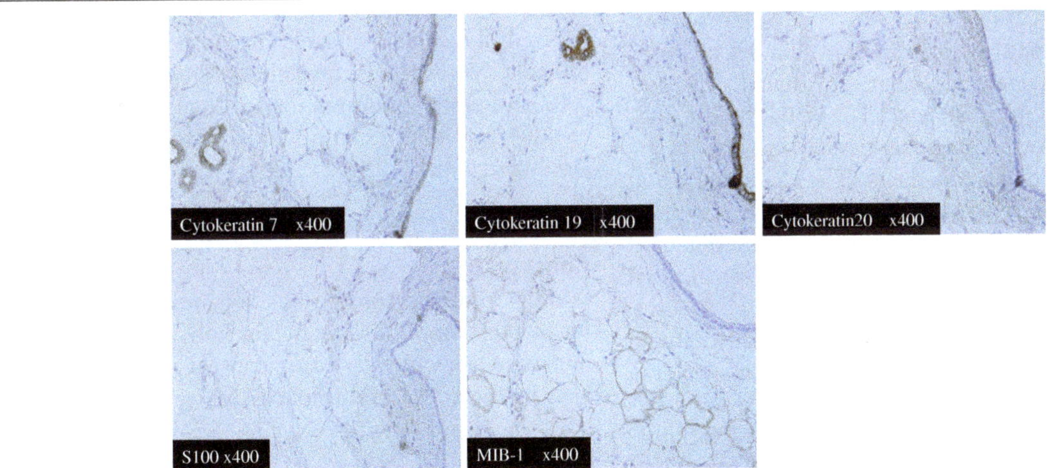

Fig. 5 Immunohistochemical stains. The epithelial cells of the ducts expressed cytokeratin 7 and cytokeratin 19, but were negative for cytokeratin 20. The adipose tissue was positive for S-100 protein and mostly negative for MIB-1

Table 2 A summary of the literature review of pancreatic hamartoma

	Age	Mean (range)	50.5 years (34 weeks - 78 years)
	Sex	M/F	18/12
	Site	Head/body & tail/diffuse	20/8/2
Clinical features	Size	Mean (range)	4.4 cm (0.9 – 19 cm)
	Treatment	PD/other	11/19
	Symptom	+/-	18/12
	Pancreatitis	+/-	4/26
	Acini	+/-	28/0*
	Islets	+/-	10/16*
	Ducts	+/-	29/0*
	Fibrous stroma	+/-	28/2
	Solid/Cystic	Solid/solid and cystic	14/14*
Histopathological features	Solitary/Multiple	Solitary/multiple	22/5*
	Immunostaining	CD34	15 cases
		CD117	9 cases
		S-100	11 cases
		CK 7/8/19	3 cases
		bcr-2	3 cases
		Ki-67	1 cases

*Lack of some cases were not demonstrated in this table

observed chronological morphological changes in the tumor. Sueyoshi et al. [14] reported transformation of the main tumor from multiple large cysts to multiple micro-cysts with solid components in two months. We suggest that this type of chronological morphological change is likely one of the clinical features of pancreatic hamartoma.

Regarding the pathological findings, almost all cases demonstrated disarranged acinar and ductal cells embedded in the fibrous stroma. The solid lesion consisted of fibrous and adipose tissue, and the cystic lesion consisted of dilated ducts. The ducts varied in size and were lined by columnar epithelium without atypical cells. The acinar cells were well differentiated without normal lobular structures. In contrast, normal islets of Langerhans were confirmed in only 9 cases. Pauser et al. [9, 10] and Yamaguchi et al. [19] defined the criteria for the diagnosis of pancreatic hamartoma as: (i) forming a well-demarcated mass, (ii) being comprised of mature acini and ducts with distorted architecture, and (iii) lacking discrete islets of Langerhans. When other case reports are taken into consideration, the presence or absence of the islet cells is still controversial.

In immunohistochemical studies, several authors reported that the acinar cells of pancreatic hamartomas were positive for exocrine markers (amylase and trypsin), and that the ductal cells were positive for epithelial markers (CAM5.2, AE1/AE3 and EMA) [7, 9, 11, 17], similar to what is observed in a normal pancreas. In the present case, cytokeratin 7 and cytokeratin 19, two typical epithelial markers, were expressed in the ductal cells. Conversely, expression of cytokeratin 20, a marker of colorectal and bile ductal epithelium, was negative. Some studies have reported negative staining for S-100 protein, α-smooth muscle actin (α-SMA), desmin and bcr-2 in the stroma cells [11, 15, 17]. In contrast, other cases, including the present case, showed positive staining for S-100 protein in the mature adipose tissue and ductal components [12, 19, 20].

Nagata et al. [11] reported that some of the disordered acinar cells, ductal epithelium, and stromal cells expressed Ki-67. In contrast, Kim et al. [15] and the present case demonstrated negative staining for MIB-1. Recently, many authors have reported that stromal spindle cells express CD34 and CD117 [9–11, 15, 17, 19, 20]. CD34 is a myeloid stem-cell marker and is thought to play an important role in maintaining stromal integrity and inhibiting tumor cell migration. CD117 is a transmembrane tyrosine kinase receptor for stem cell factors and is encoded by the proto-oncogene c-kit [10]. As mentioned above, the characteristics of pancreatic hamartoma are still unclear and controversial. This causes preoperative diagnosis to be difficult, and histological diagnosis with surgical resection is often needed. More reports are necessary to clarify the clinicopathological features of pancreatic hamartomas.

Conclusion

Pancreatic hamartoma is an extremely rare tumor of the pancreas. Recently, this disease has become clearly recognized, the clinical imaging diagnosis remains some of difficult. We suggest that the term "well-demarcated solid and cystic lesion with chronological morphological changes" could be a clinical keyword to describe pancreatic hamartomas.

Consent

Written informed consent was obtained from the patient for publication of this case report and any accompanying images. A copy of the written consent is available for review by the Editor of this journal.

Abbreviations

α-SMA: α-smooth muscle actin; AUS: abdominal ultrasound; CA19-9: carbohydrate antigen 19-9; CEA: carcinoembryonic antigen;

CT: computed tomography; ERCP: endoscopic retrograde cholangiopancreatography; EUS: endoscopic ultrasound; FAT-SAT: T2-fat saturation; HE: Hematoxylin-eosin staining; IHC: immunohistochemical staining; IPMN: Intraductal papillary mucinous neoplasm; MCN: mucinous cystic neoplasm; MPD: main pancreatic duct; MRCP: magnetic resonance cholangiopancreatography; MRI: magnetic resonance imaging; SCN: serous cystic neoplasm; SPNs: solid-pseudopapillary neoplasms; T1WI: T1-weighted imaging; T2WI: T2-weighted imaging.

Competing interests
All authors report no conflicts of interest related to this manuscript and no sources of funding.

Authors' contributions
All authors participated in clinical examinations, diagnosis, surgical operation and follow up for of this patient. HK, YM, KM, HS and SN took part in the design of this study and helped to draft the manuscript. All authors read and approved the final manuscript.

Acknowledgments
The authors are grateful to Dr. Y. Fukukura as a radiologist in Kagoshima University Hospital, Japan. We thank the Joint Research Laboratory, Kagoshima University Graduate School of Medical and Dental Sciences for the use of their facilities.

Author details
[1]Department of Digestive Surgery and Breast and Thyroid Surgery, Graduate School of Medical and Dental Sciences, Kagoshima University, 8-35-1 Sakuragaoka, Kagoshima 890-8520, Japan. [2]Department of Human pathology, Field of Oncology, Graduate School of Medical and Dental Sciences, Kagoshima University, Kagoshima, Japan. [3]Faculty of Medical School of Health Sciencesy, Graduate School of Medical and Dental Sciences, Kagoshima University, Kagoshima, Japan.

References

1. Volkan Adsay AN. Cystic lesions of the pancreas. Mod Pathol. 2007;20:S71–93.
2. Raman SP, Hruban RH, Cameron JL, Wolfgang CL, Fishman EK. Pancreatic imaging mimics: part 2, pancreatic neuroendocrine tumors and their mimics. AJR Am J Roentgenol. 2012;199:309–18.
3. Anthony PP, Faber RG, Russell RC. Pseudotumours of the pancreas. Br Med J. 1977;1:814.
4. Burt TB, Condon VR, Matlak ME. Fetal pancreatic hamartoma. Pediatr Radiol. 1983;13:287–9.
5. Flaherty MJ, Benjamin DR. Multicystic pancreatic hamartoma: a distinctive lesion with immunohistochemical and ultrastructural study. Hum Pathol. 1992;23:1309–12.
6. Izbicki JR, Knoefel WT, Müller-Höcker J, Mandelkow HK. Pancreatic hamartoma: a benign tumor of the pancreas. Am J Gastroenterol. 1994;89:1261–2.
7. Wu SS, Vargas HI, French SW. Pancreatic hamartoma with Langerhans cell histiocytosis in a draining lymph node. Histopathology. 1998;33:485–7.
8. McFaul CD, Vitone LJ, Campbell F, Azadeh B, Hughes ML, Garvey CJ, et al. Pancreatic hamartoma. Pancreatology. 2004;4:533–8.
9. Pauser U, Kosmahl M, Kruslin B, Kilmstra DS, Klöppel G. Pancreatic solid and cystic hamartoma in adults: characterization of a new tumorous lesion. Am J Surg Pathol. 2005;29:797–800.
10. Pauser U, da Silva MT, Placke J, Kilmstra DS, Klöppel G. Cellular hamartoma resembling gastrointestinal stroma tumor: a solid tumor of the pancreas expressing c-kit (CD117). Med Pathol. 2005;18:1211–6.
11. Nagata S, Yamaguchi K, Inoue T, Yamaguchi H, Ito T, Gibo J, et al. Solid pancreatic hamartoma. Pathol Int. 2007;57:276–80.
12. Durczynski A, Wiszniewski M, Olejniczak W, Polkowski M, Sporny S, Strzelczyk J. Asymptomatic solid pancreatic hamartoma. Arch Med Sci. 2011;7(6):1082–4.
13. Kersting S, Janot MS, Munding J, Suelberg D, Tannapfel A, Chromik AM, et al. Rare solid tumors of the pancreas as differential diagnosis of pancreatic adenocarcinoma. JOP. 2012;13:268–77.
14. Sueyoshi R, Okazaki T, Lane GJ, Arakawa A, Yao T, Yamataka A. Multicystic adenomatoid pancreatic hamartoma in a child: Case report and literature review. Int J Surg Case Rep. 2013;4:98–100.
15. Kim HH, Cho CK, Hur YH, Koh YS, Kim JC, Kim HJ, et al. Pancreatic hamartoma diagnosed after surgical resection. J Korean Surg Soc. 2012;83:330–4.
16. Sampelean D, Adam M, Muntean V, Hanescu B, Domsa I. Pancreatic hamartoma and SAPHO syndrome: a case report. J Gastrointestin Liver Dis. 2009;18:483–6.
17. Kawakami F, Shimizu M, Yamaguchi H, Hara S, Matsumoto I, Ku Y, et al. Multiple solid pancreatic hamartomas: A case report and review of the literature. World J Gastrointest Oncol. 2012;4:202–6.
18. Addeo P, Tudor G, Oussoultzoglou E, Averous G, Bachellier P. Pancreatic hamartoma. Surg. 2014;156:1284–5.
19. Yamaguchi H, Aishima S, Oda Y, Mizukami H, Tajiri T, Yamada S, et al. Distinctive histopathological findings of pancreatic hamartomas suggesting their "hamartomatous" nature: a study of 9 cases. Am J Surg Pathol. 2013;37:1006–13.
20. Inoue H, Tameda M, Yamada R, Tano S, Kasturahara M, Hamada Y, et al. Pancreatic hamartoma: a rare cause of obstructive jaundice. Endoscopy. 2014;46:E157–8.
21. Mandavilli SR, Port J, Ali SZ. Lymphoepithelial cyst (LEC) of the pancreas: cytomorphology and differential diagnosis on fine-needle aspiration (FNA). Diagn Cytopathol. 1999;20:371–4.
22. Tewari N, Rollins K, Wu J, Kaye P, Lobo DN. Lymphoepithelial cyst of the pancreas and elevated cyst fluid carcinoembryonic antigen: a diagnostic challenge. JOP. 2014;15:504–7.
23. Zavras N, Machairas N, Foukas P, Lazaris A, Patapis P, Machairas A. Epidermoid cyst of an intrapancreatic accessory spleen: a case report and literature review. World J Surg Oncol. 2014;12:92.
24. Salimi J, Karbakhsh M, Dolatshahi S, Ahmadi SA. Cystic teratoma of the pancreas: a case report. Ann Saudi Med. 2004;24:206–9.
25. Scheele J, Barth TF, Strassburg J, Juchems M, Kornmann M, Henne-Bruns D. Dermoid cyst of the pancreas. Int J Colorectal Dis. 2010;25:415–6.
26. Kurahara H, Shinchi H, Mataki Y, Maeda S, Takao S. A case of squamous cyst of pancreatic ducts. Pancreas. 2009;38:349–51.
27. Milanetto AC, Iaria L, Alaggio R, Pedrazzoli S, Pasquali C. Squamous cyst of pancreatic ducts: a challenging differential diagnosis among benign pancreatic cysts. JOP. 2013;14:657–60.
28. Reid MD, Choi H, Balci S, Akkas G, Adsay V. Serous cystic neoplasms of the pancreas: clinicopathologic and molecular characteristics. Semin Diagn Pathol. 2014;31:475–83.
29. Hois EL, Hibbeln JF, Sclamberg JS. CT appearance of incidental pancreatic lipomas: a case series. Abdom Imaging. 2006;31:332–8.
30. Suzuki R, Irisawa A, Hikichi T, Shibukawa G, Takagi T, Wakatsuki T, et al. Pancreatic lipoma diagnosed using EUS-FNA. A case report. JOP. 2009;10:200–3.
31. Wang H, Li K, Wang J. A large lipoma of the pancreas. ANZ J Surg. 2011;81:200.
32. Albrecht E. Uber hamartoma. Verhandlungen der Deutschen Gesellschaft fur Pathologie. 1904;7:153–7.
33. Noltenius H, Colmant HJ. Excessive hyperplasia of the exocrine pancreatic tissue and Wernicke's encephalopathy (author's transl). Med Klin. 1977;72:2155–8 [In German].

25

Intraductal papillary mucinous carcinoma of the pancreas associated with pancreas divisum

Takeshi Nishi[1,2*], Yasunari Kawabata[2], Noriyoshi Ishikawa[3], Asuka Araki[3], Seiji Yano[2], Riruke Maruyama[3] and Yoshitsugu Tajima[2]

Abstract

Background: Pancreas divisum, the most common congenital anomaly of the pancreas, is caused by failure of the fusion of the ventral and dorsal pancreatic duct systems during embryological development. Although various pancreatic tumors can occur in patients with pancreas divisum, intraductal papillary mucinous neoplasm is rare.

Case presentation: A 77-year-old woman was referred to our hospital because she was incidentally found to have a cystic tumor in her pancreas at a regular health checkup. Contrast-enhanced abdominal computed tomography images demonstrated a cystic tumor in the head of the pancreas measuring 40 mm in diameter with slightly enhancing mural nodules within the cyst. Endoscopic retrograde pancreatography via the major duodenal papilla revealed a cystic tumor and a slightly dilated main pancreatic duct with an abrupt interruption at the head of the pancreas. The orifice of the major duodenal papilla was remarkably dilated and filled with an abundant extrusion of mucin, and the diagnosis based on pancreatic juice cytology was "highly suspicious for adenocarcinoma". Magnetic resonance cholangiopancreatography depicted a normal, non-dilated dorsal pancreatic duct throughout the pancreas. The patient underwent a pylorus-preserving pancreaticoduodenectomy under the diagnosis of intraductal papillary mucinous neoplasm with suspicion of malignancy arising in the ventral part of the pancreas divisum. A pancreatography via the major and minor duodenal papillae on the surgical specimen revealed that the ventral and dorsal pancreatic ducts were not connected, and the tumor originated in the ventral duct, i.e., the Wirsung's duct. Microscopically, the tumor was diagnosed as intraductal papillary mucinous carcinoma with microinvasion. In addition, marked fibrosis with acinar cell depletion was evident in the ventral pancreas, whereas no fibrotic change was noted in the dorsal pancreas.

Conclusion: Invasive ductal carcinomas of the pancreas associated with pancreas divisum usually arise from the dorsal pancreas, in which the occurrence of pancreatic cancer may link to underlying longstanding chronic pancreatitis in the dorsal pancreas; however, the histopathogenesis of intraductal papillary mucinous neoplasm in this anomaly is a critical issue that warrants further investigation in future.

Keywords: Intraductal papillary mucinous carcinoma, Pancreas, Pancreas divisum, Ventral pancreas

* Correspondence: nishiken1027@gmail.com
[1]Deparment of Surgery, Matsue Red Cross Hospital, 200 Horo-machi, Matsue, Shimane 690-8506, Japan
[2]Department of Digestive and General Surgery, Shimane University Faculty of Medicine, 89-1 Enyacho, Izumo, Shimane 693-8501, Japan
Full list of author information is available at the end of the article

Background

Pancreas divisum, the most common congenital anomaly of the pancreas, is the result of non-fusion of the ventral and dorsal pancreatic duct systems. The incidence of pancreas divisum is reported to range from 5 to 10 % in Western countries [1–3], but only from 1 to 2 % in Asia [3–5]. About 20–45 % of patients with pancreas divisum develop clinical symptoms [2, 4], and most of these symptoms are associated with pancreatitis of the dorsal pancreas due to stenosis or a small orifice of the minor duodenal papilla that can block the outflow of pancreatic juice in the dorsal duct into the duodenum [6, 7]. Pancreatic tumors sometimes develop in patients with pancreas divisum, with an incidence of 11.1–12.5 % [8, 9]. The majority of these pancreatic tumors are ductal carcinomas, and intraductal papillary mucinous neoplasm (IPMN) is rare [8, 9]. We herein report a case of intraductal papillary mucinous carcinoma (IPMC) arising in the ventral part of pancreas divisum and review the relevant literature.

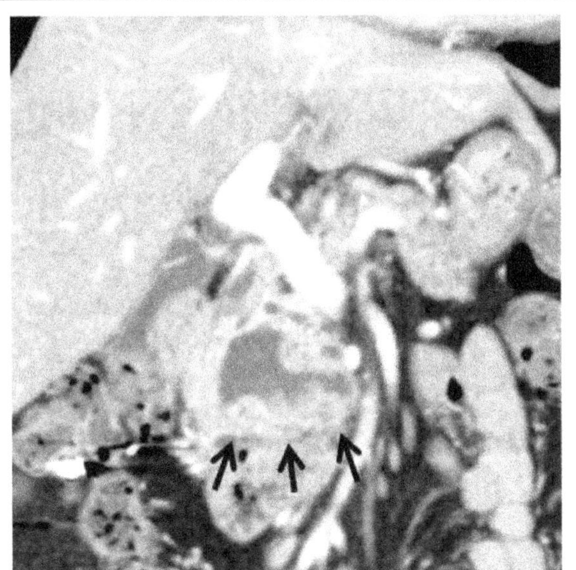

Fig. 1 Coronal image of contrast-enhanced computed tomography of the abdomen. A cystic tumor is seen in the head of the pancreas with slightly enhancing mural nodules (arrows)

Case presentation

A 77-year-old woman underwent an annual medical checkup and was diagnosed with a cystic tumor in the pancreas by computed tomography (CT) of the abdomen. The patient was referred to our hospital for further examination. Her medical history included a radical parotidectomy for a parotid gland tumor and a total knee replacement for the right leg. In addition, she was receiving treatment for hypertension and osteoporosis. On admission, she had no clinical symptoms. Her height was 154 cm and her body weight was 61 kg. There was no superficial lymphadenopathy or palpable mass in the abdomen. Her serum amylase level was 211 U/L (normal range; 30–120 U/L), and other biochemical data, including tumor marker levels, fasting plasma glucose, and hemoglobin A1c, were within normal ranges. An upper gastrointestinal endoscopy showed esophageal hiatal hernia and short-segment Barrett's esophagus. Colonoscopy showed diverticula in the sigmoid colon. Contrast-enhanced abdominal CT scanning demonstrated a cystic tumor in the head of the pancreas measuring 40 mm in diameter with slightly enhancing mural nodules within the cyst (Fig. 1). Magnetic resonance cholangiopancreatography (MRCP) revealed a cystic tumor in the head of the pancreas along with a normal, non-dilated dorsal pancreatic duct throughout the pancreas (Fig. 2). The presence of a connection between the cystic lesion and the main pancreatic duct was unclear. Endoscopic retrograde pancreatography (ERP) via the major duodenal papilla showed a cystic tumor and a slightly dilated main pancreatic duct, but the main pancreatic duct was abruptly interrupted at the head of the pancreas (Fig. 3). The major duodenal papilla was enlarged and the orifice was filled with abundant mucin (Fig. 4). The minor duodenal papilla was normal in size and ERP via the minor papilla was not possible. The diagnosis based on pancreatic juice cytology was "highly suspicious for adenocarcinoma," suggestive of an intraductal papillary mucinous carcinoma (IPMC) arising in the ventral pancreas of pancreas divisum. The patient underwent a pylorus-preserving pancreaticoduodenectomy (PPPD) with regional lymphadenectomy. The postoperative course was uneventful, except for a Grade A pancreatic fistula (staged according to the International

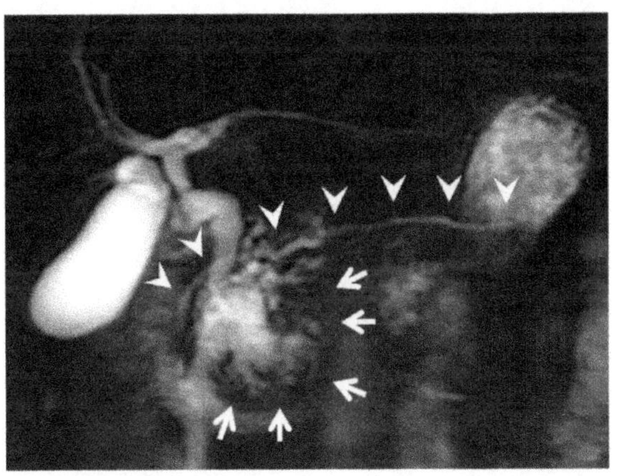

Fig. 2 Magnetic resonance cholangiopancreatography. A cystic tumor is seen in the head of the pancreas (arrows). The dorsal pancreatic duct is normal in size and clearly depicted throughout the pancreas (arrow heads)

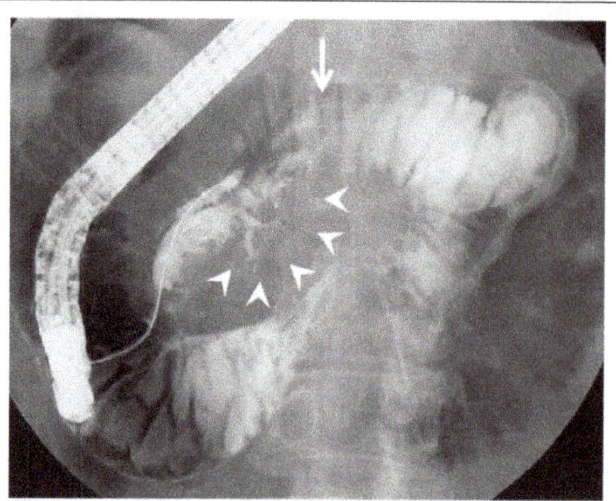

Fig. 3 Endoscopic retrograde pancreatography via the major duodenal papilla. A cystic tumor (arrow heads) and a slightly dilated main pancreatic duct, which is abruptly interrupted at the head of the pancreas (arrow), are seen

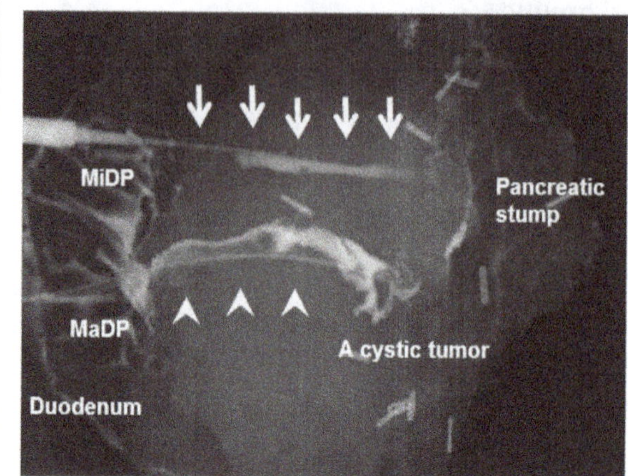

Fig. 5 Pancreatography via the major duodenal papilla (MaDP) and minor duodenal papilla (MiDP) on the surgical specimen. There is no connection between the dorsal pancreatic duct (arrows) and the ventral pancreatic duct (arrow heads). A cystic tumor is connected to the ventral pancreatic duct

Study Group on Pancreatic Fistula clinical criteria [10]), and the patient was discharged on postoperative day 29.

A pancreatography via the major and minor duodenal papillae on the surgical specimen revealed no connection between the ventral and dorsal pancreatic duct systems (Fig. 5). Macroscopically, a multilocular cystic tumor, 40 × 35 × 25 mm in size, with abundant accumulation of mucin was identified in the ventral pancreas. Microscopically, the tumor was composed of atypical epithelial cells showing nuclear enlargement, clear nucleoli, and disordered polarity (Fig. 6). They formed prominent papillary structures. The Mib-1 index was up to 80 %. The tumor cells slightly progressed into the main pancreatic duct. Finally, the tumor was determined to be a mixed type IPMC (well-differentiated adenocarcinoma) with partial microinvasion. The pancreas bearing the tumor was drained by the pancreatic duct, which opened into the major papilla, suggesting that it was the ventral pancreas. The region surrounding the IPMC was mainly composed of fibrous tissue, which was clearly distinguished from the normal pancreas (Fig. 7). The normal pancreas was relatively rich in adipose tissue and the islets of Langerhans were typically oval in shape, features consistent with the dorsal pancreas. Furthermore, the pancreatic duct in the region of the normal pancreas was linked to the minor papilla, also suggesting a dorsal pancreas origin.

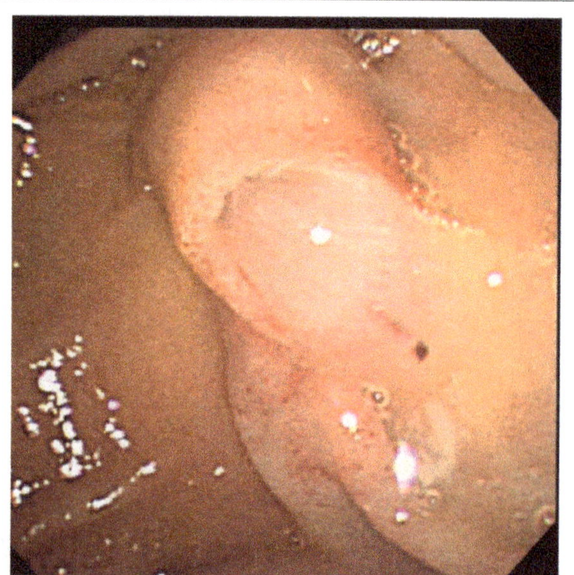

Fig. 4 Endoscopic findings of the major duodenal papilla. The major duodenal papilla is enlarged and the orifice is filled with abundant mucin

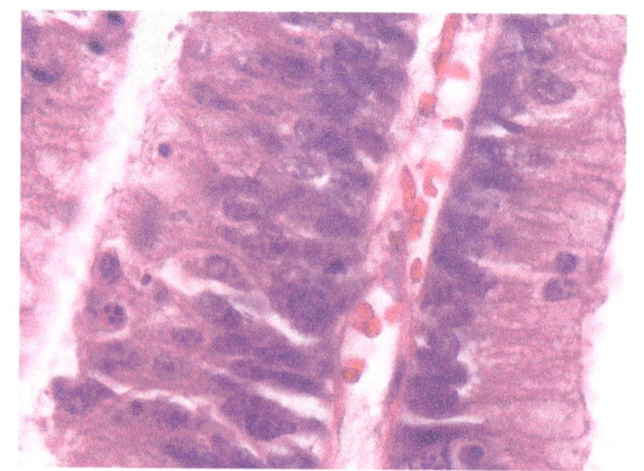

Fig. 6 Microscopic findings of the cystic tumor. The tumor is composed of atypical epithelial cells showing nuclear enlargement, clear nucleoli, and disordered polarity (hematoxylin and eosin, magnification 400x)

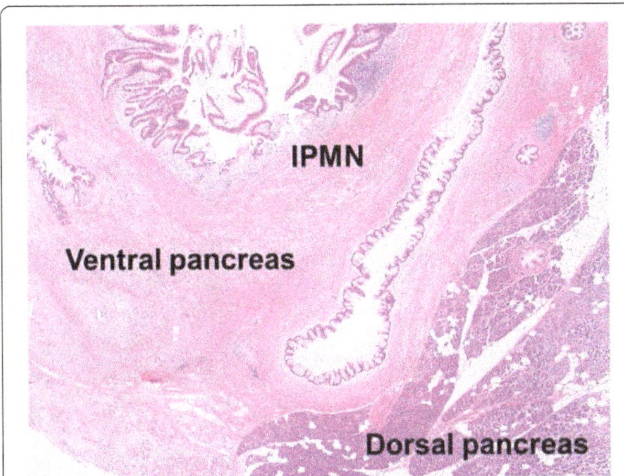

Fig. 7 Microscopic findings of the head of the pancreas. The pancreas bearing the tumor shows marked fibrosis, which is clearly distinguished from the neighboring pancreas. The normal pancreas i.e., the dorsal pancreas, is rich in adipose tissue (hematoxylin and eosin, magnification 200×)

Discussion

The pancreas is formed from the dorsal and ventral buds of the foregut. Between the 6th and 8th week of embryological life, the ventral bud rotates behind the duodenum to reach below and behind the head of the dorsal pancreas. The ventral bud forms the remainder of the head and uncinate process of the pancreas, while the dorsal bud develops into the remainder of the head and the whole of the body and tail of the pancreatic gland [6]. The two ductal systems fuse so that the pancreatic gland drains almost entirely through Wirsung's duct into the major duodenal papilla, and the distal dorsal duct regresses and drains as Santorini's duct through the minor duodenal papilla [6]. When the dorsal and ventral pancreatic duct systems fail to join during embryogenesis, the condition is called "pancreas divisum," and it results in inadequate pancreatic drainage because the bulk of the pancreatic gland drains through Santorini's duct via the minor duodenal papilla [11]. Warshaw et al. [12] have classified pancreas divisum into three types: type 1: the ventral pancreatic duct (Wirsung's duct) and dorsal pancreatic duct (Santorini's duct) are completely divided, which is the most common type, accounting for up to 70 % of cases; type 2: an absent ventral pancreatic duct, accounting for up to 20–25 % of cases; and type 3: a filamentous connection between the two duct systems. In our case, pancreas divisum was classified as type 1 based on ERP, MRCP, and pathological findings. However, there was a slight chance that it was an incomplete divisum and the connection between the ventral and dorsal pancreatic duct systems was obscured by the coexisting IPMC.

IPMN associated with pancreas divisum is rare. Recently, Zippi et al. [13] summarized 13 cases of IPMN associated with pancreas divisum. To identify potentially relevant articles related to IPMN associated with pancreas divisum, we performed a literature review by querying PubMed and MEDLINE with the search term "pancreas divisum" and "intraductal papillary mucinous tumor" or "intraductal papillary mucinous neoplasm". In addition, references from these articles were also assessed for additional relevant materials. As a result, 15 cases of IPMN associated with pancreas divisum, including our case, were identified in the English literature [8, 14–26] (Table 1). Based on these reports, the following clinical characteristics were identified: 1) female predominance (80 %), 2) predominance of type 1 (complete pancreatic divisum) (80 %), 3) tumor location in the dorsal pancreas (80 %) rather than in the ventral pancreas, and 4) a predominance of the branch-duct type (60 %) over the main-duct type. More than half of the patients presented with clinical symptoms, such as back pain or epigastric pain, and two patients' symptoms were associated with pancreatitis. In general, most cases of pancreas divisum are asymptomatic and some may present with clinical symptoms related to pancreatitis [6]. In patients with IPMN, mucin-producing tumors may cause an accumulation of mucin in the pancreatic ducts and subsequent obstructive pancreatitis. Although our patient had no symptoms, pancreatic IPMNs arising in patients with pancreas divisum may modify the clinical symptoms of the patients, because dorsal pancreatitis associated with relative stenosis of the minor papilla and pancreatitis due to IPMN may interact with each other. In our case, fibrosis of the pancreas associated with acinar cell degeneration was remarkable in the ventral pancreas, but the bulk of the pancreatic gland, i.e., the dorsal pancreas, was normal without any findings of pancreatitis. This may be the reason why our patient showed no clinical symptoms.

The treatment for IPMN with pancreas divisum depends both on the malignant potential of the IPMN and the symptoms related to pancreas divisum. Our patient showed enhancing mural nodules within the cystic tumor of the pancreas on contrast-enhanced CT examination, and pancreatic juice cytology results were highly suspicious for adenocarcinoma. A surgical resection was thus indicated for the patient according to the international consensus guidelines for IPMN proposed by International Association of Pancreatology [27]. Among reported cases of IPMN with pancreas divisum, operative procedures vary, with some patients undergoing minimally invasive surgery, such as a dorsal pancreatectomy (Table 1). With regard to the surgical management of IPMNs, the extent of pancreatic resection and lymph node dissection has not been standardized because the

Table 1 IPMNs of the pancreas associated with pancreas divisum

Authors [ref.]	Year	Patient age (years)	Sex	Type of pancreas divisum[a]	Type of IPMN	Tumor location	Tumor location based on embryology	Tumor histology	Operation	Clinical symptoms
Origuchi [14]	1996	82	F	1	Branch	Head	Dorsal	Adenoma	(Autopsy)	Icterus (due to other disease)
Thayer [15]	2002	71	F	1	MD	Head-tail	Dorsal	Carcinoma	DorP	None
Yarze [16]	2003	33	F	1	Branch	Head	Dorsal	Adenoma	PD	Epigastralgia, nausea
Sakurai [17]	2004	74	M	2	Branch	Head	Dorsal	Adenoma	PPPD	None
Sakate [18]	2004	34	M	1	Branch	Head	Ventral	Adenoma	PPPD	Back pain, epigastralgia
Kamisawa [8]	2005	63	F	1	Branch	Head	Dorsal	Unknown	Unknown	Unknown
Talbot [19]	2005	51	F	1	Branch	Head	Dorsal	Carcinoma	DorP	None
Akizuki [20][c]	2006	75	F	1	Branch	Body, Tail	Dorsal, Dorsal	Adenoma	CP & PR	Back pain
Scatton [21]	2006	45	M	1	MD	Head-tail	Dorsal	Adenoma	DorP	Episode of pancreatitis
Sterling [22]	2007	70	F	3	MD	Head-tail	Dorsal	Carcinoma[b]	None	Epigastralgia, body weight loss
Santi [23][c]	2010	74	F	1	Branch	Head, Tail	Dorsal, Ventral	Unknown	None	None
Ringold [24]	2010	65	F	1	MD	Head-tail	Dorsal	Adenoma[b]	None	None
Nakagawa [25][d]	2013	70	F	2	Branch	Head-tail	Dorsal	Unknown	None	Relapsing acute pancreatitis
Gurram [26]	2014	39	F	1	MD	Head	Ventral	Adenoma	PD	Epigastralgia
Present case		74	F	1	Mixed	Head	Ventral	Carcinoma	PPPD	None

IPMN: intraductal papillary mucinous neoplasm, [a]type of pancreas divisum according to Warshaw's classification, [b]cytological diagnosis, [c]two tumors existed in the pancreas, [d]multiple tumors existed in the pancreas, Branch: branch-duct type, MD: main-duct type, Mixed: mixed type, DorP: dorsal pancreatectomy, PD: pancreaticoduodenectomy, PPPD: pylorus-preserving pancreaticoduodenectomy, CP: central pancreatectomy, PR: partial resection

malignant potential of pancreatic IPMNs varies. Therefore, it is important to plan an adequate operation on an individual patient basis. Although organ-preserving pancreatectomy, such as duodenum-preserving pancreatic head resection, pancreatic head resection with segmental duodenectomy, or ventral pancreatectomy, could be the treatment of choice for benign or low-grade malignant lesions of the pancreas, PPPD was performed in our patient because the cystic tumor of the pancreas was strongly considered to be IPMC based on preoperative investigations and because a curative pancreatectomy provides a favorable prognosis for patients with IPMC [28, 29].

The etiologic relationship between pancreas divisum and IPMN is an extremely interesting issue. Most pancreatic ductal carcinomas arising in patients with pancreas divisum develop in the dorsal pancreas, and longstanding pancreatitis in the dorsal pancreas caused by relative stenosis of the minor duodenal papilla has been considered to be a predisposing factor for ordinal pancreatic cancer [8, 30]. In our patient, IPMC developed in the ventral pancreas. Because the ventral pancreas drains through the major papilla, ventral pancreatitis is very rare in patients with pancreas divisum [31, 32]. Although marked fibrosis with acinar cell degeneration was evident in the ventral pancreas in our patient, it might be due to chronic obstructive pancreatitis related to the accumulation of mucin in the pancreatic ducts. Talamini et al. [33] have suggested that IPMN is the cause of chronic pancreatitis and not vice versa. Although it is difficult to elucidate the etiologic relationship between pancreas divisum and IPMN, the co-existence of these two unique disorders may have no strong relevance, and the histopathogenesis of IPMNs in patients with this anomaly is a critical issue that warrants further investigation in future.

Conclusion

Longstanding obstructive pancreatitis in the dorsal pancreas due to obstruction of pancreatic juice outflow into the duodenum through the minor duodenal papilla might be a risk factor for ordinal pancreatic cancer arising in the dorsal pancreas in patients with pancreas divisum, but the relationship between pancreas divisum and IPMN is currently unclear. A large case series study would be needed to clarify the etiology of IPMN arising in patients with pancreas divisum.

Consent

Written informed consent was obtained from the patient for publication of this case report and any accompanying images. A copy of the written consent is available for review by the Editor in Chief of this journal.

Abbreviations

IPMN: Intraductal papillary mucinous neoplasm; CT: Computed tomography; MRCP: Magnetic resonance cholangiopancreatography; IPMC: Intraductal papillary mucinous carcinoma; ERP: Endoscopic retrograde pancreatography; PPPD: Pylorus-preserving pancreaticoduodenectomy.

Competing interests

The authors declare that they have no competing interests.

Authors' contributions

TN carried out the surgical procedure, designed the report, analyzed all of the reports, and drafted the manuscript. YK and SY carried out the surgical procedure and participated in designing the report. AA, NI, and RM performed the histological analysis of the surgical specimens. YT participated in designing the report and revised the manuscript for submission. All authors have read and approved the final manuscript.

Acknowledgements

We would like to thank Editage for providing editorial assistance.
This research received no specific grant from any funding agency in the public, commercial, or not-for-profit sectors.

Author details

[1]Deparment of Surgery, Matsue Red Cross Hospital, 200 Horo-machi, Matsue, Shimane 690-8506, Japan. [2]Department of Digestive and General Surgery, Shimane University Faculty of Medicine, 89-1 Enyacho, Izumo, Shimane 693-8501, Japan. [3]Department of Organ Pathology, Shimane University Faculty of Medicine, 89-1 Enyacho, Izumo, Shimane 693-8501, Japan.

References

1. DiMagno MJ, Wamsteker EJ. Pancreas divisum. Curr Gastroenterol Rep. 2011;13:150–6.
2. Cotton PB. Congenital anomaly of pancreas divisum as cause of obstructive pain and pancreatitis. Gut. 1980;21:105–14.
3. Liao Z, Gao R, Wang W, Ye Z, Lai XW, Wang XT, et al. A systematic review on endoscopic detection rate, endotherapy, and surgery for pancreas divisum. Endoscopy. 2009;41:439–44.
4. Kim MH, Lee SS, Kim CD, Lee SK, Kim HJ, Park HJ, et al. Incomplete pancreas divisum: is it merely a normal anatomic variant without clinical implications? Endoscopy. 2001;33:778–85.
5. Kamisawa T, Tu Y, Egawa N, Tsuruta K, Okamoto A. Clinical implications of incomplete pancreas divisum. JOP. 2006;7:625–30.
6. Varshney S, Johnson CD. Pancreas divisum. Int J Pancreatol. 1999;25:135–41.
7. Klein SD, Affronti JP. Pancreas divisum, an evidence-based review: part I, pathophysiology. Gastrointest Endosc. 2004;60:419–25.
8. Kamisawa T, Yoshiike M, Egawa N, Tsuruta K, Okamoto A, Funata N. Pancreatic tumor associated with pancreas divisum. J Gastroenterol Hepatol. 2005;20:915–8.
9. Takuma K, Kamisawa T, Tabata T, Egawa N, Igarashi Y. Pancreatic diseases associated with pancreas divisum. Dig Surg. 2010;27:144–8.
10. Bassi C, Dervenis C, Butturini G, Fingerhut A, Yeo C, Izbicki J, et al. Postoperative pancreatic fistula: an international study group (ISGPF) definition. Surgery. 2005;138:8–13.
11. Michael L. Exocrine Pancreas: Congenital Anomalies: Pancreas Divisum. In: Townsend CM, Beauchamp RD, Evers BM, Mattox KL, editors. Sabiston Textbook of Surgery. 18th ed. Philadelphia: Saunders; 2008. p. 1591.
12. Warshaw AL, Simeone JF, Schapiro RH, Flavin-Warshaw B. Evaluation and treatment of the dominant dorsal duct syndrome (pancreas divisum redefined). Am J Surg. 1990;159:59–66.
13. Zippi M, De Quarto A. Intraductal papillary mucinous neoplasm associated to pancreas divisum. J Gastoint Dig Syst. 2014;4:171.
14. Origuchi N, Kimura W, Muto T, Esaki Y. Mucinproducingadenoma associated with pancreas divisum and hepatic hilar carcinoma: an autopsy case. J Gastroenterol. 1996;31:455–9.
15. Thayer SP, Fernández-del Castillo C, Balcom JH, Warshaw AL. Complete dorsal pancreatectomy with preservation of the ventral pancreas: a new surgical technique. Surgery. 2002;131:577–80.
16. Yarze JC, Chase MP, Herlihy KJ, Nawras A. Pancreas divisum and intraductal papillary mucinous tumor occurring simultaneously in a patient presenting with recurrent acute pancreatitis. Dig Dis Sci. 2003;48:915.
17. Sakurai Y, Matsubara T, Imazu H, Hasegawa S, Miyakawa S, Ochiai M, et al. Intraductal papillary-mucinous tumor of the pancreas head with complete absence of the ventral pancreatic duct of Wirsung. J Hepatobiliary Pancreat Surg. 2004;11:293–8.
18. Sakate Y, Ohira M, Maeda K, Yamada N, Nishihara T, Nakata B, et al. Intraductal papillary-mucinous adenoma developed in the ventral pancreas in a patient with pancreas divisum. J Hepatobiliary Pancreat Surg. 2004;11:366–70.
19. Talbot ML, Foulis AK, Imrie CW. Total dorsal pancreatectomy for intraductal papillary mucinous neoplasm in a patient with pancreas divisum. Pancreatology. 2005;5:285–8.
20. Akizuki E, Kimura Y, Mukaiya M, Honnma T, Koito K, Katsuramaki T, et al. A case of intraductal papillary mucinous tumor associated with pancreas divisum. Pancreas. 2006;32:117–8.
21. Scatton O, Sauvanet A, Cazals-Hatem D, Vullierme MP, Ruszniewski P, Belghiti J. Dorsal pancreatectomy: an embryology-based resection. J Gastrointest Surg. 2006;10:434–8.
22. Sterling MJ, Giordano SN, Sedarat A, Belitsis K. Intraductal papillary mucinous neoplasm associated with incomplete pancreas divisum as a cause of acute recurrent pancreatitis. Dig Dis Sci. 2007;52:262–6.
23. Santi L, Renzulli M, Patti C, Cappelli A, Morieri ML. First case of 2 intraductal papillary mucinous tumors of both ventral and dorsal ducts in pancreas divisum. Pancreas. 2010;39:110–1.
24. Ringold DA, Yen RD, Chen YK. Direct dorsal pancreatoscopy with narrow-band imaging for the diagnosis of intraductal papillary mucinous neoplasm and pancreas divisum (with video). Gastrointest Endosc. 2010;72:1263–4.
25. Nakagawa Y, Yamauchi M, Ogawa R, Watada M, Mizukami K, Okimoto T, et al. Complete pancreas divisum with patulous minor papilla complicated by multifocal branch-duct intraductal papillary mucinous neoplasms. Endoscopy. 2013;45:E199–200.
26. KC, Czapla A, Thakkar S. Acute pancreatitis: pancreas divisum with ventral duct intraductal papillary mucinous neoplasms. BMJ Case Rep. 2014;Oct 7; published online.
27. Tanaka M, Fernández-del Castillo C, Adsay V, Chari S, Falconi M, Jang JY, et al. International consensus guidelines 2012 for the management of IPMN and MCN of the pancreas. Pancreatology. 2012;12:183–97.
28. Wada K, Kozarek RA, Traverso LW. Outcomes following resection of invasive and noninvasive intraductal papillary mucinous neoplasms of the pancreas. Am J Surg. 2005;189:632–7.
29. Suzuki Y, Atomi Y, Sugiyama M, Isaji S, Innui K, Kimura W, et al. Japanese multiinstitutional study of intraductal papillary mucinous tumor and mucinous cystic tumor, cystic neoplasm of the pancreas: a Japanese multiinstitutional study of intraductal papillary mucinous tumor and mucinous cystic tumor. Pancreas. 2004;28:241–6.
30. Traverso LW, Kozarek RA, Simpson T, Galagan KA. Pancreatic duct obstruction as a potential etiology of pancreatic adenocarcinoma: a clue from pancreas divisum. Am J Gastroenterol. 1993;88:117–9.
31. Saltzberg DM, Schreiber JB, Smith K, Cameron JL. Isolated ventral pancreatitis in a patient with pancreas divisum. Am J Gastroenterol. 1990;85:1407–10.
32. Sanada Y, Yoshizawa Y, Chiba M, Nemoto H, Midorikawa T, Kumada K. Ventral pancreatitis in a patient with pancreas divisum. J Pediatr Surg. 1995;30:665–7.
33. Talamini G, Zamboni G, Salvia R, Capelli P, Sartori N, Casetti L, et al. Intraductal papillary mucinous neoplasms and chronic pancreatitis. Pancreatology. 2006;6:626–34.

Cost-effectiveness of diagnostic laparoscopy for assessing resectability in pancreatic and periampullary cancer

Stephen Morris[1], Kurinchi S Gurusamy[2], Jessica Sheringham[1*] and Brian R Davidson[2]

Abstract

Background: Surgical resection is the only curative treatment for pancreatic and periampullary cancer, but many patients undergo unnecessary laparotomy because tumours can be understaged by computerised tomography (CT). A recent Cochrane review found diagnostic laparoscopy can decrease unnecessary laparotomy. We compared the cost-effectiveness of diagnostic laparoscopy prior to laparotomy versus direct laparotomy in patients with pancreatic and periampullary cancer with resectable disease based on CT scanning.

Method: Model based cost-utility analysis estimating mean costs and quality-adjusted life years (QALYs) per patient from the perspective of the UK National Health Service. A decision tree model was constructed using probabilities, outcomes and cost data from published sources. One-way and probabilistic sensitivity analyses were undertaken.

Results: When laparotomy following diagnostic laparoscopy occurred in a subsequent admission, diagnostic laparoscopy incurred similar mean costs per patient to direct laparotomy (£7470 versus £7480); diagnostic laparoscopy costs (£995) were offset by avoiding unnecessary laparotomy costs. Diagnostic laparoscopy produced significantly more mean QALYs per patient than direct laparotomy (0.346 versus 0.337). Results were sensitive to the accuracy of diagnostic laparoscopy and the probability that disease was unresectable. Diagnostic laparoscopy had 63 to 66% probability of being cost-effective at a maximum willingness to pay for a QALY of £20 000 to £30 000. When laparotomy was undertaken in the same admission as diagnostic laparoscopy the mean cost per patient of diagnostic laparoscopy increased to £8224.

Conclusions: Diagnostic laparoscopy prior to laparotomy in patients with CT-resectable cancer appears to be cost-effective in pancreatic cancer (but not in periampullary cancer), when laparotomy following diagnostic laparoscopy occurs in a subsequent admission.

Keywords: Cost-effectiveness analysis, Diagnostic laparoscopy, Pancreatic cancer, Periampullary cancer

Background

Surgical resection is generally considered to be the only curative treatment for pancreatic and periampullary cancer (which includes ampullary cancer and duodenal cancer along with cancer of the head of the pancreas). Only 15 to 20% of patients undergo potentially curative resection [1-5]. In the remaining patients, the tumours are not resectable because the cancer has spread into surrounding structures or because of disseminated disease. Despite the availability of high quality imaging including helical computed tomography (CT scanning), endoscopic ultrasound (EUS), and magnetic resonance imaging (MRI), 25% to 40% of patients who undergo laparotomy for pancreatic head cancer/periampullary cancer could not be resected, with non-resectability identified only during laparotomy [6,7].

A recent Cochrane Review of 15 studies and a total of 1015 patients found that diagnostic laparoscopy prior to laparotomy can decrease the rate of unnecessary laparotomy from 40% to 17% in patients with pancreatic and periampullary cancer found to have resectable disease from a CT scan [8]. Diagnostic or staging laparoscopy is

* Correspondence: j.sheringham@ucl.ac.uk
[1]Department of Applied Health Research, University College London, Gower Street, 1-19 Torrington Place, London WC1E 7HB, UK
Full list of author information is available at the end of the article

still relevant therefore to detect metastases not identified by high quality imaging techniques such as CT scanning. The Cochrane Review included only studies in which biopsy confirmation of metastatic spread was obtained. The specificity of diagnostic laparoscopy in all studies was 1, since the review included only studies in which diagnostic laparoscopy along with biopsy confirmation of metastatic spread was used as the index test. A review of the NHS Economic Evaluations Database [9] using the search term (laparoscop*) AND ((pancrea*) OR (periampull*)) [28 August 2013] identified 31 studies, but none of these evaluated diagnostic laparoscopy in patients who were resectable following CT scanning. This study investigates the cost-effectiveness of diagnostic laparoscopy prior to laparotomy versus direct laparotomy in patients with pancreatic and periampullary cancer who were considered to have resectable disease and be suitable for major surgery following CT scanning.

Methods

This is a model-based cost-utility analysis to estimate the mean cost per patient and the mean outcome per patient associated with diagnostic laparoscopy prior to laparotomy versus direct laparotomy in patients with pancreatic or periampullary cancers, found to have resectable disease from a CT scan. In our base case we assume that laparotomy following diagnostic laparoscopy occurs in a subsequent admission, and therefore if the laparotomy is unnecessary there is a cost saving because use of the operating theatre and the hospital stay are avoided. In a sensitivity analysis we consider a situation where the laparotomy is undertaken in the same admission as the diagnostic laparoscopy. In this case we assume the cost saving is smaller because while the hospital stay is avoided the cost of the operating theatre would still be incurred if the laparotomy is cancelled.

The outcome measure is quality-adjusted life years (QALYs), which combine length of life and quality of life [10]. QALYs are the recommended outcomes for use in economic evaluations in the UK as they are a common unit that allow for comparable decisions about resource allocation across different health conditions. The analysis is undertaken from the perspective of the UK National Health Service (NHS). Costs are calculated in 2011/12 UK£. Since diagnostic laparoscopy is unlikely to affect long term disease outcomes, a time horizon of six months for costs and outcomes was considered to be appropriate. This is sufficiently long to capture the negative impact of laparotomy on quality of life [11-13]. Due to the short time horizon, discounting of costs and benefits was unnecessary.

Model structure

The analysis uses a decision tree to describe the options being compared and the possible pathways following them (Figure 1). This is a commonly used approach in cost-effectiveness studies of health care programmes [10]. The nodes of a decision tree are points where more than one event is possible. The branches are mutually exclusive events following each node. Decision nodes, represented by squares, show the different options that might be chosen by decision-makers based on the costs and benefits they produce (e.g., to choose diagnostic laparoscopy or direct laparotomy). Chance nodes, represented by circles, show uncertain events, each of which is associated with a probability that it will occur (e.g., whether the diagnostic laparoscopy will show that the cancer is resectable or not). Terminal nodes, represented by triangles, are the endpoints of a decision tree, beyond which no further pathways are available. Each terminal node has costs and QALYs associated with it, summarising the sequence of decisions and events on a unique path leading from the initial decision node to that terminal node. These costs and QALYs are expected values, based on the probability of each event on the pathway occurring up to that point and the costs and QALYs associated with each event.

Patients enter the model with pancreatic or periampullary cancer that has been identified as being resectable following CT scanning. If they undergo diagnostic laparoscopy this may be adequate for determining resectability if histologic confirmation of metastatic disease is possible. If the diagnostic laparoscopy is adequate then it will indicate whether or not the tumour is resectable and if it is, the patient will have a laparotomy. During the laparotomy the tumour may be resected or not. If it is not resected, the patient receives palliative treatment. The laparotomy may result in complications, in some cases an additional laparotomy may be required to treat the complications, and the patient may die perioperatively. If the laparoscopy identifies the tumour as not being resectable then curative surgery is not undertaken and the patient will receive palliative treatment.

For patients undergoing direct laparotomy, it was assumed that the pathway was the same as for resectable disease being identified after adequate laparoscopy, but the probabilities, costs and QALYs associated with each pathway may be different. If the diagnostic laparoscopy was inadequate for histologic confirmation of metastatic disease, the diagnostic laparoscopy was considered to be non-informative and the subsequent pathway was assumed to be as for direct laparotomy but also incurring the costs of the diagnostic laparoscopy procedure.

Probabilities

The probabilities associated with mutually exclusive events at each chance node were obtained from published sources (Additional file 1) [8,14,15]. The probability of

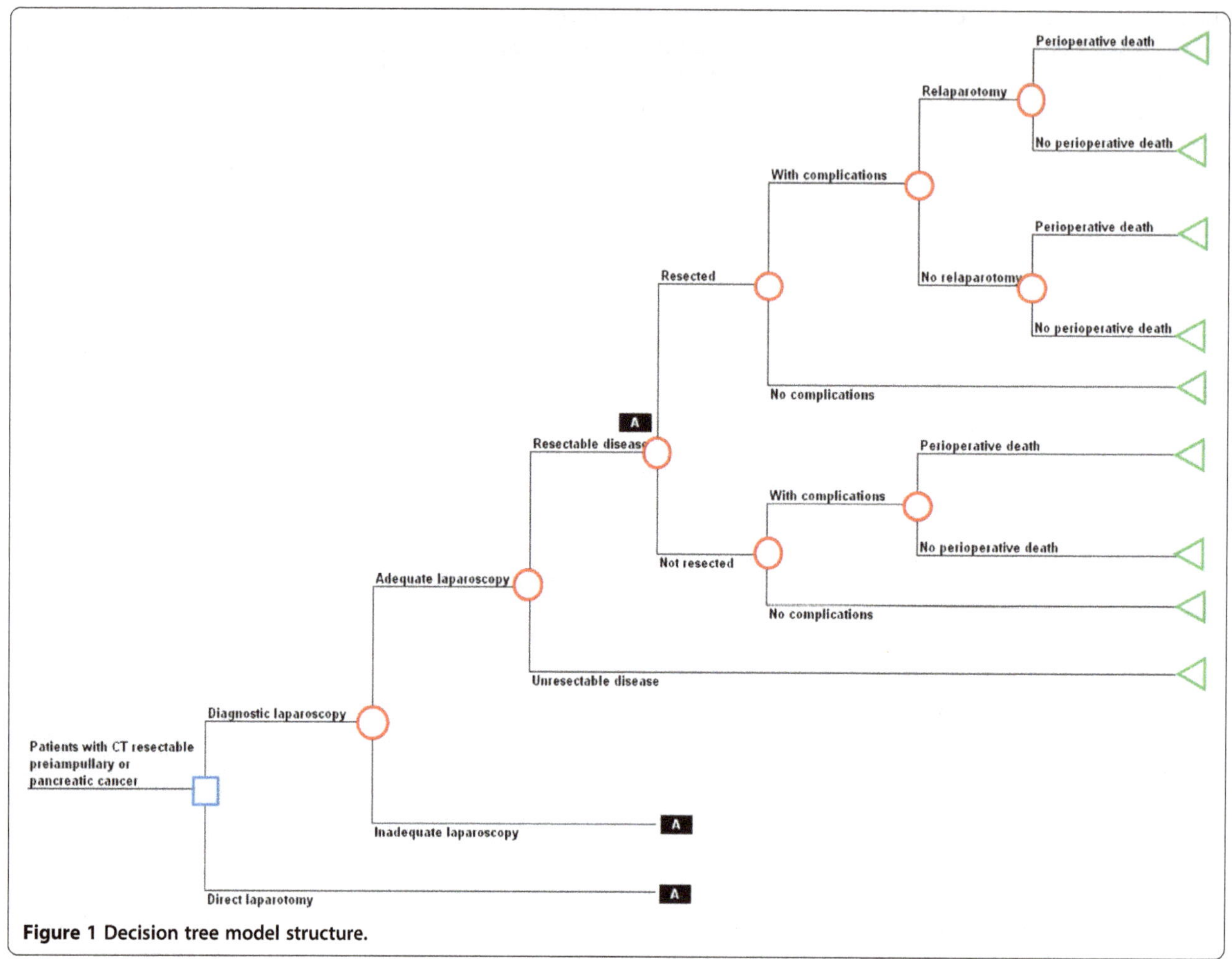

Figure 1 Decision tree model structure.

non-resectable disease with direct laparotomy was 0.403, calculated in the Cochrane Review as the median pre-test prevalence after CT scan of unresectable disease due to distant metastases or local infiltration [8]. Values in the individual studies included in the Cochrane Review ranged from 0.17 to 0.82 [8]. The Cochrane Review also calculated a post-test probability of unresectable disease of 0.173 (95% CI 0.12 to 0.24), meaning that if a patient is said to have resectable disease after diagnostic laparoscopy, there is a 0.173 probability that their cancer will be unresectable. The difference in the probability that the tumour is unresectable following adequate diagnostic laparoscopy compared with direct laparotomy is therefore 0.403-0.173 = 0.230, meaning that on average using diagnostic laparoscopy prior to laparotomy would avoid 230 unnecessary laparotomies in 1000 patients in whom laparotomy is planned for curative resection of pancreatic cancers [8] and 770 patient would have a laparotomy. The probability of undergoing laparotomy is 1−0.230 = 0.770, and the probability the tumour is unresectable among those who have a laparotomy is 0.173/0.770 = 0.225. Put another way, with direct laparotomy, 403 patients in 1000 would have unresectable disease. With diagnostic laparoscopy 230 of these patients would avoid an unnecessary laparotomy, 770 would have a laparotomy and 770*0.225 = 173 of these would have unresectable disease. The probabilities of complications with laparotomy, of relaparotomy, and of perioperative death were taken from a cohort study of 366 patients with pancreatic cancer [14]. The probability of inadequate laparoscopy was taken from one of the studies included in the Cochrane Review which reported this information [15].

Outcomes

QALYs combine length of life and quality of life, where the latter is measured by utility scores. A utility score of 1 represents full health and a utility of 0 death; negative values represent states worse than death. A review of the NHS Economic Evaluations Database [9] was undertaken using the search terms (pancrea* OR ampullary OR periampullary) AND (QALY) [23 February 2014] to identify studies reporting relevant utility scores. After reviewing the reference lists of the identified studies and removing duplicates, 5 studies containing potentially relevant utility data were identified [16-20]. The utility scores used in the model were from one study [19], selected because values were presented for different points over time, because utility scores for all the health states in the model were included in this study enabling better comparability between values, and the values reported also reflected trends in disease-specific quality of life measures found in other studies [11-13] (Additional file 1). Utility scores were measured at 2 weeks, 3 months and 6 months. QALYs were estimated using the trapezium rule for calculating the area under the curve.

Costs

The cost of diagnostic laparoscopy, including histological examination of tissue obtained at laparoscopy was assumed to be £995 (Additional file 1) [21]. This is the average value of the elective inpatient and day case cost, weighted by the proportion of patients in each group. Surgical resection with and without complications was assumed to cost £12 006 and £7083, respectively [21]. Laparotomy without resection was assumed to cost £5378 with complications and £4487 without complications [21]. The cost of repeat laparotomy was assumed to be £7083 [21].

Measuring cost-effectiveness

Cost-effectiveness was measured using monetary net benefits (MNBs). For each treatment the MNB was calculated as the mean QALYs per patient accruing to that treatment multiplied by decision-makers' maximum willingness to pay for a QALY (also referred to as the cost-effectiveness threshold, which in the UK is approximately £20 000 to 30 000 per QALY gained [22]), minus the mean cost per patient for the treatment. This approach converts the outcomes from each treatment into monetary terms and then subtracts the costs of each treatment from the monetised benefits, calculating the net benefit of each treatment in monetary terms. MNBs were calculated using the base case parameter values shown in Additional file 1; these are referred to as the deterministic results since they do not depend on chance. The treatment with the highest MNB represents good value for money and is preferred on cost-effectiveness grounds.

Sensitivity analyses

One-way sensitivity analysis was undertaken, varying the probabilities, outcomes and costs one at a time within the ranges listed in Additional file 1. The aim was to identify the threshold value for each parameter, where one exists, where the treatment with the highest MNB changed (e.g., the value at which diagnostic laparoscopy was no longer the most cost-effective option).

We undertook a probabilistic sensitivity analysis (PSA) as recommended by the National Institute for Health and Care Excellence (NICE) [22]. Distributions were assigned to parameters (Additional file 1) to reflect the uncertainty with each parameter value. A random value from the corresponding distribution for each parameter was selected. This generated an estimate of the mean cost and mean QALYs and the MNB associated with each treatment. This was repeated 5000 times and the results for each simulation were noted. The mean costs, QALYs and MNBs for each treatment were calculated from the 5000 simulations; these are referred to as the probabilistic results since they depend on chance. Using the MNBs for each of the 5000 simulations the proportion of times each treatment had the highest MNB was calculated for a range of values for the maximum willingness to pay for a QALY. These were summarised graphically using cost-effectiveness acceptability curves [10].

In the PSA we used beta distributions to model uncertainty in the probabilities and utility scores, and gamma distributions to model uncertainty in costs [23]. In cases where standard errors were required for the PSA and these were not reported in the sources used it was assumed the standard error was equal to the mean [23]. For the probability of unresectable disease with direct laparotomy after CT scanning, the parameter values for the beta distribution were based on the numbers of unresectable and resectable cancers pooled across all studies included in the Cochrane Review. For the post-test probability of unresectable disease the parameter values were calculated from the 95% confidence interval reported in the Cochrane Review. For the utilities the variance was calculated assuming a beta distribution based on 97 observations [19,20]. 95% confidence intervals around the base case values were derived using standard deviations calculated from the 5000 simulations in the PSA.

We undertook a further sensitivity analysis to investigate the cost savings associated with diagnostic laparoscopy. We considered a situation where the laparotomy following diagnostic laparoscopy was scheduled for the same admission as the diagnostic laparoscopy. When the diagnostic laparoscopy indicated the tumour was not resectable, so the laparotomy was not required, the cost of the hospital stay was avoided but the cost of the operating theatre time was not. This was assumed to cost £3524, based on 4 hours of theatre time at £881 per hour [24].

Finally, because of jaundice being a relative early presentation of ampullary cancers, the resectability rate of ampullary cancers are believed to be higher than that of pancreatic cancers [25]. We therefore reran our analyses separately based on studies from the Cochrane Review that included only patients with pancreatic cancer and only patients with periampullary cancer. As shown in the Cochrane Review, for patients with pancreatic cancer the sensitivity of diagnostic laparoscopy was 67.9%, the median pre-test probability of unresectability was 0.400 and the post-test probability of unresectable disease after negative diagnostic laparoscopy was 0.180. One study in the Cochrane Review included only patients with periampullary cancer [15]. In this study of 144 patients the sensitivity of diagnostic laparoscopy was 52.0%, the pre-test probability of unresectability was 0.174 and the post-test probability of unresectable disease after negative diagnostic laparoscopy was 0.092. We reran our models using these two sets of values holding all other values constant.

Results

Using base case values, and assuming laparotomy following diagnostic laparoscopy occurs in a subsequent admission, diagnostic laparoscopy prior to resection incurred similar costs as proceeding straight to laparotomy without prior laparoscopy (mean cost per patient £7470 (95% CI £7215 to £7724) versus £7480 (95% CI £7219 to £7741) (Table 1); the cost of the diagnostic laparoscopy (£995) was offset by avoiding the costs of unnecessary laparotomy. QALYs up to 6 months were higher for diagnostic laparoscopy compared with direct laparotomy (mean QALYs per patient 0.346 (95% CI 0.346 to 0.347) versus 0.337 (95% CI 0.337 to 0.338)) due to the negative impact of unnecessary laparotomy.

The MNB for diagnostic laparoscopy prior to laparotomy was significantly higher than those for direct laparotomy at a maximum willingness to pay for a QALY of £30 000 (£2921 (95% CI £2807 to £3035) versus £2633 (95% CI £2516 to £2750)) but at a willingness to pay for a QALY of £20 000 the MNB for diagnostic laparoscopy was numerically higher but the 95% CIs overlapped. As expected, the probabilistic results (not shown) were numerically similar to the deterministic results.

Table 1 Base case results

	Diagnostic laparoscopy	Direct laparotomy
Costs	7470 (7356, 7583)	7480 (7363, 7597)
QALYs	0.346 (0.346, 0.347)	0.337 (0.337, 0.338)
Monetary net benefit		
£20 000	−543 (−429, −656)	−738 (−621, −855)
£30 000	2921 (2807, 3035)	2633 (2516, 2750)

QALY = quality adjusted life year. Costs are in 2011/12 UK£. Figures are expected values per patient with 95% confidence intervals in brackets. The point estimates are calculated using base case values of the model parameters (deterministic results). The 95% confidence intervals are derived using standard deviations calculated from the 5000 simulations in the probabilistic sensitivity analysis. The monetary net benefit is calculated at a maximum willingness to pay for a QALY of £20 000 and £30 000. The results are calculated using base case values of the model parameters. Numbers may not sum due to rounding.

In the one-way sensitivity analysis the results were sensitive to changing the values of probability of non-resectable disease with direct laparotomy: values in the individual studies included in the Cochrane Review ranged from 0.17 to 0.82 [8]; for values <0.36 direct laparatomy had the highest MNB. Results were also sensitive to the post-test probability of unresectable disease: the Cochrane review calculated that the 95% CI of this probability was 0.12 to 0.24 [8]; at values > 0.22 direct laparatomy had the highest MNB.

The cost-effectiveness acceptability curves for each treatment show that diagnostic laparoscopy prior to laparotomy had a 63.2% probability of being cost-effective at a maximum willingness to pay for a QALY of £20 000 and a 66.2% probability at a value of £30 000 (Figure 2).

When laparotomy was scheduled for the same admission as diagnostic laparoscopy, and the cost of the hospital stay was avoided if the tumour was unresectable but the cost of the operating theatre time was not, the costs avoided by unnecessary laparotomy were smaller and the mean cost per patient of diagnostic laparoscopy prior to resection increased from £7470 to £8224, which was higher than the cost of direct laparotomy. The MNB for diagnostic laparoscopy prior to laparotomy was lower than the MNB for direct laparotomy at a willingness to pay for a QALY of both £20 000 and £30 000 (–£1297 versus -£738 and £2167 versus £2633, respectively).

When we reran our analyses separately for subgroup of studies from the Cochrane Review that included only patients with pancreatic cancer the MNB for diagnostic laparoscopy prior to laparotomy was higher than the MNB for direct laparotomy at a willingness to pay for a QALY of both £20 000 and £30 000 (–£607 versus -£751 and £2853 versus £2621, respectively). When we reran our analyses separately for patients with periampullary cancer the MNB for diagnostic laparoscopy prior to laparotomy was lower that for direct laparotomy (–£2263 versus -£1693 and £1197 versus £1734, respectively).

Discussion

Main findings

We estimated the mean cost per patient and the mean outcome per patient associated with diagnostic laparoscopy prior to resection versus direct laparotomy in patients with pancreatic and periampullary cancer found to be resectable with curative intent following CT scanning. Diagnostic laparoscopy incurred the same overall costs as direct laparotomy (mean cost per patient £7470 versus £7480) and QALYs up to 6 months were slightly higher for diagnostic laparoscopy (mean QALYs per patient 0.346 versus 0.337) due to the avoidance of unnecessary laparotomy in patients with unresectable disease. The MNBs for diagnostic laparoscopy prior to resection were significantly higher than those for direct

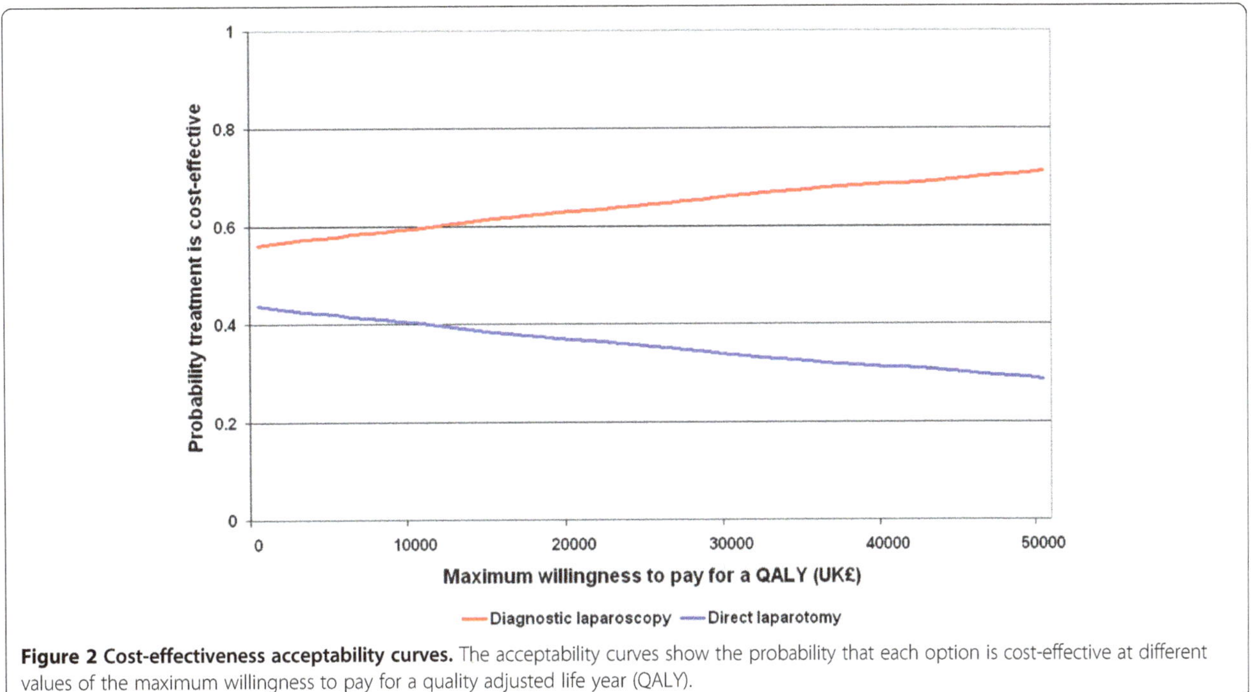

Figure 2 Cost-effectiveness acceptability curves. The acceptability curves show the probability that each option is cost-effective at different values of the maximum willingness to pay for a quality adjusted life year (QALY).

laparotomy at a maximum willingness to pay for a QALY of £30 000 but not £20 000. There is some uncertainty with this finding, with the results being sensitive to key model parameters for test accuracy (probability of unresectable disease (with curative intent) following CT scan that shows resectable disease, post-test probability of unresectable disease).

Diagnostic laparoscopy can either be performed as a separate procedure or immediately prior to laparotomy as part of larger procedure. The advantage of performing diagnostic laparoscopy as part of a larger procedure are that the patient needs only one hospital admission and one general anaesthetic. However if the patient is diagnosed as having unresectable disease at laparoscopy and the subsequent laparotomy is then cancelled, it means that operating time is wasted. If laparoscopy is performed as a separate diagnostic procedure, the patient must undergo the burden of two separate hospital admissions, time to surgery is delayed, which may increase the probability of unresectable disease, and anaesthetics but no operating time will be wasted if they are found to have unresectable disease. When laparotomy is undertaken in the same admission as diagnostic laparoscopy and the cost of the hospital stay is avoided but the cost of the operating theatre time is not, the costs of diagnostic laparoscopy are higher than those for direct laparotomy and the MNBs are lower. Diagnostic laparoscopy is not cost-effective in this scenario.

Diagnostic laparoscopy prior to laparotomy was cost-effective among patients with pancreatic cancer. It was not cost-effective in patients with periampullary cancer despite decreasing the unresectability from 17.4% to 9.2%. This subgroup analysis is based on a single study. One possible explanation of the finding is that fewer periampullary cancer patients had unresectable disease after a CT scan – 17.4% patients [15] compared to 40.0% patients [8]. As indicated in the one-way sensitivity analysis, the results of cost-effectiveness were sensitive to the proportion of patients with unresectable disease after a direct laparotomy. Since fewer unnecessary laparotomies were performed in patients with periampullary cancer, diagnostic laparoscopy may not be cost-effective. However, this has to be confirmed by other studies investigating the incidence of unresectability after direct laparotomy in patients with periampullary cancer or by further studies investigating the utility of diagnostic laparoscopy in patients with periampullary cancer.

Strengths and weaknesses

The strengths of this study are that it was based on a recently published Cochrane review that analysed in detail the available evidence for the diagnostic accuracy of laparoscopy following CT scanning for assessing resectability in pancreatic and periampullary cancer.

An extensive sensitivity analysis has also been performed, which has been useful to show that the conclusions are sensitive to key model parameters surrounding test accuracy.

The main weakness of this study is that while the base case values show diagnostic laparoscopy is cost-effective, the sensitivity analysis indicates that the conclusions will change if key model parameters vary within feasible limits. Hence, conclusions surrounding the cost-effectiveness of diagnostic laparoscopy ought to be treated with caution and further research is recommended to assess cost-effectiveness in different settings. This ought to account for the sensitivity and specificity of diagnostic laparoscopy, the proportion of people unresectable after direct laparotomy, and the costs of laparotomy and diagnostic laparoscopy.

For simplicity the model has a time horizon of 6 months and only perioperative deaths are included. The underlying mortality rate in patients with pancreatic and periampullary cancer would affect both treatment arms equally, and since we are interested in differences in costs and outcomes between the two treatment arms changing the underlying mortality rate would have no impact on relative cost-effectiveness.

The costs associated with diagnostic laparoscopy prior to laparotomy versus direct laparotomy were the same; the QALY gains associated with diagnostic laparoscopy prior to laparotomy are statistically significantly different from zero, but small (mean QALY gain per patient 0.346 - 0.337 = 0.009). This difference may be less than the minimal clinically important difference (minimal clinically important differences in health state utility values are typically in the range 0.010 to 0.048) [26]. Hence, any gains from diagnostic laparoscopy prior to laparotomy purely in terms of QALYs may be misplaced.

Comparison with other studies

This is the first study to evaluate the cost-effectiveness of diagnostic laparoscopy prior to laparotomy versus direct laparotomy in patients with pancreatic and periampullary cancer who were resectable following CT scanning.

Implications for policy and practice

The implications of this study are that when laparotomy following diagnostic laparoscopy occurs in a subsequent admission, diagnostic laparoscopy appears to be cost-effective in decreasing unnecessary laparotomy in patients with pancreatic cancer (but not in those with periampullary cancer) found to have resectable disease on CT scan, producing a small improvement in health outcomes at no extra cost. Diagnostic laparoscopy with laparotomy undertaken in the same admission is not cost-effective.

The results are sensitive to the probability of unresectable disease (with curative intent) following CT scan that shows resectable disease and the accuracy of diagnostic laparoscopy. Given that both of these are operator dependent and the probability of unresectable disease (with curative intent following CT scan) may be lower in patients with periampullary cancer, it is recommended that these probabilities are studied over a period of time to ensure that the most cost-effective option is chosen in that particular setting.

Advances in imaging techniques such as refinements to CT, MRI or positron emission tomography (PET) scans alone or in combination may provide greater diagnostic sensitivity and specificity in pancreatic cancer. However, at present, MRI and PET scans are not as widely available or performed as CT scans and diagnostic laparoscopy and there is currently no evidence that MRI and PET scans decrease unresectability rates. The cost-effectiveness of diagnostic laparoscopy therefore should be revisited if there is evidence that refined CT scanning methods or routine MRI or PET scanning shows a reduction in unresectability rates.

Further research

This study is based on a Cochrane review of the diagnostic accuracy of laparoscopy following CT scanning for assessing resectability in pancreatic and periampullary cancer. The review concluded that further diagnostic test accuracy studies with low risk of bias should be undertaken to calculate the utility of diagnostic laparoscopy more accurately. Given that the results in this study are sensitive to key model parameters for test accuracy, this research would also be beneficial for estimating whether or not diagnostic laparoscopy is cost-effective.

Further research would be useful to consider the impact that avoiding unnecessary laparotomies would have on freeing up operating theatre time and hospital beds if diagnostic laparoscopy was implemented into routine practice.

Conclusions

Diagnostic laparoscopy in patients with CT resectable pancreatic and periampullary cancer appears to be cost-effective when laparotomy following diagnostic laparoscopy occurs in a subsequent admission.

Abbreviations

CI: Confidence Intervals; CT: Computerised tomography; MNBs: Monetary net benefits; MRI: Magnetic resonance imaging; NHS: (UK) National Health Service; NICE: National Institute for Health and Care Excellence; PET: Positron Emission Tomography; PSA: Probabilistic sensitivity analysis; QALYs: Quality-Adjusted Life Years.

Competing interests

The authors declare that they have no competing interests.

Authors' contributions

SM, KSG and BRD conceived and designed the study. SM and KSG collected the data. SM and KSG analyzed the data, JS contributed to the interpretation of the analysis. All authors interpreted the data. SM wrote the first draft of the manuscript and KSG, JS and BRD provided critical revisions that were important for the intellectual content. SM, KSG, JS and BRD approved the final version of the manuscript.

Funding

This project was funded by the National Institute for Health Research National Institute for Health Research Cochrane Programme Grants Scheme (reference number 10/4001/11). The views and opinions expressed are those of the authors and do not necessarily reflect those of the National Institute for Health Research (NIHR), National Health Services (NHS), or the Department of Health.

Author details

[1]Department of Applied Health Research, University College London, Gower Street, 1-19 Torrington Place, London WC1E 7HB, UK. [2]University College London Medical School, 9th Floor, Royal Free Hospital, Rowland Hill Street, London, UK.

References

1. Conlon KC, Klimstra DS, Brennan MF. Long-term survival after curative resection for pancreatic ductal adenocarcinoma: clinicopathologic analysis of 5-year survivors. Ann Surg. 1996;223:273–9.
2. Engelken FJ, Bettschart V, Rahman MQ, Parks RW, Garden OJ. Prognostic factors in the palliation of pancreatic cancer. Eur J Surg Oncol. 2003;29:368–73.
3. Michelassi F, Erroi F, Dawson PJ, Pietrabissa A, Noda S, Handcock M, et al. Experience with 647 consecutive tumors of the duodenum, ampulla, head of the pancreas, and distal common bile duct. Ann Surg. 1989;210:544–54.
4. Shahrudin MD. Carcinoma of the pancreas: resection outcome at the University Hospital Kuala Lumpur. Int Surg. 1997;82:269–74.
5. Smith RA, Bosonnet L, Ghaneh P, Sutton R, Evans J, Healey P, et al. The platelet-lymphocyte ratio improves the predictive value of serum CA19-9 levels in determining patient selection for staging laparoscopy in suspected periampullary cancer. Surgery. 2008;143:658–66.
6. Lillemoe KD, Cameron JL, Hardacre JM, Sohn TA, Sauter PK, Coleman J, et al. Is prophylactic gastrojejunostomy indicated for unresectable periampullary cancer? A prospective randomized trial. Ann Surg. 1999;230:322–8.
7. Mayo SC, Austin DF, Sheppard BC, Mori M, Shipley DK, Billingsley KG. Evolving preoperative evaluation of patients with pancreatic cancer: does laparoscopy have a role in the current era? J Am Coll Surg. 2009;208:87–95.
8. Allen VB, Gurusamy KS, Takwoingi Y, Kalia A, Davidson BR. Diagnostic accuracy of laparoscopy following CT scanning for assessing the resectability in pancreatic and periampullary cancer. Cochrane Database of Syst Rev. 2013, Issue 6. Art. No.: CD009323. doi:10.1002/14651858.CD009323.pub2.
9. NHS Economic Evaluation Database. [http://www.crd.york.ac.uk/CRDWeb/]
10. Morris S, Devlin N, Parkin D, Spencer A. Economic analysis in health care. 2nd ed. London: Wiley; 2012.
11. van Dijkum EJ N, Kuhlmann KF, Terwee CB, Obertop H, de Haes JC, Gouma DJ. Quality of life after curative or palliative surgical treatment of pancreatic and periampullary carcinoma. Br J Surg. 2005;92:471–7.
12. Schniewind B, Bestmann B, Henne-Bruns D, Faendrich F, Kremer B, Kuechler T. Quality of life after pancreaticoduodenectomy for ductal adenocarcinoma of the pancreatic head. Br J Surg. 2006;93:1099–107.
13. Chan C, Franssen B, Dominguez I, Ramirez-Del Val A, Uscanga LF, Campuzano M. Impact on Quality of Life After Pancreatoduodenectomy: A Prospective Study Comparing Preoperative and Postoperative Scores. J Gastrointest Surg. 2012;16:1341–6.
14. Wagner M, Redaelli C, Lietz M, Seiler CA, Friess H, Buchler MW. Curative resection is the single most important factor determining outcome in patients with pancreatic adenocarcinoma. Br J Surg. 2004;91:586–94.
15. Brooks AD, Mallis MJ, Brennan MF, Conlon KC. The value of laparoscopy in the management of ampullary, duodenal, and distal bile duct tumors. J Gastrointest Surg. 2002;6:139–45.
16. Krzyzanowska MK, Earle CC, Kuntz KM, Weeks JC. Using economic analysis to evaluate the potential of multimodality therapy for elderly patients with locally advanced pancreatic cancer. Int J Radiat Oncol Biol Phys. 2007;67:211–8.
17. Murphy JD, Chang DT, Abelson J, Daly ME, Yeung HN, Nelson LM, et al. Cost-effectiveness of modern radiotherapy techniques in locally advanced pancreatic cancer. Cancer. 2012;118:1119–29.
18. Glimelius B, Hoffman K, Graf W, Haglund U, Nyrén O, Påhlman L, et al. Cost-effectiveness of palliative chemotherapy in advanced gastrointestinal cancer. Ann Oncol. 1995;6:267–74.
19. Karuna ST, Thirlby R, Biehl T, Veenstra D. Cost-Effectiveness of Laparoscopy Versus Laparotomy for Initial Surgical Evaluation and Treatment of Potentially Resectable Hepatic Colorectal Metastases: A Decision Analysis. J Surg Oncol. 2008;97:396–403.
20. Langenhoff BS, Krabbe PFM, Peerenboom L, Wobbes T, Ruers TJ. Quality of life after surgical treatment of colorectal liver metastases. Br J Surg. 2006;93:1007–14.
21. National Schedule of Reference Costs - Year 2011–12 - NHS trusts and NHS foundation trusts: NHS own costs. [https://www.gov.uk/government/publications/nhs-reference-costs-financial-year-2011-to-2012]
22. National Institute for Health and Care Excellence (NICE) Guide to the methods of technology appraisal 2013. [http://www.nice.org.uk/article/pmg9/chapter/Foreword]
23. Briggs A, Sculpher M, Claxton K. Decision modeling for health economic evaluation. Oxford: Oxford University Press; 2006.
24. Information Services Division Scotland. Theatre Services. [http://www.isdscotland.org/Health-Topics/Finance/Costs/Detailed-Tables/Theatres.asp]
25. Pancreatic Section, British Society of Gastroenterology, Pancreatic Society of Great Britain and Ireland, Association of Upper Gastrointestinal Surgeons of Great Britain and Ireland, Royal College of Pathologists, Special Interest Group for Gastro-Intestinal Radiology. Guidelines for the management of patients with pancreatic cancer periampullary and ampullary carcinomas. Gut. 2005;54 Suppl 5:v1–16.
26. Walters S, Brazier J. What is the relationship between the minimally important difference and health state utility values? The case of the SF-6D. Health Qual Life Outcomes. 2003;1:4.

Genetic mutations in *SPINK1*, *CFTR*, *CTRC* genes in acute pancreatitis

Dorota Koziel[1*], Stanislaw Gluszek[1,2], Artur Kowalik[3], Malgorzata Chlopek[3] and Liliana Pieciak[3]

Abstract

Background: Explanation of the ultimate causes of acute and chronic pancreatitis is challenging. Hence, it is necessary to seek various etiological factors, including genetic mutations that may be of importance in triggering recurrence and progression of acute to chronic pancreatitis. The aim of this study was to determine the frequency of genetic mutations in patients with acute pancreatitis and to investigate their relationship with the etiology and clinical course.

Methods: The study included 221 patients treated for acute pancreatitis and 345 healthy subjects as a control group. Peripheral blood samples were collected from each study participant and genomic DNA was isolated. Genotyping of common mutations in the SPINK1 (p.N34S and p.P55S) and CTRC (p.I259V, p.V235I, p.K247_R254del, p.E225A) genes was performed using the high-resolution melting method. Mutations in the CFTR p.F508del (delF508_CTT) were genotyped using allele-specific amplification polymerase chain reaction. All detected mutations were confirmed with direct capillary DNA sequencing.

Results: Mutations in SPINK 1, CFTR and *CTRC* were detected in 6.3 %, 2.3 % and 1.8 % of patients with acute pancreatitis versus 3.2 %, 3.8 % and 1.2 % of volunteers in the control group. No relationship was found between the detected mutations and severity of acute pancreatitis: mild acute pancreatitis, mutation of *CFTR* in 4 (2.8 %) and *CTRC* in 2 (1.4 %) patients; severe acute pancreatitis, mutation of *CFTR* and *CTRC* in 1 (2.6 %) case each. The *SPINK1* mutation was significantly more frequent in 8 (10.4 %) severe cases than in 6 (4.2 %) mild cases ($P < 0.05$), and was observed in 5/70 (7.1 %) patients with alcohol-related AP, 5/81 (6.2 %) with biliary AP, and 4/63 (6.3 %) in those without any established cause of the disease.

Conclusions: Mutation p.N34S in *SPINK1* may predispose patients to acute pancreatitis, especially in those abusing alcohol, and may promote a more severe course of the disease.

Keywords: Acute pancreatitis, Etiology, *SPINK1* mutations, *CFTR* mutations, *CTRC* mutations

Background

The most frequent causes of acute pancreatitis (AP) are gallstones and alcohol [1]. However, in a considerable number of individuals, even many attacks of gallstones and multiple episodes of alcohol abuse do not lead to acute pancreatitis [2, 3]. It was presumed that repeated acute pancreatitis and chronic pancreatitis, especially with a family history of pancreatic disease, may have a genetic background. It is considered that genetic etiology is responsible for ~25 % of all cases of chronic pancreatitis; however, it should be emphasized that ~40 % of cases are considered to be idiopathic [4].

Epidemiological investigations have confirmed high morbidity due to acute pancreatitis among adult inhabitants of the Kielce Region in Poland [5]. In 2011, pancreatic events occurred for the first time in 79.7/100,000 inhabitants. In many patients, idiopathic pancreatitis was diagnosed. The study showed that the taking of family and environmental history, which could explain the causes of the disease in some cases, was frequently omitted in the analysis of etiology [5]. This inclined us to explore further the collected epidemiological data.

In the pathogenesis of pancreatitis, various groups of genetic mutations may play an important role. Mutations

* Correspondence: dorota.koziel@wp.pl
[1]Faculty of Health Sciences, Jan Kochanowski University, Kielce, Poland
Full list of author information is available at the end of the article

in the cationic trypsinogen (*PRSS1*), anionic trypsinogen (*PRSS2*), pancreatic secretory trypsin inhibitor (*SPINK1*), cystic fibrosis transmembrane conductance regulator (*CFTR*), chymotrypsinogen (*CTRC*), calcium-sensing receptor (*CASR*) and the protein claudin-2 (*CLDN2*) genes were found in different types of pancreatitis [6–9]. The first described was a mutation of the trypsinogen gene in exon 3 (p.R122H). In other studies, other mutations in this gene were also analyzed, and related with hereditary pancreatitis, such as p.N291, p.A16V, p.R122C and p.D22G [10, 11].

The majority of studies have focused on determining the importance of various mutations in the etiology of pancreatitis. In the case of confirmed presence of a mutation, the course of acute episodes of pancreatitis is rarely investigated in the context of various environmental factors and other factors known as determinants of acute pancreatitis.

The results of studies of mutations and their contribution to the etiology of acute and chronic pancreatitis are divergent; therefore, it seems justifiable to analyze further patients with acute pancreatitis, which is a life-threatening event, and remains an important clinical challenge.

The aim of this study was to determine the frequency of genetic mutations in *SPINK1*, *CFTR* and *CTRC* genes in patients with acute pancreatitis (AP), as well as to investigate their relation with the etiology and clinical course.

Methods

The study included 221 patients with acute pancreatitis, inhabitants of the Kielce Region in Poland, who gave their informed consent for collecting genetic material. Diagnosis of mild, moderate or severe acute pancreatitis (SAP), according to the Atlanta 2012 classification, was the criterion for inclusion in the study. Diagnosis of AP was based on the joint interpretation of medical history, physical examination and targeted laboratory tests. The diagnosis was based upon satisfaction of at least 2 of the following 3 criteria: (1) upper abdominal pain of sudden onset, frequently radiating towards the back; (2) lipase or amylase activity in serum >3 times the upper limit of normal; and (3) results of imaging tests that allow one to obtain cross-sectional images: computed tomography (CT), nuclear magnetic resonance (NMR), or ultrasonography (USG). In the analysis of the etiology of AP, medical history taking can determine alcohol consumption, occurrence of concomitant diseases, drug intake, procedures performed, and endoscopic retrograde cholangiopancreatography (ERCP). Biliary etiology was confirmed based on USG, CT, NMR, and/or ERCP, only if there were indications for performance of these procedures, for example, icterus or triple elevation of alanine aminotransferase level. Endoscopic ultrasonography was performed in some patients to confirm biliary AP. Alcohol consumption was evaluated with the Short Alcohol Dependence Data (SADD) Questionnaire, and self-estimated alcohol consumption via interview. Acute pancreatitis was diagnosed if a patient gained ≥10 points on the SADD Questionnaire, or if a period of alcohol abuse lasted ≥1 year, and the daily dose was 40 g of pure ethanol.

Diagnosis of chronic pancreatitis was an exclusion criterion. The control group included adult volunteers selected by random sampling, without any apparent concomitant diseases that could have affected the structure and expression of genes to be tested in the study.

The control group consisted of 345 healthy inhabitants of the Kielce Region: 223 women and 122 men; mean age 45.1 (44 in women, 47 in men) years, in a general good state of health, with body mass index 18.5–30. The study group included 221 patients who had acute pancreatitis (88 female, 133 male); mean age 55.4 (56.2 in women, 51.4 in men). The course of AP was mild in 65.2 % of patients, moderately severe in 17.6 %, and severe in 17.2 %. The percentage of women in the study group was significantly lower compared with the control group, while the mean age was significantly higher in the study than control group.

The study was approved by the Committee on Bioethics at the Faculty of Health Sciences, Jan Kochanowski University in Kielce. Each patient and member of the control group gave their informed consent to perform the genetic testing.

DNA isolation

Peripheral blood samples were drawn from all study participants and collected in EDTA tubes. DNA was isolated using Micro AX Blood Gravity Kit (A&A Biotechnology, Gdańsk, Poland).

Quality and concentration of isolated DNA was measured by Nano Drop 2000 (Thermo Scientific, TK Biotech, Poland).

Genotyping was performed using the following molecular biology techniques: allele-specific PCR (ASA-PCR) and high-resolution melting (HRM)-PCR, and all detected mutations were confirmed by direct capillary sequencing. To validate ASA-PCR and HRM-PCR, the first 164 samples were sequenced in parallel, irrespective of genotyping results.

Mutation detection in *CFTR* gene

The p.F508del (delF508_CTT) mutation was detected using 10 μl ASA-PCR mixture containing 5 μlSybr Green Kit (Qiagen, Syngen-Biotech, Wrocław, Poland), 1 μl water, 1 μl each primer, and 1 μl DNA template.

PCR was performed in a Veriti 96 Well Thermal Cycler (Applied Biosystems, USA). The cycling profile was set at 95 °C initial denaturation for 1 min, followed by 35 cycles of 15 s at 95 °C, 15 s at 60 °C, 30 s at 72 °C, and a final extension at 72 °C for 7 min. ASA-PCR product detection and visualization were performed using a microchip electrophoresis system MCE-202 Multi NA (Shimadzu, Shim-pol, Warsaw, Poland).

Mutation detection in *SPINK1* and *CTRC* genes

Mutation detection was performed using primers (Table 1) flanking genetic regions containing the following mutations in: *SPINK1* exon 3 (p.N34S and p.P55S), and *CTRC* exon 3 and 7 (p.I259V, p.V235I, p.K247_R254del, and p.E225A).

HRM-PCR mixture was composed of 5 μl Type-it HRM PCR Kit (Qiagen, Synge-Biotech), 7 μl water, 1 μl each forward and reverse primer (Table 1), and 1 μl template DNA. PCR was performed by using Rotor Gene (Qiagen, Syngen-Biotech). Cycling conditions were: 5 min initial denaturation at 95 °C, followed by 40 cycles of 10 s at 95 °C, 30 s at 65 °C, 30 s at 65 °C, but during the first 10 cycles, we used a touchdown mode of 1 °C per cycle, 10 s at 72 °C, and a heteroduplex formation consisting of 10 s at 95 °C and 20 s at 40 °C. Melting temperature range was 75–80 °C for exon 3 *SPINK1*, and 75–95 °C for exon 7 *CTRC*. For *CTRC* exon 3, there were 37 cycles with touchdown (1 °C/cycle) and a melting range of 80–93 °C.

Polymorphisms and mutations in the HRM-PCR products were detected based on a change in the shape of a PCR product melting curve. All detected polymorphisms and mutations were then confirmed by capillary sequencing.

For capillary sequencing, the primers used – HRM-PCR products (Table 1) – were enzymatically purified using Exo SAP reagent containing phosphatase and exonuclease. The purified PCR product was sequenced with Big-Dye Terminator v3.1 Cycle Sequencing Kit (Applied Biosystems). The reaction conditions were 25 cycles of 96 °C for 10 s, 55 °C for 5 s, and 60 °C for 105 s). The reaction products were purified after sequencing by using Big Dye X Terminator Kit (Applied Biosystems). Sequencing was carried out on a 3130 Genetic Analyzer (Applied Biosystems). The resulting chromatograms were analyzed manually and compared using BLAST software from the NCBI site (Table 1).

Statistical analysis

Differences between the 2 groups were analyzed by examining the proportions of patients in each group representing a particular category (e.g., occurrence of *SPINK1* mutation), using the 1-tailed Z test for comparing 2 proportions.

The relationships between gender and occurrence of *SPINK1*, *CFTR* or *CTRC* mutations in patients with AP and in the control group were analyzed using a more conservative test. The data sets were displayed in the form of 2 × 2 contingency tables with gender as the row variable, and occurrence of mutation as the column variable. Some cell numbers were small and there were big differences between cell numbers. The null hypothesis that the specific mutation occurred equally in men and women was verified with Fisher's exact test. Odds ratios wereto compare the odds of occurrence of a specific event in the study group versus the control group, and 95 % confidence intervals were also reported.

Results

There were no significant differences in frequencies of *SPINK1*, *CFTR* and *CTRC* mutations when comparing the male and female patients. The data sets were displayed in the form of 2 × 2 contingency tables with gender as the row variable and occurrence of mutations as the column variable. Some cell numbers were small and large differences occurred between cell numbers. In such a case, Fisher's exact test was applied to analyze the relationships between the variables. The null hypothesis was that the specific mutation occurred equally in men and women (Table 2).

Table 1 Sequences of primers used for the reaction and methods used

Gene	Method		Primer sequence
CFTR ex10	allele-specific PCR	F R M	GCAAGTGAATCCTGAGCGTG
			TGGGTAGTGTGAAGGGTTCAT
			GCACCATTAAAGAAAATATCATTGG
SPINK1 ex3	HRM/capillary sequencing	F R	TTGCTATGAACTCAAGAATGGAGA
			CCGATTTTCAAAACATAACACTG
CTRC ex7	HRM/capillary sequencing	F R	CTTATGCCCTCCCGGTCTGG
			GGACAGCTGTGGAGGCAG
CTRC ex3	HRM/capillary sequencing	F R	CTGACACACAGCCCTCCC
			ATGGCCAGGTCTCAGGGTAT

Table 2 Contingency Table for analysis of the association between gender and mutation in *SPINK1, CFTR, CTRC* in the group of patients with AP and the control group of healthy individuals without a past history of acute pancreatitis

	SPINK 1			*CFTR*			*CTRC*		
	Yes	No	*p*-value	Yes	No	*p*-value	Yes	No	*p*-value
Patients with AP									
Female	5	83	NS*	4	84	NS	1	87	NS
Male	9	124		1	132		3	130	
Marginal Column Totals	14	207	-	5	216	-	4	217	-
Control group of healthy individuals									
Female	8	215	NS	6	217	NS	2	221	NS
Male	3	119		7	115		2	120	
Marginal Column Totals	11	334	-	13	332		4	341	-

NS* no statistical significance

In patients with AP, the gene mutations detected compared with the controls were as follows: *SPINK1*, 6.3 % patients versus 3.2 % controls; *CFTR*, 2.3 % patients versus 3.8 % controls; and *CTRC*, 1.8 % patients versus 1.2 % controls (Table 3).

HRM-PCR and direct sequencing detected 12 p.N32S and 2 p.P55S mis-sense mutations in *SPINK* in patients, which together constituted 6.3 % of AP cases. However, using ASA-PCR, p.F508del mutations were found in 5 (2.3 %) AP cases. HRM-PCR and direct sequencing detected 4 (1.8 %) mutations in *CTRC*. All detected mutations were of the mis-sense type, that is, 2 p.V235I, 1 p.I259V and 1 p.K247_R254del (Table 4).

In 1 patient with recurrence of moderately severe AP with alcohol etiology, we observed p.N34S mutation in *SPINK1* and p.V235I mutation in *CTRC*.

SPINK1

The *SPINK1* mutation was more common in the AP than the control group. The observed proportions were 0.063 and 0.032, respectively. The Z score was 1.777, and the corresponding *P* value was 0.03. The patients with mild AP had a significantly lower proportion of mutations in *SPINK1* than those with moderately severe or severe AP. The observed proportions were 0.042 and 0.104, respectively. The Z score was 1.8095 and the *P* value was 0.03.

In considering the causes of AP (alcoholic, biliary and idiopathic), no differences were found in the frequency of mutation in *SPINK1*. No significant differences were observed between the frequency of mutations in *SPINK1* in the subgroups with and without recurrence.

The study group without recurrent AP had a higher proportion of mutation in *SPINK1* than the control group had, and the difference was almost significant at the 0.05 level. The observed proportions were: 0.065 and 0.032, respectively. The Z score was 1.6436 and the *P* value was 0.0505 (Table 5).

CFTR

There was no significant difference in the frequency of mutation in *CFTR* in the AP and control groups. The observed proportions were: 0.023 and 0.038, respectively. The Z score was −0.9959 and the *P* value was 0.15 (Table 5).

Table 3 Clinical course of AP according to causes of the disease in the group of patients with mutation diagnosed

	Alcohol	Gallstones	Cancer	Idiopathic	Control population
	N = 70 (31.7 %)	*N* = 81 (36.7 %)	*N* = 7 (3.2 %)	*N* = 63 (28.5 %)	*N* = 345
SPINK1 n = 14 (6.3 %)					11 (3.2 %)
Mild AP	2 (2.9 %)	2 (2.5 %)	0	2 (3.2 %)	
Moderate and severe AP	3 (4.3 %)	3 (3.7 %)	0	2 (3.2 %)	
CFTR n = 5 (2.3 %)					13 (3.8 %)
Mild AP	1 (1.4 %)	2 (2.5 %)	1 (14.3 %)	0	
Moderate and severe AP		1 (1.2 %)	0	0	
CTRC n = 4 (1.8 %)					4 (1.2 %)
Mild AP	1 (1.4 %)	1 (1.2 %)	0	0	
Moderate and severe AP	1 (1.4 %)	1 (1.2 %)	0	0	

Table 4 Mutations detected in the *SPINK 1, CFTR, CTRC* genes in correlation with clinical data

Gene mutation	No. of patients	BMI	Alcohol abuse (≥40 g daily)	Cigarette smoking (currently)	Pancreatic diseases in family	Concomitant diseases	Recurrences
SPINK1 p.N34S c.101A > G exon 3	12 (5.42 %)						
1		26.0	Yes	No	No	None	Yes
2		20.2	Yes	No	No	None	No
3		29.8	No	No		None	No
4		24.0	No	No	No	cardiovascular diseases, atherosclerosis, Parkinson's disease	No
5		29.4	No	No	No	None	No
6		23.4	Yes	Yes	No	None	Yes
7		22.4	Yes	Yes	No	gallstones, gastroesophageal reflux disease, psychoorganic syndrome	No
8		27.7	No	No	No	None	No
9		26.4	No	Yes	Yes	arterial hypertension	Yes
10		25.4	No	No	No	None	Yes
11		30.1	Yes	Yes	No	arterial hypertension, type-2 diabetes	No
12		26.6	Yes	No	No	None	No
SPINK1 p.P55S c.163C>	2 (0.9 %)						
1		27.0	Yes	No	No	None	
2		19.0	No	No	No	cardiovascular diseases, gallstones	No
*CFTR*p.F508del (delF508) c.1521_1523 delCTT C > T exon 3	5 (2.3 %)						
1		20.2	No	No	Yes	cardiovascular diseases	No
2		26.4	No	No	No	arterial hypertension	Yes
3		25.6	No	No	No	arterial hypertension	No
4		19.2	No	No	No	pancreatic cancer	No
5		26.0	Yes	Yes	No	None	No
CTRC p.V235I c.703G > A exon 7	2 (0.9 %)						
1		23.4	Yes	Yes	No	None	No
2		22.9	Yes	Yes	No	None	Yes
p.I259V c.775A > C exon 7	1 (0.5 %)						
1		27.0	No	No	Yes		Yes
p.K247_R254 delc.738_761del24 exon 7	1 (0.5 %)						
1		26.2	No	No	No	None	No

CTRC

There was no significant difference in the frequency of mutation in *CTRC* in the AP and control groups. The observed proportions were: 0.018 and 0.012, respectively. The Z score was 0.6396 and the P value was 0.26 (Table 5).

Discussion

SPINK1 is a specific trypsin inhibitor and an acute phase protein that is secreted by the acinar cells. SPINK1 protein plays a role in the prevention of premature activation of zymogen that is catalyzed by trypsin within the pancreatic duct system or the acinar tissue. A reactive

Table 5 Frequency and odds ratios (95 % CI) of mutations in *SPINK1, CFTR, CTRC* in the individual groups with acute pancreatitis and in the control group

	No.	*SPINK1** 14/221 (6.3 %)		*OR * (95 % CI)*	*P value*	*CFTR*** 5/221 (2.3 %)	*OR (95 % CI)*	*P value*	*CTRC*** 4/221 (1.8 %)		*OR (95 % CI)*	*P value*
Severity of the course												
Mild AP	144	6 (4.2 %)		2.05 (0.85-5.1)	$P < 0.005$	4 (2.8 %)	0.59 (0.16- 1.80)	NS	2 (1.4 %)		1.57 (0.29-8.52)	NS
Moderate AP	39	7 (17.9 %)	8 (10.4 %)			0			2 (1.4 %)	1,4 %		
Severe AP	38	1 (2.6 %)				1 (2.6 %)			1 (2.6 %)			
Etiology of AP												
Alcohol	70	5 (7.1 %)		2.33 (0.61- 7.57)	NS	1 (1.4 %)	0.37 (0.01-2.55)	NS	2 (2.9 %)		2.50 (0.22- 17.84)	NS
Gallstones	81	5 (6.2 %)		1.99 (0.53- 6.45)		3 (3.7 %)	0.98 (0.18- 3.7)		2 (2.5 %)		2.15 (0.19-15.33)	
Idiopathic	63	4 (6.3)		2.05 (0.46- 7.23)		0	0 (0–1.78)		0		0 (0–8.365)	
Cancer	7	0		0 (0–23.88)		1 (14.3 %)	4.2 (20.09- 39.08)		0		0 (0–85.65)	
Reccurrences of AP												
Yes	82	5 (6.1 %)		1.97 (0.52- 6.37)	NS	1 (1.2 %)	0.32 (0.01- 2.16)	NS	2 (2.4 %)		2.13 (0.19- 15.135)	NS
No	139	9 (6.5 %)		2.10 (0.75- 5.72)		4 (2.9 %)	0.76 (0.18- 2.51)		2 (1.4 %)		1.24 (0.111-8.8	
Control group	345	11 (3.2 %)*				13 (3.8 %)**			4 (1.2 %)**			

Indicates that the odds of SPINK1 mutations are 2.05 times higher in the AP group than in the control group. The limits (0.847; 5.096) for OR 95 % confidence interval are not very wide, so the OR estimate has rather good precision. The association between the group and the SPINK1mutations occurrence is not significant at the 0.05 level because 95 % confidence interval for the OR contains 1. However, right-sided F exact test rejects the null hypothesis that OR = 1 in favour of the alternative hypothesis that true odds ratio is higher than 1 ($p = 0.0466$). This means that the odds of SPINK1 in the AP group are higher than in the control group, and this conclusion is statistically significant at the 0.05 level

NS no statistical significance

**SPINK1* mutation in the acute pancreatitis group (AP) is more frequent than in the control group: $p < 0.005$

**The differences between the *CFTR, CTRC* mutations in the acute pancreatitis group (AP) and in the control group are insignificant

site in the protein serves as a specific target substrate for trypsin. *SPINK1* polymorphisms are common in the general population (~2 %) and are significantly associated with pancreatitis [12]. The results of studies of p.N34S *SPINK1* mutation in acute pancreatitis are divergent. Tukiainen et al. [13] evaluated the frequency of mutation in *SPINK1* in 371 patients with acute pancreatitis, including 207 with the mild form and 164 with the severe form. The control group comprised 459 individuals. The p.N34S mutation occurred in 29 patients (7.8 %) and 12 individuals (2.6 %) in the control group. In the majority of patients, the disease had an alcohol-related etiology ($n = 229$; 61 %). The frequency of p.N34S mutation was higher in the group with severe disease (15/164; 9.1 %) and with alcoholic etiology (21/229; 9.2 %). The differences were not statistically significant. No differences between age and number of attacks were observed in the groups examined. The researchers concluded that the p.N34S mutation in *SPINK1* may increase susceptibility to acute pancreatitis. O'Reilly et al. [14] confirmed the relationship between this mutation and AP. The abovementioned mutation occurred significantly more often in patients with AP. The authors suggest that this mutation predisposes to premature protease activation in the development of pancreatitis. In turn, Aounet al. [15] found that p.N34S mutation in *SPINK1* was not associated with the first attack of pancreatitis; however, it increased the risk of recurrence. In the present study, the frequency of *SPINK1* mutations in 221 patients with pancreatitis was 6.3 %, which was significantly higher than in the control group ($P = 0.03$). This mutation also occurred significantly more frequently in the patients with moderate and severe forms of AP ($P = 0.03$), compared with those with a mild course of the disease. Our study confirmed the importance of this mutation as a predisposing factor for AP, and was simultaneously responsible for the more severe course of the disease. No differences were observed in the frequency of mutations in individual subgroups according to the cause (alcoholic, biliary, idiopathic, and others). Thus, our observations and those of other researchers suggest that *SPINK1* mutations predispose to severe pancreatitis. Such a relationship was not found in studies of Polish patients with CP. However, it should be stated that the group examined was several times smaller than that investigated in the present study [16].

The studies conducted to date suggest that the spectrum of mutations in *SPINK1* is geographically varied: the IVS 3 + 2 T > C mutation is more frequent in Chinese children with Idiopathic chronic pancreatitis (ICP), whereas p.N34S is more frequent among western populations. The role of IVS3 + 2 T > C mutation has not been finally recognized. It may exert an effect on gene transcription; or it may be the cause of translocation of the entire exon 3 where there is a binding site for trypsin, damaging the splicing donor site, and in the final phase, causing disorder in the protease/antiprotease balance in the pancreas. Further studies are necessary to explain the molecular mechanisms [17].

In the present study, the p.N34S mutation in *SPINK1* was most frequently observed (5.4 % in patients with AP and 0.3 % in the control group), and more rarely, p.P55S mutation (0.9 % and 0.6 % in the control group). The IVS3 + 2 T > C mutation in *SPINK1* often occurred in the study by Wanga et al. [11] – 57.3 % of cases; however, they did not find any p.N34S mutation in *SPINK1*. Kume et al. [18] observed these mutations in 13–17 % of Japanese patients. The IVS3 + 2 T > C mutation in *SPINK1* was often noted in Korean patients with idiopathic and familial pancreatitis [19]. Studies conducted in western countries indicated that this mutation occurred in only 1 (1 %) of 96 patients, and in 3 (2.7 %) of 112 pediatric patients with ICP [20]. Pfutzer et al. [21] showed that N34S mutation in *SPINK1* was seen in 40 % (23/57) of American children with ICP, while Truninger et al. [10] found it in 43 % (6/14) of German patients with early onset of ICP.

Wang et al. [11] observed that the frequency of mutation in *SPINK1* (57.3 %) was higher than that described by Witt et al. (19–40 %). Mystakidis et al. [22] did not find any mutation in *SPINK1* in a group of 30 patients with pancreatitis after ERCP, and concluded that this mutation does not play any important role in the pathogenesis of this type of pancreatitis. Nevertheless, we consider that more comprehensive studies should be carried out to confirm these results. In our study, no patients developed post-ERCP pancreatitis.

Recent studies have suggested an important role for CFTR in the development of pancreatitis, particularly through its role in intraluminal pH regulation from bicarbonate secretion and the flushing of ductal proteins. Secretory granules of pancreatic acinar cells co-release protons with digestive enzymes during normal pancreatic secretion. Diminished ductal bicarbonate secretion and consequent reduced alkalinization of the acinar lumen may promote the development of pancreatitis since acidification of the pancreatic lumen can lead to a loss of tight junction integrity, allowing the leakage of digestive enzymes into the pancreatic duct lumen and interstitial space [23]. Stressors, such as oxidative damage, overloading the protein-folding capacity of the endoplasmic reticulum, trigger the unfolded protein response [24].

Obstructive tubulopathy of the pancreas is the result of *CFTR* dysfunction and plays a primary role in the development of CP; however, the precise process of the course of the inflammation has not been fully established. The function of *CFTR* in the pancreas is important for the dilution and alkalinization of protein-rich secretions, and therefore, plays a preventive role in the formation of protein plugs in the pancreatic ducts. Partial loss of *CFTR* function may be related to idiopathic and alcohol-related pancreatitis. Recently, Schneider et al. [25] have described that the co-occurrence of R75Q mutation in *CFTR* and variants of *SPINK1* was considerably higher in patients with ICP, compared with the control group (8.75 % vs. 0.38 %). Using the patchclamp technique, they found that *CFTR* may be the cause of disturbed secretion of bicarbonates and increased risk of pancreatitis. A large number of *CFTR* mutations and the presence of specific *CFTR* genotype are associated with pancreatitis. In the present study, there was no significant difference in the proportions of mutations in *CFTR* in the AP group (5/221; 2.3 %) and control group (13/345; 3.8 %). The observed proportions were: 0.023 and 0.038, respectively. The Z score was −0.9959 and the *P* value was 0.15866. No relationship was confirmed in mutations with severe AP: mild AP mutation of *CFTR* in 4 (2.8 %) patients, and in the SAP mutation of *CFTR* in 1 (2.6 %) patient. Rosendahl et al. [26] examined 660 patients with chronic pancreatitis and noted that the accumulation of *CFTR* variants in chronic pancreatitis was lower than described previously; nevertheless, the presence of these variants may have increased the risk of development of the disease by 2.7–4.5-fold. The studies confirmed a complex genetic interaction with CP, and a smaller effect of *CFTR* variants in the development of the disease.

The mechanisms by which *CTRC* protects against pancreatitis have been established; however, the importance of *CTRC* variants in terms of risk for RAP and CP is less clear [27]. The *CTRC* mutations may predispose to CP through ineffective trypsin degradation, ineffective carboxypeptidase activation, and induction of endoplasmic reticulum [27]. The *CTRC* mutation is related with chronic pancreatitis in European and Asian populations. Wang et al. [11] did not find mutations in Chinese children with idiopathic pancreatitis, and indicated that *CTRC* mutation may vary geographically and ethnically. In our own studies, *CTRC* mutation occurred with a similar frequency in the study group with AP (4/221; 1.8 %) and in the control group (4/345; 1.2 %). No differences were observed between individual subgroups of AP severity. No p.A73T mutations in *CTRC* were found in the patient or control group. The p.K247_R254del mutation in *CTRC* was confirmed in 1 patient with AP and 3 healthy individuals. The remaining mutations examined, p.E225A, p.V235I and p.I259V in *CTRC*, occurred singly in the group of patients with AP and in the healthy volunteers.

Chang et al. [28] evaluated a Chinese cohort of cases of CP and associated additional mutations with CP, but did not replicate the previous findings. Rosendahl et al. [26] showed that the rare p.R254W and p.K247_R254del variants were significantly over-represented in cases of pancreatitis in Germany.

Conclusions

The N34S mutation of *SPINK1* may predispose to AP, especially in patients who abuse alcohol, and may result in a more severe course of the disease. The accumulation of various mutations and environmental factors may be of importance in the development of AP.

Abbreviations

AP: Acute pancreatitis; CP: Chronic pancreatitis; *PRSS1*: Cationic trypsinogen gene; *PRSS2*: Anionic tripsinogen; *SPINK1*: The pancreatic secretory trypsin inhibitor gene; *CFTR*: The cystic fibrosis transmembrane conductance regulator gene; *CTRC*: The chymotrypsinogen gene; *CASR*: The calcium-sensing receptor gene; *CLDN2*: The protein claudin-2; SAP: Severe acute pancreatitis; CT: Images computed tomography; NMR: Nuclear magnetic resonance; USG: Ultrasonography; ERCP: Endoscopic retrograde cholangiopancreatography; HRM: High resolution melting; ASA-PCR: Allele-specific PCR; ICP: Idiopathic chronic pancreatitis..

Competing interests

The authors declare that they have no competing interests. We guarantee that this paper is original and has not been published in any form to date, nor is it under consideration by any other editorial boards.

Authors' contributions

DK and SG were responsible for the project conception, patients' recruitment, and collection of clinical data. DK, SG and AK designed the study, interpreted genetic and clinical data, and wrote the manuscript. AK designed the genetic analysis, assisted by MCH and LP. MCH and LP conducted the genetic studies, which were analyzed and interpreted by AK, MCH and LP. All authors read and approved the final manuscript.

Author details

[1]Faculty of Health Sciences, Jan Kochanowski University, Kielce, Poland. [2]Clinic General Oncological and Endocrinological Surgery, Regional Hospital, Kielce, Poland. [3]Department of Molecular Diagnostics, Holy Cross Cancer Centre, Kielce, Poland.

References

1. Kozieł D, Kozłowska M, Deneka J, Matykiewicz J, Głuszek S. Retrospective analysis of clinical problems concerning acute pancreatitis in one treatment center. Prz Gastroenterol. 2013;8:320–6.
2. Yadaw D, Eigenbrodt ML, Briggs MJ, Williams DK, Wiseman EJ. Pancreatitis: prevalence and risk factors among male veterans in a detoxification program. Pancreas. 2007;34:390–8.
3. Whitcomb DC. Genetic risk factors for pancreatic disorders. Gastroenterology. 2013;144:1292–302.
4. Keller J, Layer P. Idiopathic chronic pancreatitis. Best Pract Res Clin Gastroenterol. 2008;22:105–13.
5. Gluszek S, Koziel D. Prevalence and progression of acute pancreatitis in the świętokrzyskie voivodeship population. Pol Przegl Chir. 2012;84:618–25.
6. Solomon S, Whitcomb DC. Genetics of pancreatitis: an update for clinicians and genetic counselors. Curr Gastroenterol Rep. 2012;14:112–7.
7. Chandak GR, Idris MM, Reddy DN, Mani KR, Bhaskar S, Rao GV, et al. Absence of PRSS1 mutations and association of SPINK1 trypsin inhibitor mutations in hereditary and non-hereditary chronic pancreatitis. Gut. 2004;53:723–8.
8. Koziel D, Kowalik A, Piecak L, Chlopek M, Gluszek S. The frequency of *SPINK 1*, *PRSS1* and *CFTR* mutations in acute pancreatitis [abstract]. Pancreatology. 2013;13(3S):S55.
9. Koziel D, Gluszek S, Kowalik A, Chlopek M. Genetic factors in acute pancreatitis [abstract]. Pancreatology. 2014;14(3S):96.

10. Truninger K, Kock J, Wirth HP, Muellhaupt B, Arnold C, von Weizsäcker F, Seifert B, Ammann RW, Blum HE. Muellhaupt B. Trypsinogen gene mutations in patients with chronic or recurrent acute pancreatitis. Pancreas. 2001;22:18–23.
11. Wang W, Sun XT, Weng XL, Zhou DZ, Sun C, Xia T, Hu LH, Lai XW, Ye B, Liu MY, Jiang F, Gao J, Bo LM, Liu Y, Liao Z, Li ZS. Comprehensive screening for *PRSS1*, *SPINK1*, *CFTR*, *CTRC* and *CLDN2* gene mutations in Chinese paediatric patients with idiopathic chronic pancreatitis: a cohort study. BMJ. 2013;3, e003150.
12. Ravi Kanth V, Nageshwar RD. Genetics of acute and chronic pancreatitis: an update. World J Gastrointest Pathophysiol. 2014;5:427–37.
13. Ooi CY1, Durie PR. Cystic fibrosis transmembrane conductance regulator (CFTR) gene mutations in pancreatitis. J Cyst Fibros. 2012;11:355–62.
14. Lugea A, Tischler D, Nguyen J, Gong J, Gukovsky I, French SW, Gorelick FS, Pandol SJ. Adaptive unfolded protein response attenuates alcohol-induced pancreatic damage. Gastroenterology. 2011;140:987–97.
15. Aoun E, Muddana V, Papachristou GI, Whitcomb DC. SPINK1 N34S is strongly associated with recurrent acute pancreatitis but is not a risk factor for the first or sentinel acute pancreatitis event. Am J Gastroenterol. 2010;105:446–51.
16. Gasiorowska A, Talar-Wojnarowska R, Czupryniak L, Smolarz B, Romanowicz-Makowska H, Kulig A, Malecka-Panas E. The prevalence of cationic trypsinogen (PRSS1) and serine protease inhibitor, Kazal type 1 (SPINK1) gene mutations in Polish patients with alcoholic and idiopathic chronic pancreatitis. Dig Dis Sci. 2011;56:894–901.
17. Witt H, Luck W, Becker M. A signal peptide cleavage site mutation in the cationic trypsinogen gene is strongly associated with chronic pancreatitis. Gastroenterology. 1999;117:7–10.
18. Kume K, Masamune A, Kikuta K, Shimosegawa T. [−215G > A; IVS3 + 2 T > C] mutation in the SPINK1 gene causes exon 3 skipping and loss of the trypsin binding site. Gut. 2006;55:1214.
19. Oh HC, Kim MH, Choi KS, Moon SH, Park Do H, Lee SS, Seo DW, Lee SK, Yoo HW, Kim GH. Analysis of PRSS1 and SPINK1 mutations in Korean patients with idiopathic and familial pancreatitis. Pancreas. 2009;38:180–3.
20. Witt H1, Luck W, Hennies HC, Classen M, Kage A, Lass U, Landt O, Becker M: **Mutations in the gene encoding the serine protease inhibitor, Kazal type 1 are associated with chronic pancreatitis.** *Nat Genet.* 2000, **25**:213–6.
21. Pfützer RH1, Barmada MM, Brunskill AP, Finch R, Hart PS, Neoptolemos J, Furey WF, Whitcomb DC: **SPINK1/PSTI polymorphisms act as disease modifiers in familial and idiopathic chronic pancreatitis.** *Gastroenterology* 2000, **119**:615–23.
22. Mystakidis K, Kouklakis G, Papoutsi A, Souftas VD, Efremidou E, Kapetanos D, Pitiakoudis M, Lyratzopoulos N, Karagiannakis A, Pantelios A. Is post-ERCP pancreatitis a genetically predisposed complication? Gastroenterol Res Pract. 2012;2012:473960.
23. Tukiainen E, Kylänpää ML, Kemppainen E, Nevanlinna H, Paju A, Repo H, Stenman UH, Puolakkainen P. Pancreatic secretory trypsin inhibitor (SPINK1) gene mutations in patients with acute pancreatitis. Pancreas. 2005;30:239–42.
24. O'Reilly DA, Witt H, Rahman SH, Schulz HU, Sargen K, Kage A, Cartmell MT, Landt O, Larvin M, Demaine AG, McMahon MJ, Becker M, Kingsnorth AN. The SPINK1 N34S variant is associated with acute pancreatitis. Eur J Gastroenterol Hepatol. 2008;20:726–31.
25. Schneider A1, Larusch J, Sun X, Aloe A, Lamb J, Hawes R, Cotton P, Brand RE, Anderson MA, Money ME, Banks PA, Lewis MD, Baillie J, Sherman S, Disario J, Burton FR, Gardner TB, Amann ST, Gelrud A, George R, Rockacy MJ, Kassabian S, Martinson J, Slivka A, Yadav D, Oruc N, Barmada MM, Frizzell R, Whitcomb DC: **Combined bicarbonate conductance-impairing variants in CFTR and SPINK1 variants are associated with chronic pancreatitis in patients without cystic fibrosis.** *Gastroenterology* 2011, **140**:162–71.
26. Rosendahl J, Landt O, Bernadova J, Kovacs P, Teich N, Bödeker H, Keim V, Ruffert C, Mössner J, Kage A, Stumvoll M, Groneberg D, Krüger R, Luck W, Treiber M, Becker M. CFTR, SPINK1, CTRC and PRSS1 variants in chronic pancreatitis: is the role of mutated CFTR overestimated? Gut. 2013;62(4):582–92.
27. Zhou J, Sahin-Tóth M. Chymotrypsin C mutations in chronic pancreatitis. J Gastroenterol Hepatol. 2011;26:1238–46.
28. Chang YT, Wei SC, PC L, Tien YW, Jan IS, Su YN, Wong JM, Chang MC. Association and differential role of PRSS1 and SPINK1 mutation in early-onset and late-onset idiopathic chronic pancreatitis in Chinese subjects. Gut. 2009;58:885.

Ischemic acute pancreatitis with pancreatic pseudocyst in a patient with abdominal aortic aneurysm and generalized atheromatosis

Ileana Cocota[1*], Radu Badea[2], Traian Scridon[3] and Dan L Dumitrascu[4]

Abstract

Background: Ischemic pancreatitis is a rare medical entity. The pancreatic tissue is susceptible to ischemia with the possibility of developing acute pancreatitis. The abdominal aortic aneurysm can be one possible cause of pancreatic hypoperfusion.

Case presentation: We report the case of a 68-year-old man, Caucasian, with a history of a cluster of severe cardiovascular conditions, who presented epigastric pain of variable intensity for about 2 weeks. The pain occurred after intense physical effort, and was associated with anorexia and asthenia. The palpation revealed epigastric pain and palpable pulsatile mass above the umbilicus. Laboratory tests showed increased serum and urine amylases. The abdominal contrast-enhanced CT scan evidenced acute lesions of the pancreas and a caudal pancreatic pseudocyst of 39x24 mm. An abdominal aortic aneurysm was also described (which extended from the kidney level to the bilateral femoral level) with a maximum diameter of 60.5 mm and generalized atheromatosis. By corroborating clinical, anamnestic, laboratory and imaging data, the case was diagnosed as moderately severe acute ischemic pancreatitis, pancreatic pseudocyst, abdominal aortic aneurysm, generalized atheromatosis. The pancreatic pseudocyst was resorbed in eight months. Surgery for the abdominal aneurysm was performed after the resorption of the pseudocyst. The patient died after aortic surgery because of a septic complication.

Conclusion: Ischemic pancreatitis is a rare condition but should be considered in a patient with upper abdominal pain and elevated amylase in the context of an abdominal aortic aneurysm and generalized atheromatosis.

Keywords: Ischemic pancreatitis, Pancreatic pseudocyst, Abdominal aortic aneurysm, Atherosclerosis

Background

The most frequent etiological factors of acute pancreatitis are gallstone disease and alcohol consumption, followed by hyperlipemia, pancreatic malformations, autoimmunity, etc. [1]. Pancreatic ischemia is a rare cause for acute pancreatitis and in most cases it develops only into mild or moderate forms, but there are also forms with extensive pancreatic necrosis that can progress to pancreatic abscesses [1]. Ischemic acute pancreatitis should be treated as any other form of acute pancreatitis, removing, of course, the cause of pancreatic hypoperfusion whenever possible.

* Correspondence: ileanacocota@yahoo.com
[1]2nd Medical Department, Cluj-Napoca, Romania
Full list of author information is available at the end of the article

Case presentation

We present the case of a 68-year-old male patient, Caucasian, living in an urban environment, who was admitted in emergency for epigastric pain. His personal history included duodenal ulcer 20 years ago, coronary heart disease, heart failure diagnosed 6 years ago, with PTCA and stent implantation in the anterior interventricular branch of the left coronary artery 5 years ago, exertional angina pectoris, dilated cardiomyopathy, hypertension risk grade III, hypertensive cardiomyopathy, type 2 diabetes (controlled by oral therapy). The epigastric pain had set on suddenly 2 weeks before, after an intense physical effort (and with inadequate hydration) and radiated to the back. The pain had variable intensity during its evolution, initially described as being of great intensity, later as having an average intensity and was accompanied by anorexia and asthenia. The patient reported associated progressive exertional dyspnea and chest pain with angina characteristics when making intensive efforts.

The patient denied any history of gallstone disease and any high-fat, high-calorie intake or alcohol consumption. He was on a therapeutic regimen containing angiotensin-converting enzyme inhibitor (Prestarium 5 mg once daily), beta blocker (Carvedilol 6,25 mg twice daily), antiplatelet (Aspirin 75 mg once daily), nitrate (Isosorbide mononitrate 40 mg once daily), statin (Rosuvastatin 10 mg once daily) and biguanide (Metformin 800 mg once daily); was compliant to this therapy. As a risk factor he was an ex-smoker, but did not present any familial risk factor.

Clinical findings on hospital admission: apyrexia; asthenia; no pulmonary findings; rhythmic heart sounds, heart rate = 56 beats/min, blood pressure = 140/85 mmHg; no peripheral swelling; abdomen with tenderness in the epigastric area and palpable pulsatile mass above the umbilicus, no defense or muscle stiffness, Murphy and Blumberg signs were negative; normal bowel movements; the diuresis was normal.

The blood tests showed: ESR = 20 mm/h, normal blood count, increased serum (158 UI/l, 1.5 × normal) and urinary amylase (1053 UI/l, 2 × normal), serum glucose = 119 mg/dl, hepatic and renal functions unaltered, normal triglycerides and cholesterol.

The chest x-ray showed no pathological changes.

The abdominal ultrasound followed by abdominal contrast-enhanced ultrasound (CEUS) revealed a 40 mm pancreatic pseudocyst with sediment (Figure 1) and the dilation of an abdominal aortic aneurysm (diameter > 55 mm), (Figure 2), liver steatosis, no gallstones, spleen and kidneys with normal ultrasound appearance.

The CT examination with contrast substance (Ioperamidum) described the spindle-shaped aneurysm of the abdominal aorta dilation beginning from the renal level, extending to 169 mm, until the iliac bifurcation and continuing on both iliac arteries, 40 mm left and 20 mm right respectively. The maximum diameter of the aortic aneurysm was 60.5 mm, with calcified circumferential atheromatosis, diffuse on its whole length; a parietal circumferential thrombosis with a maximum thickness of 27 mm and a minimum of 7 mm was also present; the diameter of the circulated lumen was 19 mm in the distal portion of the aorta, and 29/32 mm respectively below the kidneys. At the level of the renal arteries the aorta had an antero-posterior caliber of 36 mm and a latero-lateral diameter of 42 mm, with thrombosis of 5 mm postero-laterally. No signs of dissection or rupture of the aneurysm were evidenced. Calcified atheromas were described at the level of the splenic artery, and also at the level of the superior mesenteric artery ostium and bilateral renal arteries (Figure 3). On suprarenal and throracic sections, the aorta had a normal caliber.

The CT examination with contrast substance highlighted a round-oval lesion of 39/24 mm, with a slightly heterogeneous structure, partially with fluid content, at the level of the pancreas tail. In the omental bursa and near the tail of the pancreas there was fluid collection and

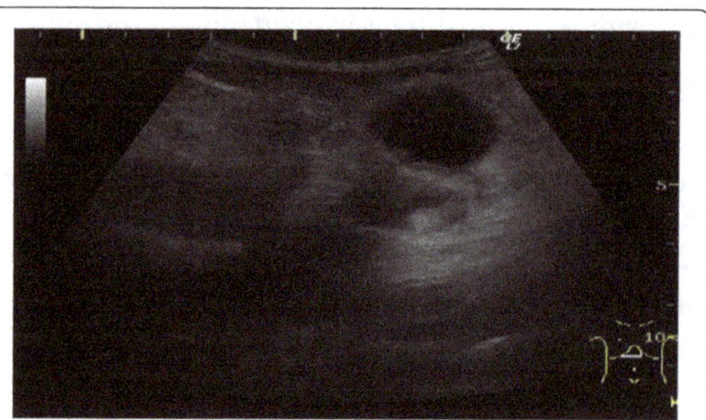

Figure 1 Abdominal ultrasound: pancreatic pseudocyst.

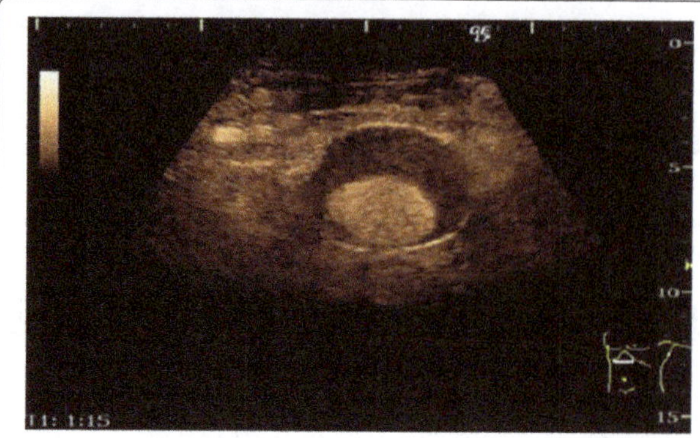

Figure 2 Abdominal contrast-enhanced ultrasound: abdominal aortic aneurysm.

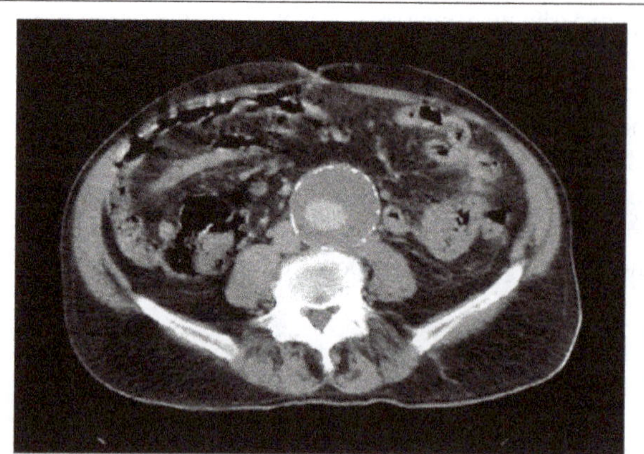

Figure 3 Abdominal CT with contrast: partially thrombosed aneurysm of the abdominal aorta.

fatty infiltration. Otherwise, the pancreas had a normal aspect, and the duct of Wirsung was not dilated. The remaining abdominal organs were normal on the CT scan. (Figure 4). Based on the clinical and anamnestic data (patient denied alcohol consumption or a high fat intake; gallstones were absent; pain appeared after an intensive physical effort), together with the laboratory and imaging data, the case was interpreted as moderately severe ischemic acute pancreatitis [2], pancreatic pseudocyst, partially thrombosed aneurysm of the abdominal aorta, general atheromatosis.

Taking into account the presence of ischemic acute pancreatitis and partially thrombosed aortic aneurysm, a superior gastrointestinal endoscopy was recommended in order to exclude ischemic gastropathy but the patient refused to undergo this procedure.

The cardiovascular surgery examination and the general surgery consultation recommended the abdominal aortic aneurysm surgery to be postponed for 2–3 months, waiting for spontaneous resolution of the pancreatic pseudocyst.

The patient followed a standard therapy including dietary restrictions, hydroelectrolytic rebalancing, proton pump inhibitors, antispasmodics, antibiotics, pancreatic enzymes together with the cardiologic treatment (angiotensin-converting-enzyme inhibitor, beta blockers, antiplatelet therapy, nitrates, statin) and oral antidiabetic drugs. The evolution was favorable with slow normalization of pancreatic enzymes.

After 2 months, the patient returned for follow-up examination. His clinical condition was improved, he did not present abdominal tenderness. Biological findings: ESR = 20 mm/h; normal pancreatic enzymes. The repeated abdominal contrast CT scan showed no significant changes in size for the pancreatic pseudocyst and the abdominal aortic aneurysm (Figure 5).

This time gastroscopy was performed, showing no pathological changes.

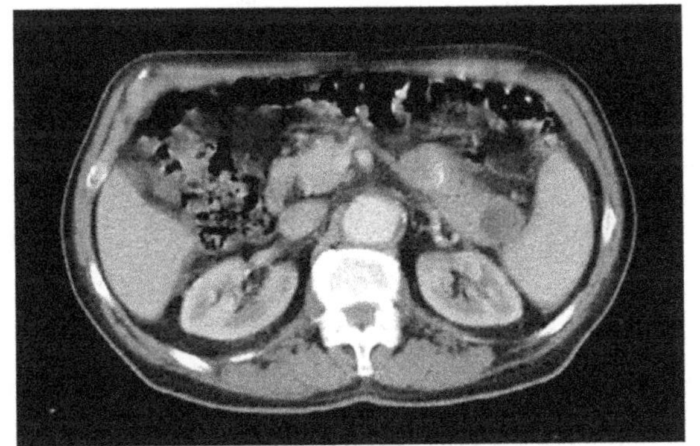

Figure 4 Abdominal CT with contrast: caudal pancreatic pseudocyst.

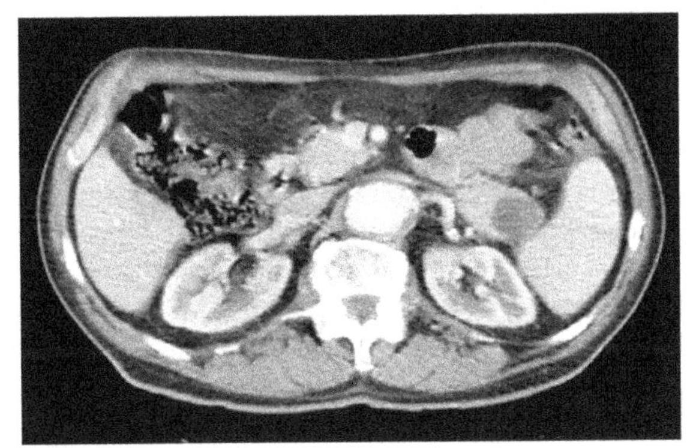

Figure 5 Abdominal CT with contrast: caudal pancreatic pseudocyst (after 2 months).

A cardiovascular surgery consultation was performed again, and the patient was scheduled for aortobifemoral endoluminal prosthesis. Meanwhile the follow–up showed that the pancreatic pseudocyst had resorbed in eight months. (Figure 6). Surgery was delayed due to an intercurrent respiratory infection of the patient (bronchitis).

Surgery for the abdominal aneurysm was performed after the resorption of the pseudocyst. The cure of the aortic aneurysm was performed by bypass grafting with dacron aorto-bifemoral prosthesis. After surgery, a complication appeared, namely a periprosthetic retroperitoneal abscess. Another surgical intervention was therefore necessary, but severe septic shock occurred, leading to the patient's death.

Discussion

The arterial vascularization of the pancreas is ensured by branches of the hepatic artery and superior mesenteric artery for the head of the pancreas, and branches

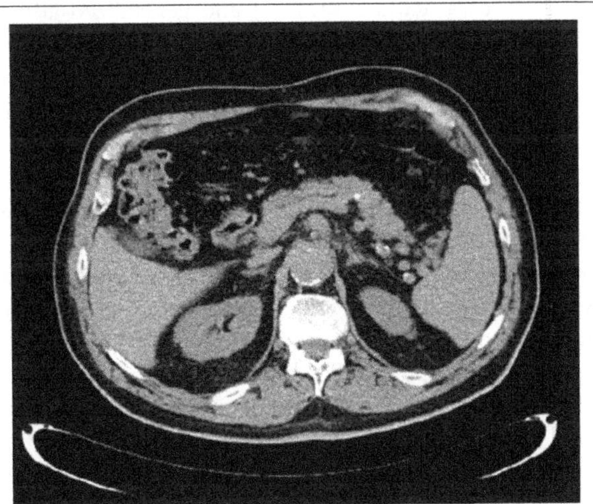

Figure 6 Abdominal CT native: normal pancreatic structure (after eight months).

from the splenic artery for the body and the tail of the pancreas. It is known that the pancreatic tissue is susceptible to ischemia with the possibility of developing acute pancreatitis [1]. The appearance of oxygen-derived free radicals that affect the microvascularization, leading to endothelial dysfunction, increase of the permeability for active proteases, affecting intracellular homeostasis, as well as activating the polymorphonuclear cells, represent important mechanisms in the pathogenesis of ischemic pancreatitis [3]. Ischemic acute pancreatitis may have different presentations: in some cases it can be expressed as a prolonged increase of serum and urinary amylases, accompanied by minimal symptoms, which in most cases are solved spontaneously; but in some cases complications may occur, i.e. pancreatic necrosis and abscess formation [1].

Cases of acute pancreatitis after cardiogenic shock determined by cardiac tamponade have been described [4], supported also by postmortem studies [5] or studies on experimental animals [6]. Cases of ischemic acute pancreatitis after cardiac arrest followed by reversible resuscitation [7], but also as a complication of intra-aortic balloon counterpulsation have also been published [8]. Ischemic pancreatitis after aortic dissection of an abdominal aortic aneurysm has been reported [9,10], and even as a rare complication of surgical treatment of thoraco-abdominal aortic aneurysm [11-13].

Generalized atheromatosis with significant impairment of splanchnic circulation was also considered a cause, which determines the appearance of pancreatic necrosis of an ischemic type [11]. A case of acute ischemic pancreatitis was reported in an individual who had performed intense physical exercise without appropriate fluid intake [14].

Our patient – in the context of the partially thrombosed aneurysm of the abdominal aorta (which extended from kidney level to femoral arteries) and generalized atheromatosis (with calcified, raw atheroma, at the level of the splenic artery, superior mesenteric artery ostium and renal arteries), he had undertaken intense physical effort, with an increased need for oxygen at the level of the muscles, to the detriment of the splanchnic territory, i.e. pancreatic, causing the onset of ischemic acute pancreatitis. We have also excluded any other possible causes of pancreatitis. In the case described, the pathogenetic mechanism of pancreatitis is explained by the arterial steal phenomenon, aneurysm of the aorta causing pancreatic hypoperfusion, especially in the presence of generalized atheromatosis.

Because the surgical treatment of an aortic aneurysm itself can suffer complications with the appearance of pancreatitis of an ischemic type, the intervention was delayed until the normalization of pancreatic enzymes and the limitation of the lesions. Surgery for the abdominal aneurysm was performed after the resorption of the pseudocyst. But postoperative complications occurred - periprosthetic retroperitoneal abscess and severe septic shock, which led to the patient's death.

This case has several particular features. The diagnosis of a partially thrombosed aneurysm of the abdominal aorta could be established only after the presentation for abdominal pain caused by ischemic recurrent acute pancreatitis, i.e. after an unusual complication. Both the thrombosed aneurysm of the abdominal aorta and the generalized atheromatosis were simultaneously detected, which significantly affected the pancreatic circulation, each of these entities being able to cause ischemic pancreatitis. It should be mentioned that even the surgery for abdominal aortic aneurysm itself may cause pancreatic ischemia and an ischemic episode of pancreatitis; therefore, aorto-bifemoral endoluminal prosthesis was delayed until the normalization of serum pancreatic enzymes.

Conclusions

Ischemic pancreatitis is a rare condition but should be taken into consideration for patients with upper abdominal pain, elevated amylases and significant cardiovascular diseases with extended atheromatosis. The diagnosis relies on the exclusion of other more common causes of pancreatitis.

Consent

Written informed consent was obtained from the patient's family for the publication of this case report. A copy of the written consent is available for review by the Editor-in-Chief of this journal.

Abbreviations

PTCA: Percutaneous transluminal coronary angioplasty; ESR: Erythrocyte sedimentation rate; CT: Computed tomography; CEUS: Abdominal contrast-enhanced ultrasound.

Competing interests

The authors declare that they have no competing interests.

Authors' contributions

IC and DLD prepared the manuscript. DLD and RB provided abdominal ultrasound examinations. RB provided the abdominal contrast-enhanced ultrasound examinations. IC, DLD and TS cared for the patient and provided advice on the clinical aspects of the case report. All authors read and approved the final version of the manuscript.

Author details

[1]2nd Medical Department, Cluj-Napoca, Romania. [2]Department of Clinical Imaging Ultrasound, "Iuliu Hatieganu" University of Medicine and Pharmacy, Cluj-Napoca, Romania. [3]Heart Institute "Prof. Dr. Nicolae Stancioiu", "Iuliu Hatieganu" University of Medicine and Pharmacy, Cluj-Napoca, Romania. [4]2nd Medical Department, "Iuliu Hatieganu" University of Medicine and Pharmacy, Cluj-Napoca, Romania.

References

1. Sakorafas GH, Tsiotou AG. Etiology and pathogenesis of acute pancreatitis: current concepts. J Clin Gastroenterol. 2000;30:343–56.
2. Banks PA, Bollen TL, Dervenis C, Gooszen HG, Johnson CD, Sarr MG, et al. Classification of acute pancreatitis—2012: revision of the Atlanta classification and definitions by international consensus. Gut. 2013;62:102–11.
3. Sakorafas GH, Tsiotou AG, Sarr MG. Ischemia/reperfusion-induced pancreatitis. Dig Surg. 2000;17:3–14.
4. Hanumantharaya D, Dave U, Aprim Y, Al-Sarireh B, Middleton L. Ischemic pancreatitis in a patient with cardiogenic shock. Internet J Gastroenterol. 2010;9 Suppl 2:7.
5. Warshaw AL, O' Hara PJ. Susceptibility of the pancreas to ischemic injury in shock. Ann Surg. 1978;188:197–201.
6. Reilly PM, Toung TJ, Miyachi M, Schiller HJ, Bulkley GB. Haemodynamics of pancreatic ischemia in cardiogenic shock in pigs. Gastroenterology. 1997;113:938–45.
7. Piton G, Barbot O, Manzon C, Moronval F, Patry C, Navellou JC, et al. Acute ischemic pancreatitis following cardiac arrest: a case report. J Pancreas. 2010;11 Suppl 5:456–9.
8. Rizk AB, Rashkow AM. Acute pancreatitis associated with intra-aortic balloon pump placement. Cathet Cardiovasc Diagn. 1996;38:363–4.
9. Umeda I, Hayashi T, Ishiwatari H, Yoshida M, Miyanishi K, Sato Y, et al. A case of severe acute pancreatitis and ischemic gastropathy caused by acute aortic dissection. Jpn J Gastroenterol. 2011;108 Suppl 1:103–10.
10. Vibert E, Becquemin JP, Rotman N, Mellière D. Acute pancreatitis after surgical treatment of abdominal aortic aneurysm. Ann Chir. 2002;127 Suppl 2:101–6.
11. Sakorafas GH, Sakorafas GH, Tsiotos GG, Bower TC, Sarr MG. Ischemic necrotizing pancreatitis. Two case reports and review of the literature. Int J Pancreatol. 1998;24 Suppl 2:117–21.
12. Drissi M, Madani M, Hatim A, Ibat D, Athmani M, Taberkant M, et al. Severe acute pancreatitis after surgical treatment of a ruptured abdominal aortic aneurysm. Ann Vasc Surg. 2009;23 Suppl 6:785–7.
13. Baydin A, Genc S, Aygun D, Eden AO, Yardan T, Bahcivan M. Acute pancreatitis after acuteaortic dissection: report of a case and review of the literature. Fırat Med J. 2008;13 Suppl 4:271–3.
14. Mast JJ, Morak MJM, Brett BT, Van Eijck CHJ. Ischemic acute necrotizing pancreatitis in a marathon runner. J Pancreas. 2009;10 Suppl 1:53–4.

Permissions

All chapters in this book were first published in GASTROENTEROLOGY, by BioMed Central; hereby published with permission under the Creative Commons Attribution License or equivalent. Every chapter published in this book has been scrutinized by our experts. Their significance has been extensively debated. The topics covered herein carry significant findings which will fuel the growth of the discipline. They may even be implemented as practical applications or may be referred to as a beginning point for another development.

The contributors of this book come from diverse backgrounds, making this book a truly international effort. This book will bring forth new frontiers with its revolutionizing research information and detailed analysis of the nascent developments around the world.

We would like to thank all the contributing authors for lending their expertise to make the book truly unique. They have played a crucial role in the development of this book. Without their invaluable contributions this book wouldn't have been possible. They have made vital efforts to compile up to date information on the varied aspects of this subject to make this book a valuable addition to the collection of many professionals and students.

This book was conceptualized with the vision of imparting up-to-date information and advanced data in this field. To ensure the same, a matchless editorial board was set up. Every individual on the board went through rigorous rounds of assessment to prove their worth. After which they invested a large part of their time researching and compiling the most relevant data for our readers.

The editorial board has been involved in producing this book since its inception. They have spent rigorous hours researching and exploring the diverse topics which have resulted in the successful publishing of this book. They have passed on their knowledge of decades through this book. To expedite this challenging task, the publisher supported the team at every step. A small team of assistant editors was also appointed to further simplify the editing procedure and attain best results for the readers.

Apart from the editorial board, the designing team has also invested a significant amount of their time in understanding the subject and creating the most relevant covers. They scrutinized every image to scout for the most suitable representation of the subject and create an appropriate cover for the book.

The publishing team has been an ardent support to the editorial, designing and production team. Their endless efforts to recruit the best for this project, has resulted in the accomplishment of this book. They are a veteran in the field of academics and their pool of knowledge is as vast as their experience in printing. Their expertise and guidance has proved useful at every step. Their uncompromising quality standards have made this book an exceptional effort. Their encouragement from time to time has been an inspiration for everyone.

The publisher and the editorial board hope that this book will prove to be a valuable piece of knowledge for researchers, students, practitioners and scholars across the globe.

List of Contributors

Long Cheng, Zhulin Luo, Ke Xiang, Zhu Huang, Lijun Tang and Fuzhou Tian
Department of General Surgery, Chengdu Military General Hospital, Jinniu District, Chengdu, Sichuan Province, PR China, 610083

Jiandong Ren
Department of Pharmacy, Chengdu Military General Hospital, Chengdu, Sichuan Province, People's Republic of China

Guoliang Yao, Yonggang Fan and Jingming Zhai
Department of General Surgery, The First Affiliated Hospital of Henan University of Science and Technology, 24 Jinghua Road, Luoyang 471003, People's Republic of China

Haruhisa Nakao, Norimitsu Ishii, Yuji Kobayashi, Kiyoaki Ito and Masashi Yoneda
Division of Gastroenterology, Department of Internal Medicine, Aichi Medical University School of Medicine, Nagakute 480-1195, Japan

Kenji Wakai
Department of Preventive Medicine, Nagoya University Graduate School of Medicine, Nagoya 466-8550, Japan

Mitsuru Mori and Masanori Nojima
Department of Public Health, Sapporo Medical University School of Medicine, Sapporo 060-0061, Japan

Yasutoshi Kimura
Department of Surgery, Surgical Oncology and Science, Sapporo Medical University, Sapporo 060-8543, Japan

Takao Endo
Sapporo Shirakaba-dai Hospital, Sapporo 062-0052, Japan

Masato Matsuyama
Hepatobiliary and Pancreatic Section, Gastroenterological Division, Cancer Institute Hospital, Tokyo 135-8550, Japan

Kozue Nakamura
Department of Food and Nutrition, Gifu City Women's College, Gifu 501-2592, Japan

Akiko Tamakoshi
Department of Public Health, Hokkaido University Graduate School of Medicine, Sapporo 060-8638, Japan

Mami Takahashi
Central Animal Division, National Cancer Center Research Institute, Tokyo 104-0045, Japan

Kazuaki Shimada
Department of Hepatobiliary and Pancreatic Surgery, National Cancer Center Hospital, Tokyo 104-0045, Japan

Takeshi Nishiyama, Shogo Kikuchi and Yingsong Lin
Department of Public Health, Aichi Medical University School of Medicine, Nagakute 480-1195, Japan

Omar Banafea, Jinfang Zhao, Ruifeng Zhao and Liangru Zhu
Division of Gastroenterology, Union Hospital, Tongji Medical College, Huazhong University of Science and Technology, No. 1277 Jiefang Avenue, Wuhan 430022, Hubei Province, China

Fabian Pius Mghanga
Department of Nuclear Medicine, Union Hospital, Tongji Medical College, Huazhong University of Science and Technology, Hubei Province Key Laboratory of Molecular Imaging, Wuhan 430022, China

Shuixiang He
Department of Gastroenterology, the first affiliated hospital of Xi'an Jiao Tong university, Xi'an, China

Yong Gu
Department of Gastroenterology, the first affiliated hospital of Xi'an Jiao Tong university, Xi'an, China
Digestive System Department, Shaanxi Provincial Crops Hospital of Chinese People's Armed Police Force, Xi'an, China

Limei Wang, Zhiguo Liu, Hui Luo, Qin Tao, Rongchun Zhang, Xiangping Wang, Rui Huang, Linhui Zhang, Yanglin Pan and Xuegang Guo
Xijing Hospital of Digestive Diseases, Fourth Military Medical University, Xi'an, Shannxi, China

Lina Zhao
Department of Radiotherapy, Xijing Hospital, Xian, China

Zhipeng Hua, Yongjie Su and Xuefeng Huang
Department of Hepatobiliary Surgery, Zhongshan Hospital of Xiamen University, Hubing South Road, Xiamen, Fujian, China

Zhengyu Yin, Xiaoming Wang and Pingguo Liu
Department of Hepatobiliary Surgery, Zhongshan Hospital of Xiamen University, Hubing South Road, Xiamen, Fujian, China
Fujian Provincial Key Laboratory of Chronic Liver Disease and Hepatocellular Carcinoma (Xiamen University Affiliated ZhongShan Hospital), Xiamen, China

Kang Zhang
Fujian Provincial Key Laboratory of Chronic Liver Disease and Hepatocellular Carcinoma (Xiamen University Affiliated Zhong Shan Hospital), Xiamen, China

Jianhua Wan, Yuping Ren, Zhenhua Zhu, Liang Xia and Nonghua Lu
Department of Gastroenterology, The First Affiliated Hospital of Nanchang University, 17 Yongwaizheng Street, Nanchang, Jiangxi 330006, People's Republic of China

Kwangho Yang
Department of Surgery, Division of Hepato-Biliary-Pancreatic Surgery and Transplantation, Pusan National University Yangsan Hospital, 20, Geumo-ro, Mulgeum-eup, Yangsan, Gyeongsangnam-do 50612, South Korea
Research Institute for Convergence of Biomedical Science and Technology, Pusan National University Yangsan Hospital, 20, Geumo-ro, Mulgeum-eup, Yangsan, Gyeongsangnam-do 50612, South Korea

Sung Pil Yun and Hyung Il Seo
Department of Surgery, Biomedical Research Institute, Pusan National University Hospital, 179, Gudeok-Ro, Seo-Gu, Busan 602-739, South Korea

Suk Kim
Department of Radiology, Biomedical Research Institute, Pusan National University Hospital, 179, Gudeok-Ro, Seo-Gu, Busan 602-739, South Korea

Nari Shin
Department of Pathology, Pusan National University Yangsan Hospital, 20, Geumo ro, Mulgeum-eup, Yangsan, Gyeongsangnam-do 50612, South Korea

Do Youn Park
Department of Pathology, Biomedical Research Institute, Pusan National University Hospital, 179, Gudeok-Ro, Seo-Gu, Busan 602-739, South Korea

Fei-hu Zhang, Kai-liang Fan, Xiao-bin Dong, Ning Han, Hao Zhao and Li Kong
Department of Emergency Center, Affiliated Hospital of Shandong University of Traditional Chinese Medicine, Jingshi Road No.16369, Jinan, Shandong Province 250011, China

Yu-han Sun
Department of Traditional Chinese Medicine, Jinan Municipal Organs Hospital, Jianguoxiaojingsan Road No.35, Jinan, Shandong Province 250001, China

Jingzhu Zhang, Lu Ke, Qi Yang, Guotao Lu, Baiqiang Li, Zhihui Tong, Weiqin Li and Jieshou Li
Research Institute of General Surgery, Jinling Hospital, Medical School of Nanjing University, 305 East Zhongshan Road, Nanjing 210002, China

Jianfeng Tu
Research Institute of General Surgery, Jinling Hospital, Medical School of Nanjing University, 305 East Zhongshan Road, Nanjing 210002, China
Zhejiang Provincial People's Hospital, People's Hospital of Hangzhou Medical College, Shangtang road 158#, Hangzhou 310014, China

Yue Yang
Hangzhou Medical College, Binwen road 481#, Hangzhou 310053, China

Hiroaki Nagano, Masayuki Nakajo, Yoriko Kajiya and Atsushi Tani
Departments of Radiology, Nanpuh Hospital, 14-3 Nagata, Kagoshima 892-8512, Japan

Sadao Tanaka
Departments of Pathology, Nanpuh Hospital, 14-3 Nagata, Kagoshima 892-8512, Japan

Mari Toyota and Toru Niihara
Departments of Gastroenterology, Nanpuh Hospital, 14-3 Nagata, Kagoshima 892-8512, Japan

Masaki Kitazono and Toyokuni Suenaga
Departments of Surgery, Nanpuh Hospital, 14-3 Nagata, Kagoshima 892-8512, Japan

Yoshihiko Fukukura and Takashi Yoshiura
Department of Radiology, Kagoshima University Graduate School of Medical and Dental Sciences, 8-35-1 Sakuragaoka, Kagoshima-shi, Kagoshima 890-8544, Japan

Anne Katrin Berger, Georg Martin Haag, Dirk Jäger and Christoph Springfeld
Department of Medical Oncology, National Center for Tumor Diseases (NCT), Heidelberg University Hospital, Im Neuenheimer Feld 460, 69120 Heidelberg, Germany

Martin Ehmann
Pharmacy Department, Heidelberg University Hospital, Heidelberg, Germany

Anne Byl
NCT Clinical Cancer Registry, German Cancer Research Center, Heidelberg, Germany

Seung Kook Cho, Saehyun Jung, Kyong Joo Lee and Jae Woo Kim
Department of Internal Medicine, Yonsei University Wonju College of Medicine, 20 Ilsan-ro, Wonju-si 26426, Republic of Korea

Xiaoyao Li, Lu Ke, Jie Dong, Bo Ye, Lei Meng, Wenjian Mao, Qi Yang, Weiqin Li and Jieshou Li
Surgical Intensive Care Unit (SICU), Department of General Surgery, Jinling Hospital, Medical School of Nanjing University, Nanjing, China

Ke Chen, Xiao-long Liu, Yu Pan and Xian-fa Wang
Department of General Surgery, Sir Run Run Shaw Hospital, School of Medicine, Zhejiang University, 3 East Qingchun Road, Hangzhou 310016, Zhejiang Province, China

Hendi Maher
School of Medicine, Zhejiang University, 866 Yuhangtang Road, Hangzhou 310058, Zhejiang Province, China

Sana Chams, Skye El Sayegh, Mulham Hamdon, Sarwan Kumar and Vesna Tegeltija
Department of Internal Medicine, Wayne State University School of Medicine Rochester Hills, MI, USA

Jun Cao, Chunyan Peng, Xiwei Ding, Yonghua Shen, Han Wu and Ruhua Zheng
Department of Gastroenterology, Nanjing Drum Tower Hospital, The Affiliated Hospital of Nanjing University Medical School, Nanjing, China

Lei Wang and Xiaoping Zou
Department of Gastroenterology, Nanjing Drum Tower Hospital, The Affiliated Hospital of Nanjing University Medical School, Nanjing, China
Zhongshan Road 321, Department of Gastroenterology, Nanjing Drum Tower Hospital, The Affiliated Hospital of Nanjing University Medical School, Nanjing 210008, Jiang Su Province, China

Lu Hao
Department of Gastroenterology, Hainan Branch of Chinese PLA General Hospital, Hainan, China

Lin He, Ya-Wei Bi, Di Zhang, Xiang-Peng Zeng, Jun Pan, Dan Wang, Ting-Ting Du, Jin Huan Lin, Wen-Bin Zou and Hong-Lei Guo
Department of Gastroenterology, Gongli Hospital, The Second Military Medical University, Shanghai, China

Teng Wang, Lei Xin, Hui Chen, Zhuan Liao, Zhao-Shen Li and Liang-Hao Hu
Department of Gastroenterology, Gongli Hospital, The Second Military Medical University, Shanghai, China
Department of Gastroenterology, Changhai Hospital, The Second Military Medical University, Shanghai, China

Jun-Tao Ji
Department of Gastroenterology, Changhai Hospital, The Second Military Medical University, Shanghai, China

Li-Sheng Wang and Zheng-Lei Xu
Department of Gastroenterology, The Second Clinical Medical College (Shenzhen People's Hospital), Jinan University, Guangdong, China

Ting Xie
Department of Gastroenterology, Zhongda Hospital, Southeast University, Nanjing, China

Bai-Rong Li
Department of Gastroenterology, Air Force General Hospital, Beijing, China

Feiyang Wang
Department of General Surgery, Shanghai Jiaotong University Affiliated First People's Hospital, Shanghai 200080, China
Department of Pancreatic Surgery, Union Hospital, Tongji Medical College, Huazhong University of Science and Technology, Wuhan 430022, China

Zibo Meng, Yushun Zhang and Heshui Wu
Department of Pancreatic Surgery, Union Hospital, Tongji Medical College, Huazhong University of Science and Technology, Wuhan 430022, China

Shoukang Li
Department of Thoracic Surgery, Union Hospital, Tongji Medical College, Huazhong University of Science and Technology, Wuhan 430022, China

Xiao Shen, Lu Ke, Lei Zou, Baiqiang Li, Zhihui Tong and Weiqin Li
Surgical Intensive Care Unit (SICU), Department of General Surgery, Jinling Hospital, Medical School of Nanjing University, No. 305 Zhongshan East Road, Nanjing 210002, Jiangsu Province, China

Jing Sun, Ning Li and Jieshou Li
Department of General Surgery, Jinling Hospital, Medical School of Nanjing University, No. 305 Zhongshan East Road, Nanjing 210002, Jiangsu Province, China

Marco Chiarelli and Martino Gerosa
Department of Surgery, Ospedale Alessandro Manzoni, Lecco, Via dell'Eremo 9/11, 23900 Lecco, LC, Italy

Angelo Guttadauro and Francesco Gabrielli
Department of Surgery, University of Milan-Bicocca, Istituti Clinici Zucchi, Via Zucchi, 24, 20900 Monza, MB, Italy

Alessandro Marando
Department of Pathology, Ospedale Alessandro Manzoni, Lecco, Via dell'Eremo 9/11, 23900, Lecco LC, Italy

Matilde De Simone and Ugo Cioffi
Department of Surgery, University of Milan, Milan, Italy

Levina S. Pakasi and Laurentius A. Lesmana
Digestive Disease & GI Oncology Center, Medistra Hospital, Jakarta, Indonesia

Cosmas Rinaldi A. Lesmana
Digestive Disease & GI Oncology Center, Medistra Hospital, Jakarta, Indonesia
Department of Internal Medicine, Hepatobiliary Division, Cipto Mangunkusumo Hospital, University of Indonesia, Jakarta, Indonesia

Sri Inggriani and Maria L. Aidawati
Department of Radiology, Medistra Hospital, Jakarta, Indonesia

Miaozun Zhang, Ren Fang, Ronggao Chen, Jiafei Yan, Weiwei Jin and Harsha Ajoodhea
Department of General Surgery, Sir Run Run Shaw Hospital, School of Medicine, Zhejiang University, 3 East Qingchun Road, Hangzhou 310016, Zhejiang Province, China

Yiping Mou, Xiaowu Xu and Renchao Zhang
Department of General Surgery, Zhejiang Provincial People's Hospital, Wenzhou Medical University, 158 Shangtang Road, Hangzhou 310014, Zhejiang Province, China

Daisuke Matsushita, Hiroshi Kurahara, Yuko Mataki, Kosei Maemura, Satoshi Iino, Masahiko Sakoda, Shinichi Ueno and Shoji Natsugoe
Department of Digestive Surgery and Breast and Thyroid Surgery, Graduate School of Medical and Dental Sciences, Kagoshima University, 8-35-1 Sakuragaoka, Kagoshima 890-8520, Japan

Michiyo Higashi
Department of Human pathology, Field of Oncology, Graduate School of Medical and Dental Sciences, Kagoshima University, Kagoshima, Japan

Hiroyuki Shinchi
Faculty of Medical School of Health Sciencesy, Graduate School of Medical and Dental Sciences, Kagoshima University, Kagoshima, Japan

Takeshi Nishi
Deparment of Surgery, Matsue Red Cross Hospital, 200 Horo-machi, Matsue, Shimane 690-8506, Japan
Department of Digestive and General Surgery, Shimane University Faculty of Medicine, 89-1 Enyacho, Izumo, Shimane 693-8501, Japan

Yasunari Kawabata, Seiji Yano and Yoshitsugu Tajima
Department of Digestive and General Surgery, Shimane University Faculty of Medicine, 89-1 Enyacho, Izumo, Shimane 693-8501, Japan

Noriyoshi Ishikawa, Asuka Araki and Riruke Maruyama
Department of Organ Pathology, Shimane University Faculty of Medicine, 89-1 Enyacho, Izumo, Shimane 693-8501, Japan

Stephen Morris and Jessica Sheringham
Department of Applied Health Research, University College London, Gower Street, 1-19 Torrington Place, London WC1E 7HB, UK

Kurinchi S Gurusamy and Brian R Davidson
University College London Medical School, 9th Floor, Royal Free Hospital, Rowland Hill Street, London, UK

Dorota Koziel
Faculty of Health Sciences, Jan Kochanowski University, Kielce, Poland

Stanislaw Gluszek
Faculty of Health Sciences, Jan Kochanowski University, Kielce, Poland
Clinic General Oncological and Endocrinological Surgery, Regional Hospital Kielce, Poland

Artur Kowalik, Malgorzata Chlopek and Liliana Pieciak
Department of Molecular Diagnostics, Holy Cross Cancer Centre, Kielce, Poland

Ileana Cocota
2nd Medical Department, Cluj-Napoca, Romania

Radu Badea
Department of Clinical Imaging Ultrasound, "Iuliu Hatieganu" University of Medicine and Pharmacy, Cluj-Napoca, Romania

Traian Scridon
Heart Institute "Prof. Dr. Nicolae Stancioiu", "Iuliu Hatieganu" University of Medicine and Pharmacy, Cluj-Napoca, Romania

Dan L Dumitrascu
2nd Medical Department, "Iuliu Hatieganu" University of Medicine and Pharmacy, Cluj-Napoca, Romania

Index

www.ingramcontent.com/pod-product-compliance
Lightning Source LLC
Chambersburg PA
CBHW082039190326
41458CB00010B/3405